Coronary Angioscopy

*I dedicate this book to my beloved
wife, Sakiko.*
*"Life isn't worth living, unless it is lived
for someone else" was her way of life.*

Kyoichi Mizuno

Preface

This book provides a long-awaited perspective on state-of-the-art coronary angioscopy. Angioscopy is a relatively new diagnostic tool that permits nonoperative imaging of coronary structures through the use of fiber optic systems. Direct visualization of the internal surface of a vessel provides detailed information about the characteristics of a plaque or thrombus. Coronary angioscopy is playing an ever-expanding role in research and in clinical practice because it provides a precise, full-color, three-dimensional image of the interior surface of the morphology of coronary arteries.

Angioscopy allows coronary macropathology during ongoing ischemia in living individuals, information that hitherto was unavailable except during autopsy. The ability to discriminate colors in angioscopy makes it relatively easy to distinguish between a thrombus and a plaque even if a clot is very small. Furthermore, angioscopy can also distinguish between the type of plaque (yellow versus white) and type of thrombus (red versus white).

It is important to learn the biological and scientific facts through angioscopy, which is useful for the recognition of vascular pathogenesis, diagnostic evaluation, and treatment. Here, it is relevant to recall the proverbs "A picture is worth a thousand words", "Seeing is believing", and "One eyewitness is better than many hearsay witnesses".

We hope that this book will provide professionals in the field with a useful, comprehensive guide to modern coronary diagnostic and coronary care. The book is divided into 3 parts and 19 chapters including an overview, angioscopic procedures, and angioscopic findings after stent- and drug-based therapies. We wish to thank all the authors, who are well-known researchers in angioscopy. We also thank the editorial staff of Springer Japan, especially Ms. Tomoka Taya and Ms. Sachiko Hayakawa.

Tokyo, Japan Kyoichi Mizuno
Chiba, Japan Masamichi Takano

as follows: $n_1\sin\theta$. The NA is also used to indicate a view angle for the optical waveguide. The standard NA of silica glass optical fiber is around 0.20. The high-NA silica glass optical fiber contains large amount of high-refractive-index material, in particular Ge in its core. The high-NA silica fiber has up to 0.35 of NA. The NA of the plastic optical fiber is ranging from 0.5 to 0.63.

1.1.3 Pixel Separation Method for Image Transmission

Optical images that contain information of color and figure can be transmitted through rigid optics, such as an objective lens and telescope, in general. Despite the optical fiber of which refractive-index distribution forms a quadratic function being equivalent to a series of convex lenses, this fiber is not able to deliver images precisely because of mode transformation, i.e., turbulent wave front by the bending of the optical fiber as well as imprecision of refractive-index distribution on radial direction of the optical fiber. Therefore, a picture element (pixel) separation method should be used to transmit images by the optical fiber. Each pixel in the picture can be delivered through an individual optical fiber. Figure 1.2 shows example of an image set at various pixel sizes. Obviously, fine pixel resolution is better for diagnostic use, but it is restricted by other factors, in particular the diameter of the optical fiber (image guide). The required amount of pixels is dependent on an observation area and desired resolution for an observation. Three or six thousand pixels have been used in the coronary angioscopic imaging.

1.2 Optical Image Guides

1.2.1 Silica-Based Optical Waveguide

The production technology of silica-based image guide had been established by Japanese engineer Atsushi Utsumi who had been working with Mitsubishi Cable, Co. Ltd [2]. A cross-sectional schematic structure of his waveguide is illustrated in Fig. 1.3, comparing it to conventional optical fiber bundle used in a fiber endoscope. The optical fiber bundle is basically a human-work assembling fiber, which contains several thousands of independent pixel fibers. Because the optical fiber bundle was expensive and its pixel size is limited to 20,000–40,000 pixels, a CCD endoscope had been replaced. In contrast, the silica-based image guide is a unified fiber, which contains several thousands of independent core in a common clad region. Since this silica-based image guide can be fabricated by a wiredrawing process corresponding to fit large-lot production, it should be very thin and inexpensive. Despite pixel size being limited to approximately 10 k, this silica-based image guide has been used in an angioscope due to its thinness and inexpensiveness. Technical challenges

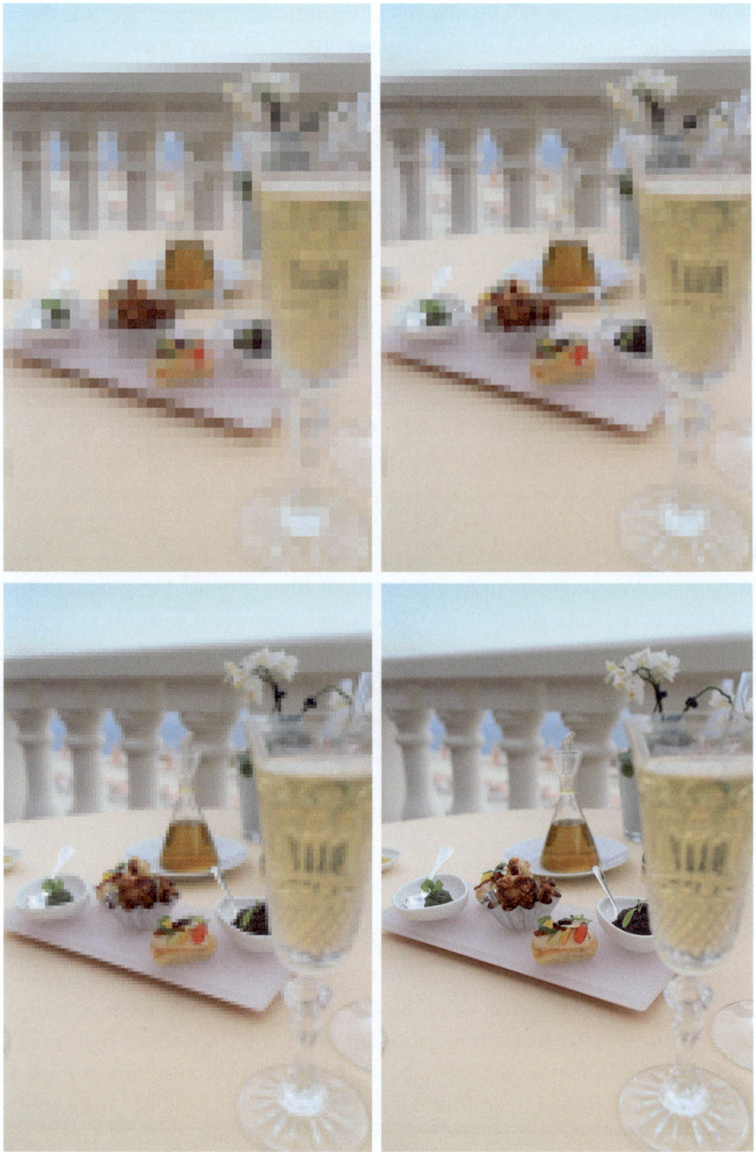

Fig. 1.2 Effect of pixel size on image quality. Number of pixels are 2.2 k, 5 k, 20 k, and 18 M, respectively, *left* to *right*

in the fabrication of this image guide are core diameter stability/distribution and optimization to suppress optical leakage between each core. When the core diameter distribution is scattered, some core has a specific color due to the mode difference in small amount of the transmission mode (see 1.1.2). Moreover, because the clad

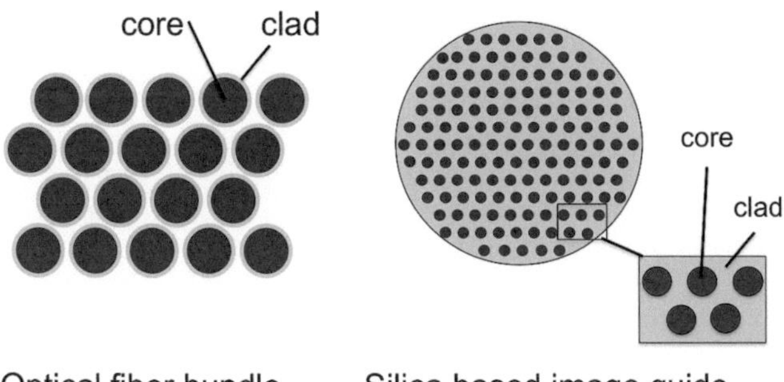

Fig. 1.3 The schematic structures of the silica-based image guide and optical fiber bundle

region is common for all cores, the optical leakage exists as close-set pixel to pixel. This leakage reduces image quality to be a bleary image. A few Japanese optical fiber fabricators only can produce a high-quality silica-based image guide so far.

1.2.2 Specifications of Optical Image Guides

The specification of the silica-based image guides for the coronary angioscope is summarized in Table 1.1 with one particular new image guide made of a plastic material. The information of this table is based on specification catalogs from each fabricator [3–5]. The author also tries to predict and indicate undisclosed information in Table 1.1. Three thousand or six thousand pixels are employed in general. The minimum bending radius should be less than 15 mm for the coronary angioscope. The outer diameter of the image guide should be less than around 0.4 mm because of both stiffness and size. The glass fibers need a coating layer to avoid a scratch of the fiber outside to keep their bending capability because of the brittle fracture characteristics of glass materials. The angioscope image taken in the 1990s was dark and not sharp because of low pixel density (equal to low pixel size in the image) using a low-NA image guide in the early years [6, 7]. The standard pixel size in an angioscope image in the 1990s was 3000, but a 6000 pixel image is generally used in recent years. The recent advance of high-NA silica-based image guide can make bright and sharp angioscopic image by increasing pixel density as well as suppressing cross leakage. Another advantage of the high-NA image guide is a wide view angle of the image. Since edge distortion is observed in the wide view angle image, in general, an observer feels spatial effect even from a two-dimensional image. One particular waveguide made of plastic material in Table 1.1 has the obvious capability to be applied in the coronary angioscope but has not been applied yet. The cost of plastic fiber might be less than tenth part of the silica-based image guide. Moreover, plastic material has lower stiffness than silica glass. These characteristics are helpful to make ideal coronary angioscope.

Table 1.1 Image guide specifications applicable to the angioscope

Image fiber	Material	Pixels	Fiber diameter [mm]	Outer diameter [mm]	Numerical aperture	Min. bend. radius [mm]	References
Maker A1	Silica glass	1,600	0.16	0.21	a	20 (10; temp.)	[3]
Maker A2	Silica glass	3,000	0.20	0.25	a	25 (15; temp.)	[3]
Maker A3	Silica glass	6,000	0.28	0.34	a	30 (15; temp.)	[3]
Maker B1	Silica glass	3,000	0.25	0.31	a	b	[4]
Maker B2	Silica glass	6,000	0.34	0.41	a	b	[4]
Maker C	Plastic	7,400	0.45	–	0.5	c	[5]

[a]NAs ranging 0.30–0.35 were predicted
[b]Similar bending capability was estimated as those of Maker A
[c]Below 10 mm radius was predicted based on single plastic optical fiber performance

1.3 Structure of Angioscope and Visualization Equipment

1.3.1 Structure of the Angioscope

The structure of the angioscope using the silica-based optical image guide is schematically illustrated in Fig. 1.4. To illuminate the diagnostic location, the illumination light beam that has higher NA than that of the image guide to cover the viewing region is emitted via plastic optical fibers. The arrangement of the illumination fibers against the image guide is important to recognize a stereoscopic feeling by the illumination shadow. Basically, since the angioscope cross section is a small area, the ideal illumination is hard to attain. The objective lens at the tip of the image guide is necessary to make image formation. Selfoc® microlens that is equivalent to a precise convex lens with a cylindrical shape is employed to attain thinner shape angioscope. The possible diagnostic range from the surface of the angioscope is ruled from the minimum focal point of the Selfoc® microlens to the detectable limit decided by the illumination and image-sensing capability. Several millimeters to 20 mm from the tip should be the possible diagnostic range. All components of the angioscope described in Fig. 1.4 are dielectric material, so that the safety requirements of electricity upon contact with the human body in particular to avoid microshock are easily attained.

1.3.2 Structure of Imaging Optics and Light Source

The illumination light source and imaging optics are described in Fig. 1.5. The image-sensing device and imaging optics are located at the distal end of the angio-

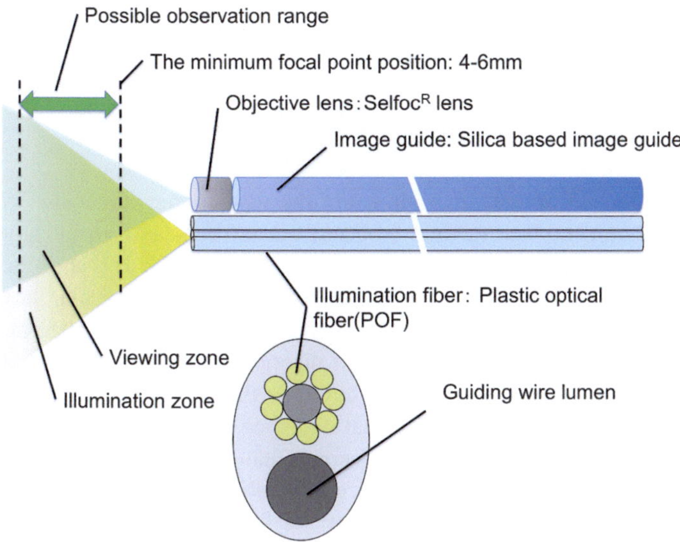

Fig. 1.4 The structure of the angioscope. Viewing area and illumination area are shown with possible observation range. The head structure of a monorail-type angioscope is also shown

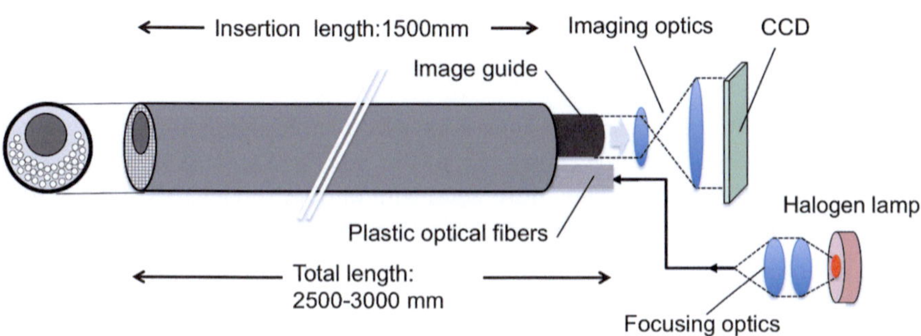

Fig. 1.5 The structure of the imaging optics and illumination light source. The simple thin angioscope is shown

scope, that is, out of a body. This is one of the advantages of the angioscope using the silica-based image guide. The CCD camera capability improved drastically in recent years so that the angioscope image quality has been improved strongly. The wide dynamic range as well as gain control system is helpful to get an effective image on the inhomogeneous illumination distribution depending on the view angle discussed in Sect. 1.4.2. The white-light illumination based on a halogen lamp is employed. The efficient coupling of this incoherent light source to thin fibers is difficult. But in the case of using white laser light based on He-Cd laser, a speckle pattern is presented to degenerate image quality.

1.4 Consideration of Particular Circumstance on Angioscopic Diagnosis

1.4.1 Refractive Matching by Flush Fluid

Figure 1.6 indicates optical environment of the angioscopic diagnosis. Transparent flush fluid should replace opaque blood to get intravascular visualization. Since reflective index of this flush fluid is approximately the same as that of the vascular wall/plaque [8], there is almost no normal reflection on the vascular surface. This decreased normal reflection on the objective surface blurs the sharpness of the angioscopic image. In contrast, diffuse reflection light from nearby vascular or plaque surface governed image information, so that the angioscopic image color reflects vascular and/or plaque information. Therefore, the angioscopic image is suited for diagnosis inside of the plaque rather than its shape.

Figure 1.7 demonstrates the influence of flush fluid environment on the view angle. The view angle narrows in the case of flush fluid environment due to the change of reflection angle on the boundary between the objective lens surface and the fluid. Narrower view angle may reduce the three-dimensional feeling.

1.4.2 View Angle on Angioscopic Imaging

Figure 1.8 explains the characteristics of an effective observation zone at various observation angles against the center axis of the vascular lumen. The coaxial view is ideal to get all circumference information with bird's-eye view. Meanwhile, this image is lacking three-dimensional appearances except in the case of severe stenosis or occlusion. The quasi-coaxial and skew view offers localized precise information,

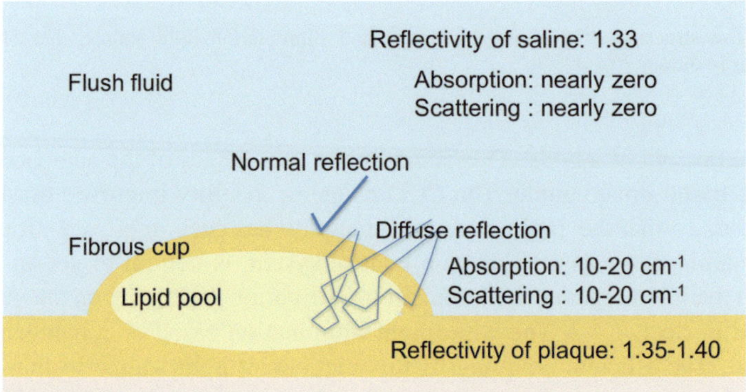

Fig. 1.6 Specific optical environments on angioscopic visualization. Refractive-index matching is attained on the boundary between the lumen surface and flush fluid

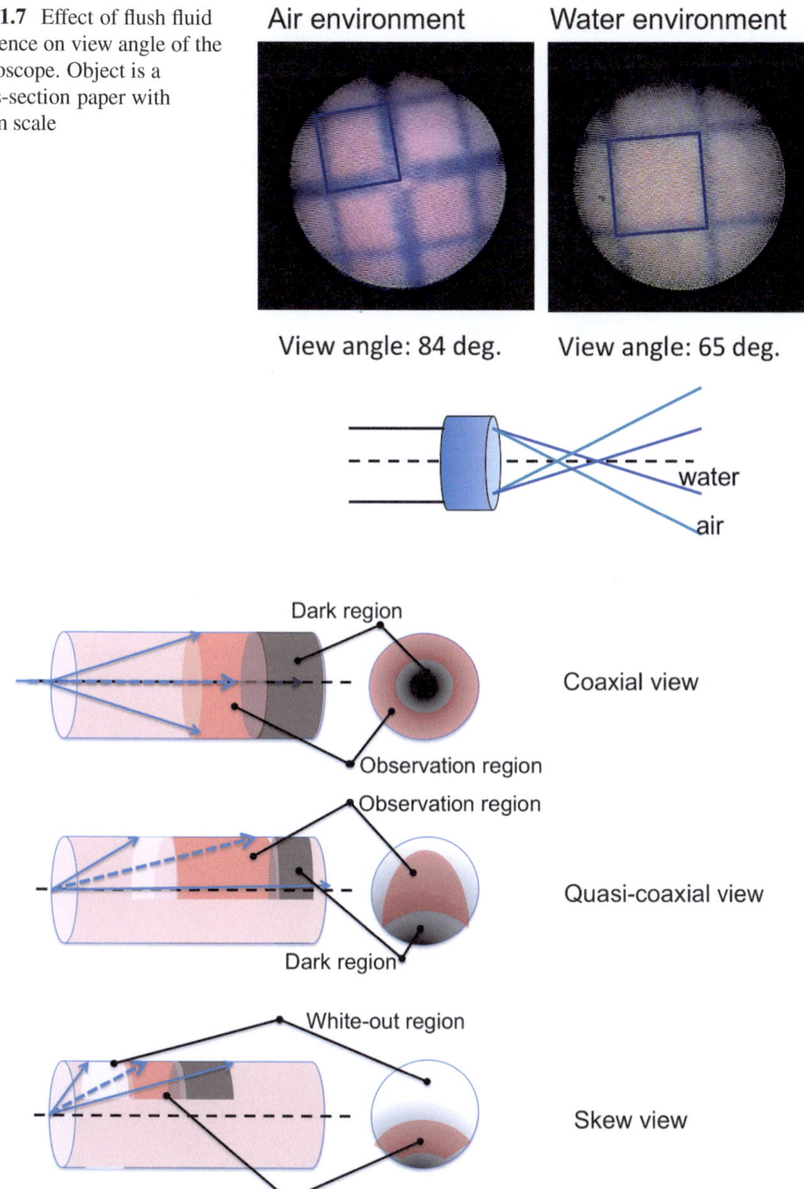

Fig. 1.7 Effect of flush fluid existence on view angle of the angioscope. Object is a cross-section paper with 1 mm scale

Fig. 1.8 Effect of observation angle against lumen longitudinal axis. Effective observation area, *white*out area, and *dark* area are indicated as *red*, *white*, and *black color*, respectively. *Dotted arrow* and *solid arrow* indicate the observation center axis and limit line of the observation zone. The angle between objective (vascular surface) and observation axis is not a right angle

but it cannot get circumference information in the vascular lumen. Moreover, a marked inhomogeneous illumination condition is found in these view angles, so that the over-illumination zone erases image information, i.e., whiteout. This kind of view angle issue is a unique problem in long and thin lumen observation of coronary angioscope.

References

1. Ghatak A, Thyagarajan K. Optical fibers. In: Trager F, editor. Springer handbook of lasers and optics. New York: Springer; 2007.
2. Mizuno K, Arai T, Satomura K, Shibuya T, Arakawa K, Okamoto Y, Miyamoto A, Kurita A, Kikuchi M, Nakamura H, Utsumi A, Takeuchi K. New percutaneous transluminal coronary angioscope. J Am Coll Cardiol. 1989;13:363–8.
3. Datasheet from Fujikura Co. Ltd. (Japan), Model FIGH-016-160S, Model FIGH-03-200S, and FIGH-06-280S.
4. Datasheet from Mitsubishi Cable Co. Ltd. (Japan), Model ML-003 and ML-006.
5. Datasheet from AsashiKASEI E-Materials Co. Ltd. (Japan), Model MBI-450S.
6. Mizuno K, Miyamoto A, Satomura K, Kurita A, Arai T, Sakurada M, Yanagida S, Nakamura H. Angioscopic coronary macro morphology in patients with acute coronary disorders. Lancet. 1991;337:809–912.
7. Mizuno K, Satomura K, Miyamoto A, Arakawa K, Shibuya T, Arai T, Kurita A, Nakamura H, Ambrose J. Angioscopic evaluation of coronary artery thrombi in acute coronary syndromes. New Engl J Med. 1992;326:287–91.
8. Prince MR, Deutsch TF, Mathews-Roth MM, Margolis R, Parrish JA, Oseroff AR. Preferential light absorption in atheromas in vitro: implications for laser angioplasty. J Clin Invest. 1986;78:295–302.

Chapter 2
The Role of Multiple Imaging Modalities to Disclose the Mechanism of ACS Angioscopy in Comparison to Other Imaging Modalities Including OCT, IVUS and CTA

Yukio Ozaki, Masanori Okumura, Tevfik F. Ismail, Sadako Motoyama, Hiroyuki Naruse, Takashi Muramatsu, Hideki Kawai, Masayoshi Sarai, and Jagat Narula

Abstract *Aims*: Whilst pathological and optical coherence tomography (OCT) studies have indicated that ACS lesions have either ruptured fibrous (RFC-ACS) or intact (IFC-ACS) fibrous caps, CT angiographic (CTA) characteristics of RFC-ACS include low-attenuation plaques and positive plaque remodelling. However, features associated with IFC-ACS have not been previously described. The aim of this study was to assess the CTA characteristics of IFC-ACS lesions.

Methods and Results: Of the 66 patients with ACS or stable angina that consented to multiple imaging procedures, 57 culprit lesions in 57 patients were evaluated with sufficient image quality of angioscopy, OCT, IVUS and CTA. Whilst intraluminal thrombus was assessed by OCT or angioscopy, culprit lesions were classified further by OCT-based demonstration of fibrous cap integrity. Of 35 culprit lesions with ACS, OCT revealed IFC with thrombus in 10 (29 %) and RFC in the remaining 25 (71 %); all 22 lesions with stable angina had intact fibrous caps. Fibrous caps were significantly thinner in RFC-ACS than in IFC-ACS and stable angina (45 ± 12 μm, 131 ± 57 μm, 321 ± 146 μm, respectively; $p = 0.001$). CT-verified low-attenuation plaques were more frequently observed in RFC-ACS than in IFC-ACS and stable angina (88 %, 40 %, 18 %; $p = 0.001$) lesions. Similarly, positive remodelling was

Y. Ozaki, M.D., FACC, FESC (✉) • M. Okumura, M.D. • H. Naruse, M.D.
T. Muramatsu, M.D. • M. Sarai, M.D.
Department of Cardiology, Fujita Health University Hospital, 1-98 Dengaku, Kutsukake, Toyoake, Aichi, Japan
e-mail: ozakiyuk@fujita-hu.ac.jp

T.F. Ismail, MBBS, MRCP
Royal Brompton Hospital, London, UK

S. Motoyama, M.D. • H. Kawai, M.D. • J. Narula, M.D., FACC
Mount Sinai School of Medicine, New York, NY, USA

© Springer Japan 2015
K. Mizuno, M. Takano (eds.), *Coronary Angioscopy*,
DOI 10.1007/978-4-431-55546-9_2

more predominantly seen in RFC-ACS than in IFC-ACS and stable angina (96 %, 20 %, 14 %; $p = 0.001$). However, none of the specific CT angiography features clearly distinguished IFC-ACS from stable lesions.

Conclusion: This report is derived from our previous study proposing for the first time that nondisrupted culprit lesions (IFC-ACS) would represent pathological plaque erosions. IFC-ACS lesions based on OCT and angioscopy features demonstrated less low-attenuation plaque and less positive remodelling than RFC-ACS by CT angiography. Since there are no unique CT features of IFC-ACS lesions to enable their clear distinction from stable lesions, it will be difficult to develop CT-based non-invasive imaging techniques to allow the clear identification of subjects at high risk of developing ACS due to IFC.

Keywords Plaque erosion • Plaque rupture • Acute coronary syndrome • CT • intact fibrous caps (IFC) • Intravascular ultrasound • Optical coherence tomography

2.1 Introduction

Histopathological characterisation of the culprit lesion in acute coronary syndromes (ACS) demonstrates either ruptured fibrous caps (RFC) or intact fibrous caps (IFC). The latter lesions are often referred to as plaque erosions and are responsible for up to one-third of culprit lesions in ACS patients [1–14]. The culprit lesions associated with RFC-ACS have been better characterised by CT angiography and demonstrate positive remodelling of the vessel at the lesion site and frequently carry low-attenuation plaques [15–23]. Plaque rupture has demonstrated nearly 85–90 % diagnostic accuracy for association with culprit lesions, and the presence of low-attenuation plaque defined as <30 HU has 75 % sensitivity and 95 % specificity [23]. It has been proposed that the presence of these two features (plaque rupture and low-attenuation plaque) in the absence of ACS may confer a greater than 20-fold higher hazard ratio for subsequent development of ACS over time [24].

Unlike RFC-ACS, IFC-ACS occur preferentially in younger subjects and women, who often do not demonstrate traditional coronary risk factors except active smoking [9]. Histopathologically, these lesions are not positively remodelled, often impose limited luminal occlusion and are hyaluronan proteoglycan rich [4]. Upon optical coherence tomography (OCT), such lesions are characterised by loss of endothelial lining with lacerations of the superficial intimal layers [25]. However, no information is available about the non-invasive CT angiographic characteristics of these lesions. We sought to characterise these lesions by CT angiography.

In the present study, we sought to describe the CT angiographic features of ACS lesions associated with IFC. For this purpose, we classified the ACS lesions into RFC-ACS and IFC-ACS based on the findings of the integrity of the fibrous caps using OCT as well as the presence of luminal thrombus identified by coronary angioscopy and OCT. The CT characteristics of the culprit lesions with IFC were compared with lesions of patients with RFC-ACS and stable coronary disease. All imaging evaluations including OCT, IVUS, angioscopy and CT angiography were performed before PCI for culprit lesions.

2.2   Methods

2.2.1   Study Design, Inclusion and Exclusion Criteria

Coronary angioscopy, optical coherence tomography (OCT), intravascular ultrasound (IVUS) and CT angiography (CTA) were performed prospectively to characterise culprit lesions and to examine the role of CT in the non-invasive prediction of lesions likely to be complicated by IFC-ACS. Patients with ACS showing non-ST-segment elevation myocardial infarction (NSTEMI) or unstable angina pectoris (UA) and stable angina pectoris were studied. Only native coronary artery lesions were included in the study. Patients were excluded from the study when they had contraindications to anticoagulation and antiplatelet therapy. Lesions located in totally occluded, tortuous vessels and in the left main stem were excluded from the study due to the difficulty in performing precise intracoronary imaging. The study was approved by local ethics committees and was carried out according to the guidelines of the Declaration of Helsinki. Written informed consent was obtained from all patients.

2.2.2   Definitions of RFC-ACS and IFC-ACS

RFC-ACS was identified by the OCT-verified presence of fibrous cap disruption (i.e. fibrous cap discontinuity) or an ulceration of the plaque, and IFC-ACS was defined as the presence of an intact fibrous cap (i.e. the absence of plaque rupture) by OCT associated with the presence of thrombus by angioscopy or OCT [25].

The possible ischaemic location in the culprit vessel was screened by the ECG and echo data, followed by CT angiography [23, 24]. Subsequently, IVUS, OCT and angioscopy were performed in the entire vessel as far as possible, via motorised IVUS and OCT, and manual angioscopy from the very distal segment of the culprit coronary artery. We obtained diagnostic quality images from distal to proximal segments of the coronary artery in 57 out of 66 consecutive patients. A single culprit lesion per patient was assessed to avoid the effect of intra-cluster correlation (ICC) in this study. In the 57 patients, 57 culprit lesions were interrogated, of which 25 lesions were associated with RFC, 10 with IFC and 22 with stable angina lesions.

2.2.3 CT Image Acquisition and Analysis

Whilst CT angiography was performed by Aquilion (Toshiba Co., Japan), the reconstructed image data was transferred to a computer workstation for post-processing (ZIO M900, Amin/ZIO, Tokyo, Japan). Coronary plaque was reported as either calcified or non-calcified plaques (NCP). Furthermore, based on our previous report [26], we divided the NCP into 2 categories: low-attenuation plaques (NCP <30 HU, corresponding to IVUS lipid cores) and intermediate-attenuation plaques (30 HU < NCP <150 HU, corresponding to IVUS fibrous plaques).

2.2.4 Intracoronary Imaging Procedures

Selective coronary angiography was performed after the intracoronary injection of nitrates following the introduction of guiding catheter after the administration of intravenous heparin at 100 IU/kg. After the passage of a 0.014-in. guidewire across the lesion, optical coherence tomography (OCT) and intracoronary angioscopy were carefully performed followed by mechanical intravascular ultrasound (IVUS) with motorised pullback [27, 28]. Since STEMI was not included in this study, no culprit lesion had totally occluded. IVUS, OCT and angioscopy were repeated after stenting to obtain optimal stent deployment including adequate lesion coverage, stent expansion and stent apposition [29]. Following the passage of a 0.014-in. guidewire across the lesion, a proximal occlusion balloon catheter with an over-the-wire (OTW) was positioned proximal to the lesion. While a 0.014-in. guidewire was exchanged to a 0.016-in. OCT image wire (LightLab Imaging, Westford, MA) through OTW, OCT image wire was carefully passed through the lesion. Whilst Ringer's solution or low molecular dextran were continuously flushed through the lumen to remove blood flow, motorized pullback was started at a rate of 1.0 mm/s for a length of 30 mm. The images were saved in the OCT image system digitally for subsequent analysis [29–35].

Coronary angioscopy (Vecmova, Clinical Supply, Gifu, Japan) was performed after the OCT examination during the injection of low molecular dextran, whilst blood was cleared away from the view by this injection [27, 36]. Following OCT and coronary angioscopy, a mechanical IVUS imaging catheter (40 MHz, 2.5Fr, Boston Scientific, Natick, MA) was introduced over a 0.014-in. guidewire and positioned distal to the lesion [27, 28]. Lesion geometry was then imaged by using a motorised pullback (0.5 mm/s). We performed all the three intracoronary imaging examinations within 15 min. The position of all the three imaging catheters was documented by simultaneous fluoroscopy during the imaging procedures to facilitate the review process and to ensure corresponding images were obtained with all the imaging modalities [27, 28].

2.2.5 Intracoronary Imaging Image Analysis

The corresponding image from multiple imaging modalities was identified using the distance from landmarks such as side branches and calcium deposits as well as angiographic and simultaneous fluoroscopic recordings [27, 28]. In OCT images, calcification within plaques was identified by the presence of well-delineated and low-backscattering heterogeneous regions and fibrous plaques identified by the presence of homogeneous high-backscattering areas [29–35, 37, 38]. Lipid necrotic pools were identified as areas less well delineated than calcifications (i.e. diffusely bordered) and exhibiting lower signal density and more heterogeneous backscattering than fibrous plaques. The latter are associated with overlying signal-rich bands, corresponding to the fibrous cap [29–35, 37, 38]. Thin-cap fibrous atheroma (TCFA) was defined as areas where cap thickness was less than 65 μm and lipid pool greater than two quadrants [3, 10, 29–35, 37]. When the precise fibrous cap thickness could not be obtained (e.g. the absence of a well-defined lipid core or the presence of thrombus interfering with the assessment), the measurements were performed in the nearest adjacent OCT slice. Thrombi were identified as masses protruding into the vessel lumen. Whilst red thrombi consisting mainly of red blood cells were observed as high-backscattering protrusions with signal-free shadowing by OCT, white thrombus containing mainly platelets and white blood cells was characterised by signal-rich and low-backscattering billowing projections protruding into the lumen [34].

On coronary angioscopy, thrombi were defined as intraluminal masses adherent to the intima. Thrombi were categorised as nonmobile mural (closely adherent to the vessel wall), mobile (protruding into the lumen) or totally occlusive. Yellow plaques were defined as areas of homogeneous yellow lesions clearly identifiable from the normal white wall. Yellow plaque was further classified into light and deep yellow plaque [27].

IVUS-verified cross-sectional luminal area was defined as the integrated area central to the intimal leading edge echo [27, 28]. The total vessel cross-sectional area (vessel area) was defined as the area inside the interface between the plaque-media complex and adventitia (area inside the external elastic membrane) [27, 28]. Plaque area was defined as vessel area minus luminal area. Our intra- and interobserver reproducibility data for each imaging modality (i.e. OCT, angioscopy, IVUS and CT angiography) have been previously reported [23, 27–29].

2.2.6 Quantitative Coronary Angiography (QCA)

QCA analyses were performed using the computer-based edge-detection Coronary Angiography Analysis System (CAAS II, Pie Medical, Maastricht, NL) [28, 39, 40]. Interpolated reference vessel diameter (RD), minimal lumen diameter (MLD) and percentage diameter stenosis were obtained using the guiding catheter as a scaling device from the QCA system [28, 39, 40]. OCT, coronary angioscopy, IVUS and QCA analyses were performed at the independent core laboratory of the Fujita Health University [40].

2.3 Results

2.3.1 Clinical and Angiographic Characteristics

Clinical characteristics were compared in 57 patients, including 25 with RFC-ACS, 10 with IFC-ACS and 22 stable angina patients (Table 2.1). No significant difference was found between the three groups with respect to age and traditional risk factors, except gender and smoking habits. The incidence of female gender was higher in patients with IFC than those with RFC and stable angina ($p = 0.007$). Current smokers were also more common in the IFC group than the other two groups ($p = 0.001$). Qualitative and quantitative angiographic features including lesion location, ACC/AHA lesion type and QCA measurements were similar in the 57 culprit lesions including 25 RFC, 10 IFC and 25 stable lesions (Table 2.1). Whilst multiple plaque ruptures were found in the same vessel in 2 of 25 patients with RFC-ACS, multiple target lesions for PCI were observed in 3 of 22 patients with stable angina. Taking into account intracluster correlation (ICC), we only performed statistical estimations in single lesion in one patient-based analysis (Tables 2.1 and 2.2).

2.3.2 Culprit Lesion Characteristics by OCT in RFC-ACS, IFC-ACS and Stable Angina

Intracoronary imaging findings are shown in Table 2.2. Whilst OCT revealed that fibrous cap thickness was significantly thinner in RFC lesions than other lesions (45 ± 12, 131 ± 57, 321 ± 146 μm, respectively; $p < 0.001$), the prevalence of lesions with lipid pools greater than 2 quadrants was higher in RFC lesions than in IFC and stable angina lesions (92 %, 40 %, 23 %; $p < 0.001$). TCFA was more commonly observed in the RFC group than in the IFC or stable angina groups (92 %, 20 %, 9 %; $p < 0.001$). Thrombus was more frequently observed in RFC and IFC lesions compared with the stable lesions by OCT (Table 2.2) (Figs. 2.1, 2.2 and 2.3).

2.3.3 Coronary Angioscopic Features of Culprit Lesions

Whilst thrombus was seen in most cases in the RFC group and all lesions in the IFC group, thrombus was rather rare in the stable angina group (88 %, 100 %, 14 %, respectively; $p = 0.001$). Although differences in the prevalence of yellow plaque

Table 2.1 Baseline clinical and angiographic characteristics in 57 lesions of 57 patients with RFC-ACS, IFC-ACS and stable angina

	RFC-ACS	IFC-ACS	Stable angina	*p*-value
Patients (n)	**25**	**10**	**22**	
Age (years)	63.7 ± 10.1	61.5 ± 8.2	62.6 ± 8.2	
Male (*n*, %)	25 (100)	8 (80)	22 (100)	0.007
Clinical presentation (*n*, %)				
NSTEMI	15 (60)	4 (40)	–	–
UAP	10 (40)	6 (60)	–	–
Stable angina pectoris	–	–	22 (100)	–
Diabetes (*n*, %)	8 (32)	3 (30)	8 (36)	0.922
Hypertension (%)	12 (48)	6 (60)	13 (59)	0.692
Hypercholesterolemia (%)	12 (48)	6 (60)	10 (45)	0.739
Smokers (*n*, %)				
Nonsmoker	10 (38)	1 (9)	7 (35)	0.001
Ex-smoker	9 (46)	2 (18)	12 (60)	–
Current smoker	6 (17)	7 (73)	3 (5)	–
Culprit lesions (n)	**25**	**10**	**22**	
Coronary artery (*n*, %)				
RCA/ LAD/ LCX	11/13/1	4/5/1	5/14/3	0.522
ACC/AHA lesion type (*n*)				
A/B1/B2/C	0/13/12/0	1/4/5/0	2/11/9/0	0.839
QCA				
RD pre (mm)	2.55 ± 0.52	2.46 ± 0.46	2.64 ± 0.58	0.666
MLD pre (mm)	0.94 ± 0.20	1.09 ± 0.22	0.96 ± 0.25	0.179
Lesion length (mm)	20.7 ± 7.0	22.5 ± 7.2	22.9 ± 9.4	0.647
Non-culprit lesions in non-culprit vessel assessed by CT angiography				
Non-culprit lesions (n)	**19**	**8**	**12**	
Average lesion severity (%)	42 ± 19 %	32 ± 12 %	46 ± 20 %	0.265
NCP ≤ 30 HU (*n*, %)	7 (37 %)	2 (25 %)	1 (8 %)	0.208
Spotty calcification (*n*, %)	5 (26 %)	2 (25 %)	2 (16 %)	0.815
Positive remodelling (*n*, %)	10 (53 %)	1 (13 %)	2 (16 %)	0.044

(containing lipids) did not reach statistically significant levels between the three groups, it tended to be more common in RFC and IFC lesions as compared to the stable lesions (84 %, 70 %, 55 %; $p = 0.088$) (Table 2.2).

2.3.4 IVUS Comparison Between RFC, IFC and Stable Plaques

Whilst IVUS demonstrated that vessel and lumen areas were similar between the three types of lesions, plaque size tended to be greater in the RFC group than in the

Table 2.2 Comparison of OCT, coronary angioscopy, IVUS and CTA findings in 57 lesions with RFC-ACS, IFC-ACS and stable plaque aetiology

	RFC-ACS	IFC-ACS	Stable Angina	*p*-value
Lesion (n)	**25**	**10**	**22**	–
OCT				
Fibrous cap thickness (μm)	$45 \pm 12^{A1)*}$	$131 \pm 57^{B1)*}$	$321 \pm 146^{C1)*}$	**0.001**
Lipid angle >2 quads (*n, %*)	23 (92 %)	4 (40 %)	5 (23 %)	0.001
TCFA (*n, %*)	23 (92 %)	2 (20 %)	2 (9 %)	0.001
Thrombus (*n, %*)	25 (100 %)	10 (100 %)	4 (18 %)	0.001
Coronary angioscopy				
Thrombus (*n, %*)	22 (88 %)	10 (100 %)	3 (14 %)	0.001
Mural thrombus (n, %)	*13 (52 %)*	*7 (70 %)*	*3 (14 %)*	–
Protruding thrombus (n, %)	*9 (36 %)*	*3 (30 %)*	*0 (0 %)*	–
Yellow plaque (*n, %*)	21 (84 %)	7 (70 %)	12 (55 %)	0.088
Light yellow plaque (n, %)	*5 (16 %)*	*3 (30 %)*	*5 (23 %)*	–
Deep yellow plaque (n, %)	*18 (68 %)*	*4 (40 %)*	*7 (31 %)*	–
White plaque (*n, %*)	4 (16 %)	3 (30 %)	10 (45 %)	0.088
IVUS				
Vessel area pre (mm^2)	14.8 ± 3.2	12.8 ± 2.1	12.6 ± 5.1	0.133
Lumen area pre (mm^2)	2.0 ± 0.8	2.5 ± 0.8	1.9 ± 0.8	0.132
Plaque area pre (mm^2)	12.9 ± 3.0	10.2 ± 2.1	10.7 ± 4.9	0.083
Prox. ref. vessel area (mm^2)	14.3 ± 2.9	13.5 ± 1.9	14.1 ± 5.0	0.862
Distal ref. vessel area (mm^2)	11.7 ± 2.9	11.8 ± 1.8	12.6 ± 5.3	0.781
Remodelling index	$1.14 \pm 0.12^{A2)*}$	$1.00 \pm 0.08^{B2)*}$	$0.95 \pm 0.11^{C2)*}$	**0.001**
CTA				
NCP $\leq$30 HU (LAP; *n, %*)	22 (88 %)	4 (40 %)	4 (18 %)	0.001
NCP from 30 to 150 HU (*n, %*)	25 (100 %)	10 (100 %)	22 (100 %)	–
Spotty calcification (*n, %*)	20 (80 %)	2 (20 %)	5 (23 %)	0.001
Large calcification (*n, %*)	3 (12 %)	1 (10 %)	13 (59 %)	0.001
Remodelling index (%)	$1.15 \pm 0.06^{A3)*}$	$1.02 \pm 0.08^{B3)*}$	$0.99 \pm 0.09^{C3)*}$	**0.001**
Positive remodelling (PR; *n, %*)	24 (96 %)	2 (20 %)	3 (14 %)	0.001
LAP and PR (*n, %*)	22 (88 %)	1 (10 %)	0 (0 %)	0.001

Multiple comparisons also revealed significant differences in fibrous cap thickness; $p < 0.05$ in A1)* vs. B1)*, A1)* vs. C1)*, B1)* vs. C1)*: Remodelling index by IVUS; $p < 0.05$ in A2)* vs. B2)*, A2)* vs. C2)*: Remodelling index by CTA; $p < 0.05$ in A3)* vs. B3)*, A3)* vs. C3)*

IFC and stable angina groups (12.9 ± 3.0, 10.2 ± 2.1, 10.7 ± 4.9 mm^2; $p = 0.083$). Remodelling index was significantly greater in RFC lesions than that in IFC and stable lesions (1.14 ± 0.12, 1.00 ± 0.08, 0.95 ± 0.11; $p = 0.001$) (Table 2.2).

2.3.5   CTA Findings in RFC and IFC Culprit Lesions

The characteristics of the 25 RFC, 10 IFC and 22 stable angina culprit lesions are presented in Table 2.2. Whilst low-attenuation plaques were more frequent in the RFC than in the IFC or stable angina groups (88 %, 40 %, 18 %; $p = 0.001$),

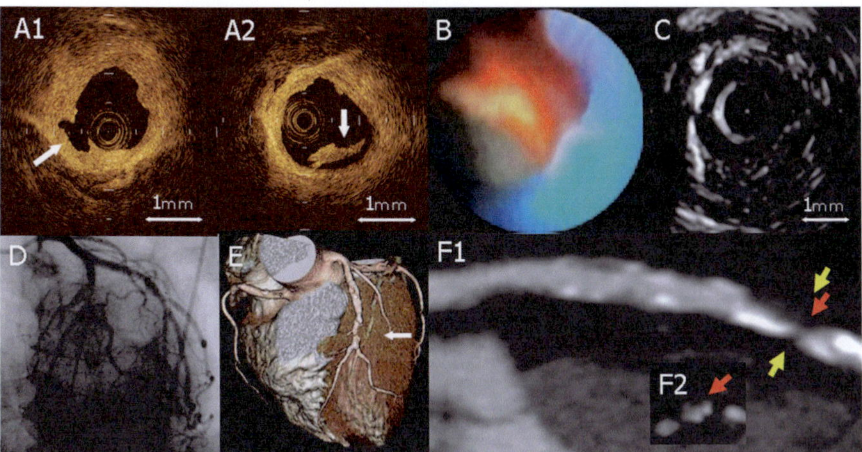

Fig. 2.1 Ruptured fibrous cap (RFC-ACS) plaque. OCT (**a**1, **a**2), coronary angioscopy (**b**), IVUS (**c**), angiography (**d**), volume rendering (**e**), curved MPR (**f**1) and the cross-sectional images (**f**2) were obtained in a culprit lesion with plaque rupture in 67-year-old male presenting with ACS. OCT revealed fibrous cap disruption (**a**1) and thrombus formation in adjacent slices (**a**2). Coronary angioscopy (**b**) showed yellow plaque and red thrombus formation through the blue coronary angioscopy guide catheter. IVUS (**c**) indicates two focal calcium deposits $<90°$. Angiography (**d**) and volume-rendered CT images (**e**) disclose a significant stenosis in the middle segment of the left anterior descending coronary artery. Curved MPR CT images (**f**1) reveal positive remodelling associated with focal calcium deposits. Curved MPR and the cross-sectional images (**f**2) display the presence of soft plaque with an attenuation of <30 HU [13]

intermediate-attenuation plaque was present in all culprit lesions in all three groups. Whilst spotty calcification was more frequently observed in RFC lesions than in IFC and stable lesions (80 %, 20 %, 23 %; $p = 0.001$), large calcification was more frequently observed in stable lesions than in RFC and IFC lesions (59 %, 12 %, 10 %, $p = 0.001$). Remodelling index was significantly greater in RFC culprit lesions than that in IFC culprit lesions and stable angina culprit lesions (1.15 ± 0.06, 1.02 ± 0.08, 0.99 ± 0.09; $p = 0.001$). Positive remodelling was more frequent in RFC lesions than that in IFC or stable lesions (96 %, 20 %, 14 %, $p = 0.001$). However, remodelling index, the incidence of positive remodelling and spotty calcification by CTA were not significantly different between IFC and stable lesions (Table 2.2).

2.4   Discussion

2.4.1   Clinical and Imaging Features of IFC-ACS

In our group of ACS patients presenting with NSTEMI or unstable angina, 30 % were not associated with fibrous cap rupture. The prevalence of current smokers and the proportion of females were higher in these patients compared to the RFC group [9, 10].

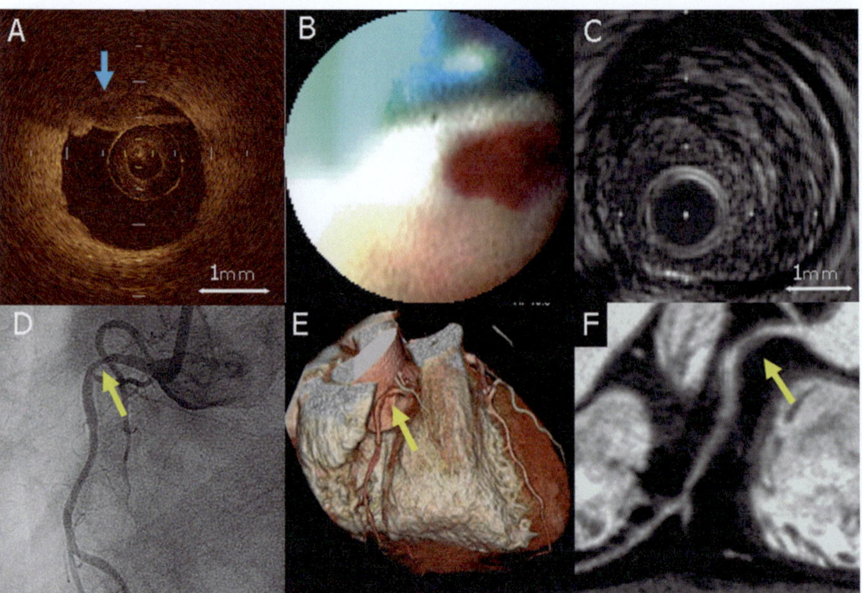

Fig. 2.2 Intact fibrous cap (IFC-ACS) plaque. OCT (**a**), coronary angioscopy (**b**), IVUS (**c**), angiography (**d**), volume-rendered (**e**) and curved MPR (**f**) images were derived from a culprit lesion with intact fibrous caps in a 63-year-old male presenting with an ACS. OCT revealed no evidence of fibrous cap rupture (**a**) but the presence of thrombus formation. Coronary angioscopy (**b**) showed red thrombus formation through the blue coronary angioscopy guide catheter. IVUS (**c**) reveals a soft and homogenous plaque with poor echo-reflectivity. Angiography (**d**) and the volume-rendered CT images (**e**) disclose a significant stenosis in the proximal segment of the right coronary artery. Curved MPR CT images (**f**) indicate the absence of positive remodelling and a non-calcified plaque [13]

The cap thickness measured by OCT in the IFC group (131 ± 57 μm) was significantly greater than the RFC group (45 ± 12 μm); cap thickness was maximum in the stable lesions (321 ± 146 μm, $p = 0.001$). This underscores the importance of fibrous cap thickness in plaque stability. A lipid pool angle encroaching >2 quadrants was substantially less frequent in the IFC group (40 %) compared with the RFC group (92 %, $p = 0.001$), but similar to the stable angina group (23 %, $p = 0.197$). Non-invasive CTA imaging confirmed the lack of lipid-rich plaques in the IFC group. Low-attenuation plaque was significantly less common in IFC-ACS group compared with RFC (40 % and 88 %, $p = 0.01$), but similar to stable angina (40 % and 18 %, $p = 0.186$). Positive remodelling was less common in IFC than that in the RFC group (20 % and 96 %, $p = 0.001$), but no different to that in the stable angina group (20 % and 14 %, $p = 0.645$). Spotty calcification was less frequent in IFC than in RFC lesions (20 % and 80 %, $p = 0.001$), but similar to stable lesions (20 % and 23 %, $p = 0.862$). Large calcification was less frequent in IFC than in stable lesions (10 %, 59 %, $p = 0.01$), but not different from RFC (10 %, 12 %, $p = 0.866$).

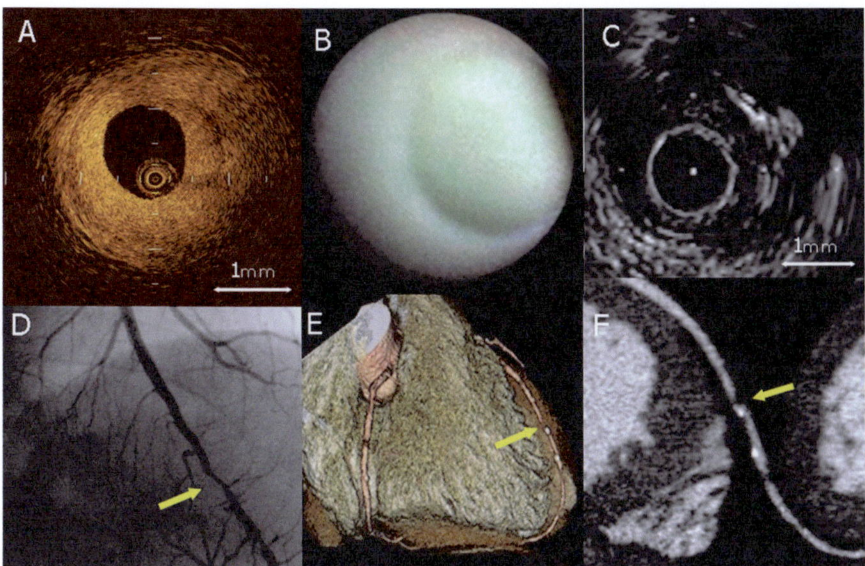

Fig. 2.3 Stable plaque. OCT (**a**), coronary angioscopy (**b**), IVUS (**c**), angiography (**d**), volume-rendered (**e**) and curved MPR (**f**) images were obtained from a culprit lesion with stable plaque in a 57-year-old male presenting with stable angina. OCT revealed a thick fibrous cap (**a**) with smooth lumen. Coronary angioscopy (**b**) showed a pale white and smooth surface to the plaque. IVUS (**c**) revealed focal calcium deposits in the plaque. Angiography (**d**) and volume-rendered CT images (**e**) disclose a significant stenosis in the distal segment of the left anterior descending coronary artery. The curved MPR CT image (**f**) indicates the absence of positive remodelling with focal calcium deposits [13]

Although distinct morphological features of IFC plaques from RFC and stable plaques were seen by OCT, no such unique characteristics were discernable by CTA. These lesions, although distinct from RFC plaques due to the presence of positive remodelling and low-attenuation plaque in the latter, were not clearly different from stable angina plaques.

2.4.2 Impact of IFC on ACS

Approximately one-third of lesions responsible for major coronary thrombi on pathological analysis are secondary to plaque erosions [4, 10]. Kolodgie and colleagues reported that unlike ruptured plaques, eroded plaques showed constrictive remodelling and did not necessarily demonstrate voluminous plaques nor necrotic cores [9]. These lesions revealed a unique proteoglycan substrate, which facilitates endothelial sloughing and thrombogenicity [9]. On the other hand, the ruptured plaques were histopathologically characterised by large plaque volumes and large

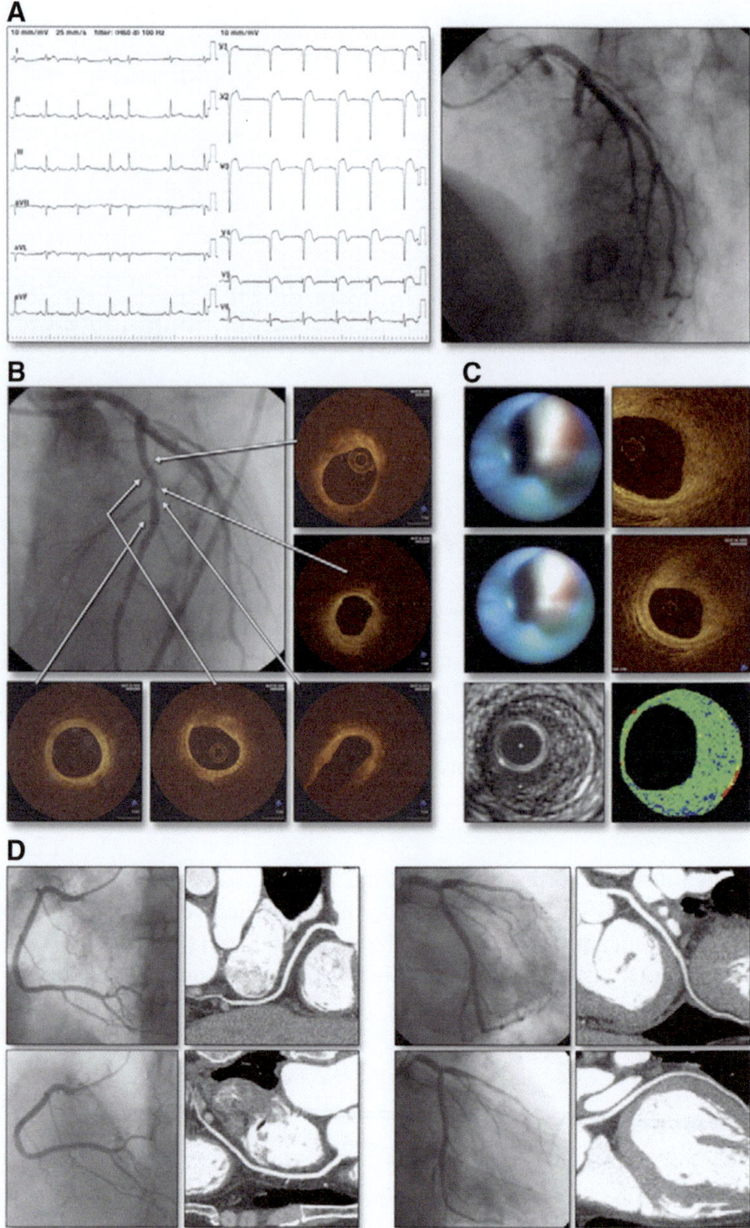

Fig. 2.4 Management of acute coronary syndrome with an intact fibrous cap (ACS-IFC) in a patient at Fujita Health University Hospital in reference [41]. Severe chest discomfort and shortness of breath developed in a 66-year-old man after 12 h of intermittent and stuttering retrosternal discomfort. He presented to a local hospital; his blood pressure was 96/57 mmHg, his heart rate was 84 beats/min and an electrocardiogram revealed ST-segment elevation in precordial leads (**a**). The coronary risk factors included dyslipidemia and 46-pack-year smoking history.

necrotic cores that were covered by attenuated fibrous caps often inflamed with monocyte-macrophage infiltration [3]. In addition, small calcified concretions in fibrous caps have been shown to contribute to plaque ruptures [6, 7]. Although the ruptured plaques were generally voluminous, they did not always impinge on the vascular lumen and expanded outwardly by the process of positive remodelling [4, 5]. On the other hand, it is reasonable to presume that nondisrupted culprit lesions (IFC-ACS) in our study would represent plaque erosions. As the underlying plaques in the IFC group were not lipid rich or positively remodelled, CTA strategies similar to those used for the identification of ruptured plaques would not be helpful for the prediction of plaque erosion before the occurrence of an event.

2.4.3   Role of Multiple Imaging Modalities to Disclose the Mechanism of ACS

The combination of invasive and non-invasive imaging modalities can contribute to understanding the mechanisms of plaque vulnerability in humans, because various imaging modalities have their strengths and weaknesses (Table 2.3). OCT is able to provide high-resolution images using the back reflection of near-infrared light from optical interfaces in tissue, though its penetration depth is limited to 2 mm. Angioscopy can define the surface characteristics of the ruptured plaque, but is unable to interrogate the interior of the plaque. Whilst greyscale IVUS provides information about plaque morphology to a resolution greater than 100 μm, the lack of high resolution may not allow estimation of fibrous cap thicknesses. The strategy of using a combination of different modalities allows their individual limitations to be effectively mitigated, and a study such as ours may define the ideal combination

---

Fig. 2.4 (continued) An emergent coronary angiography was performed 4 h after the onset of chest pain, which revealed total occlusion of the proximal segment of left anterior descending coronary artery (**a**). Then intravenous administration of heparin (10,000 IU) and half-dose alteplase was started, and he was transferred to a tertiary cardiovascular care centre for a percutaneous coronary intervention. Repeat coronary angiography (8 h after the onset of chest pain) demonstrated no thrombus or stenosis at the original site of total occlusion. Optical coherence tomography (OCT), angioscopy, greyscale intravascular ultrasound and integrated backscatter intravascular ultrasound (**b, c**) were performed. On arrival, CK-MB was 399 (normal: 0.6–3.5) ng/ml, and troponin I was 60.80 (normal: 0.00–0.06) ng/ml. Coronary angioscopy showed faint red thrombus formation through the blue coronary angioscopy guide catheter, whereas OCT did not show a typical red thrombus with a high-backscattering protrusion mass with signal-free shadowing, but some signal reduction was observed from 12 to 3 o'clock positions (**c**). Multiple slices of OCT images revealed an intact fibrous cap (**b**). Intravascular ultrasound and integrated backscatter intravascular ultrasound demonstrated predominantly a fibrous plaque (*green*) and negligible lipid-rich component (*blue*) (**c**). No intervention was undertaken. Predischarge curved multiplanar reconstruction computed tomography images confirmed the absence of positive remodelling and no significant stenosis at the site of the original occlusion (**d**) and mainly normal coronary arteries [42]

Table 2.3 Comparison of imaging detection for coronary vulnerable plaque

	CTA	Greyscale IVUS (40 MHz)	VH-IVUS (20 MHz)	IB-IVUS (40 MHz)	OCT	CAS
Axial resolution (μm)	500	100	200	75	10	50
Lipid pool	+	+/−	+	+	+	+/−
TCFA	−	−	+	+	++	+
Thrombus	+/−	+/−	−	−	+	++
Intimal injury	−	+/−	+/−	+/−	++	+

CTA indicates CT angiography, *IVUS* intravascular ultrasound, *VH* virtual histology, *IB* integrated backscatter, *OCT* optical coherence tomography, *CAS* coronary angioscopy, *TCFA* thin-cap fibroatheroma

++ indicates excellent; +, good; +/−, possible; −, impossible

Although non-invasive CTA could display whole main coronary trees, its image resolution is lower than intracoronary imaging devices, IVUS and OCT, which provide cross-sectional images of the vessels. Whilst OCT is able to provide high-resolution images, greyscale IVUS provides information of plaque morphology with deep penetration depth. Whilst TCFA is identified by OCT and a colour map of VH-IVUS and IB-IVUS, that is recognised as yellow plaque on the images of CAS (see Sect. 2.4.3)

of imaging modalities for maximum gain. Only a few studies have examined the mechanisms underlying plaque vulnerability in vivo using multiple invasive imaging modalities [13, 25, 27, 32, 37], especially CT angiography (Table 2.3).

2.4.4 OCT-Based Clinical Term "IFC-ACS" Versus Pathology Term "Plaque Erosion"

Whilst Jia and his colleagues recently reported that OCT can help discriminate between plaque rupture and erosion clinically, they propose the word "OCT erosion" [14]. However, we believe that a pathological term such as "erosion" may not be appropriate, and, as we proposed, the acute coronary syndromes should be clinically classified on the basis of OCT as those associated with an intact fibrous cap (IFC-ACS) and ruptured fibrous cap (RFC-ACS) [13, 41]. This is not a mere semantic difference but makes the clinical classification as the basis for diagnosis and management. Therefore, in the clinical setting, "IFC-ACS" can be better than the pathology term "plaque erosion" (i.e. OCT erosion) [13, 14, 41].

2.4.5 Clinical Implication of IFC-ACS

IFC-ACS would represent pathological plaque erosions in our study [13]. We recently performed OCT imaging after aspiration thrombectomy and identified plaque erosion as the cause in 31 patients presenting with ST-segment elevation myocardial infarction (Fig. 2.4) [42]. Of the 31 patients, 12 (39 %) patients were treated with dual antiplatelet therapy without stenting and the remaining 19 (61 %) patients underwent stenting [42]. At a two-year follow-up, no difference was found between the two. These observations support an alternative treatment strategy for patients with acute coronary events and OCT-verified intact fibrous cap ACS (IFC-ACS), where nonobstructive lesions might be managed without stenting. This no-stenting management is shown in a case from Fujita Health University Hospital [42]. The recent editorial by Dr. Eugene Braunwald also indicates that the OCT-based clinical description may bring an important change in the treatment paradigm for the management of ACS [43].

2.4.6 Conclusions

This report is derived from our previous study proposing for the first time that nondisrupted culprit lesions (IFC-ACS) in our study would represent plaque erosions (i.e. pathological term). The IFC-ACS lesions based on OCT and angio-scopic characteristics demonstrated less low-attenuation plaque and less positive remodelling than ruptured plaques by CT angiography. Since there are no unique CT features of non-ruptured culprit lesions (IFC-ACS) to enable their clear distinction from stable lesions, it will be difficult to develop CT-based non-invasive imaging techniques to allow the clear identification of subjects at high risk of developing ACS due to IFC.

References

1. Davies MJ. The composition of coronary-artery plaques. N Engl J Med. 1997;336:1312–4.
2. Burke AP, Farb A, Malcom GT, Liang YH, Smialek J, Virmani R. Coronary risk factors and plaque morphology in men with coronary disease who died suddenly. N Engl J Med. 1997;336:1276–82.
3. Virmani R, Kolodgie FD, Burke AP, Farb A, Schwartz SM. Lessons from sudden coronary death: a comprehensive morphological classification scheme for atherosclerotic lesions. Arterioscler Thromb Vasc Biol. 2000;20:1262–75.
4. Kolodgie FD, Virmani R, Burke AP, Farb A, Weber DK, Kutys R, et al. Pathologic assessment of the vulnerable human coronary plaque. Heart. 2004;90:1385–91.
5. Naghavi M, Libby P, Falk E, Casscells SW, Litovsky S, Rumberger J, et al. From vulnerable plaque to vulnerable patient: a call for new definitions and risk assessment strategies: Part II. Circulation. 2003;108:1772–8.
6. Narula J, Willerson JT. Prologue: detection of vulnerable plaque. J Am Coll Cardiol. 2006;47:C1.
7. Muller JE, Tawakol A, Kathiresan S, Narula J. New opportunities for identification and reduction of coronary risk: treatment of vulnerable patients, arteries, and plaques. J Am Coll Cardiol. 2006;47:C2–6.
8. Narula J, Finn AV, Demaria AN. Picking plaques that pop. J Am Coll Cardiol. 2005;45:1970–3.

9. Schaar JA, Muller JE, Falk E, Virmani R, Fuster V, Serruys PW, et al. Terminology for high-risk and vulnerable coronary artery plaques. Report of a meeting on the vulnerable plaque, June 17 and 18, 2003, Santorini, Greece. Eur Heart J. 2004;25:1077–82.

10. Virmani R, Burke AP, Farb A, Kolodgie FD. Pathology of the vulnerable plaque. J Am Coll Cardiol. 2006;47:C13–8.

11. Farb A, Burke AP, Tang AL, Liang TY, Mannan P, Smialek J, et al. Coronary plaque erosion without rupture into a lipid core. A frequent cause of coronary thrombosis in sudden coronary death. Circulation. 1996;93:1354–63.

12. Arbustini E, Dal Bello B, Morbini P, Burke AP, Bocciarelli M, Specchia G, et al. Plaque erosion is a major substrate for coronary thrombosis in acute myocardial infarction. Heart. 1999;82:269–72.

13. Ozaki Y, Okumura M, Ismail TF, Motoyama S, Naruse H, Hattori K, et al. Coronary CT angiographic characteristics of culprit lesions in acute coronary syndromes not related to plaque rupture as defined by optical coherence tomography and angioscopy. Eur Heart J. 2011;32:2814–23.

14. Jia H, Abtahian F, Aguirre AD, Lee S, Chia S, Lowe H, et al. In vivo diagnosis of plaque erosion and calcified nodule in patients with acute coronary syndrome by intravascular optical coherence tomography. J Am Coll Cardiol. 2013;62(19):1748–58.

15. McPherson DD, Sirna SJ, Hiratzka LF, Thorpe L, Armstrong ML, Marcus ML, et al. Coronary arterial remodeling studied by high-frequency epicardial echocardiography: an early compensatory mechanism in patients with obstructive coronary atherosclerosis. J Am Coll Cardiol. 1991;17:79–86.

16. Schoenhagen P, Ziada KM, Kapadia SR, Crowe TD, Nissen SE, Tuzcu EM. Extent and direction of arterial remodeling in stable versus unstable coronary syndromes : an intravascular ultrasound study. Circulation. 2000;101:598–603.

17. Varnava AM, Mills PG, Davies MJ. Relationship between coronary artery remodeling and plaque vulnerability. Circulation. 2002;105:939–43.

18. Hassani SE, Mintz GS, Fong HS, Kim SW, Xue Z, Pichard AD, et al. Negative remodeling and calcified plaque in octogenarians with acute myocardial infarction: an intravascular ultrasound analysis. J Am Coll Cardiol. 2006;47:2413–9.

19. Schuijf JD, Bax JJ, Jukema JW, Lamb HJ, Warda HM, Vliegen HW, et al. Feasibility of assessment of coronary stent patency using 16-slice computed tomography. Am J Cardiol. 2004;94:427–30.

20. Schroeder S, Kopp AF, Baumbach A, Meisner C, Kuettner A, Georg C, et al. Noninvasive detection and evaluation of atherosclerotic coronary plaques with multislice computed tomography. J Am Coll Cardiol. 2001;37:1430–5.

21. Hoffmann MH, Shi H, Schmitz BL, Schmid FT, Lieberknecht M, Schulze R, et al. Noninvasive coronary angiography with multislice computed tomography. JAMA. 2005;293:2471–8.

22. Hoffmann U, Moselewski F, Nieman K, Jang IK, Ferencik M, Rahman AM, et al. Noninvasive assessment of plaque morphology and composition in culprit and stable lesions in acute coronary syndrome and stable lesions in stable angina by multidetector computed tomography. J Am Coll Cardiol. 2006;47:1655–62.

23. Motoyama S, Kondo T, Sarai M, Sugiura A, Harigaya H, Sato T, et al. Multislice computed tomographic characteristics of coronary lesions in acute coronary syndromes. J Am Coll Cardiol. 2007;50:319–26.

24. Motoyama S, Sarai M, Harigaya H, Anno H, Inoue K, Hara T, et al. Computed tomographic angiography characteristics of atherosclerotic plaques subsequently resulting in acute coronary syndrome. J Am Coll Cardiol. 2009;54:49–57.

25. Kubo T, Imanishi T, Takarada S, Kuroi A, Ueno S, Yamano T, et al. Assessment of culprit lesion morphology in acute myocardial infarction: ability of optical coherence tomography compared with intravascular ultrasound and coronary angioscopy. J Am Coll Cardiol. 2007;50:933–9.

26. Motoyama S, Kondo T, Anno H, Sugiura A, Ito Y, Mori K, et al. Atherosclerotic plaque characterization by 0.5-mm-slice multislice computed tomographic imaging. Circ J. 2007;71:363–6.

27. de Feyter PJ, Ozaki Y, Baptista J, Escaned J, Di Mario C, de Jaegere PP, et al. Ischemia-related lesion characteristics in patients with stable or unstable angina. A study with intracoronary angioscopy and ultrasound. Circulation. 1995;92:1408–13.
28. Ozaki Y, Violaris AG, Kobayashi T, Keane D, Camenzind E, Di Mario C, et al. Comparison of coronary luminal quantification obtained from intracoronary ultrasound and both geometric and videodensitometric quantitative angiography before and after balloon angioplasty and directional atherectomy. Circulation. 1997;96:491–9.
29. Ozaki Y, Okumura M, Ismail TF, Naruse H, Hattori K, Kan S, et al. The fate of incomplete stent apposition with drug-eluting stents: an optical coherence tomography-based natural history study. Eur Heart J. 2010;31:1470–6.
30. Prati F, Regar E, Mintz GS, Arbustini E, Di Mario C, Jang IK, et al. Expert review document on methodology, terminology, and clinical applications of optical coherence tomography: physical principles, methodology of image acquisition, and clinical application for assessment of coronary arteries and atherosclerosis. Eur Heart J. 2010;31:401–15.
31. Barlis P, Serruys PW, Gonzalo N, van der Giessen WJ, de Jaegere PJ, Regar E. Assessment of culprit and remote coronary narrowings using optical coherence tomography with long-term outcomes. Am J Cardiol. 2008;102:391–5.
32. Gonzalo N, Garcia-Garcia HM, Regar E, Barlis P, Wentzel J, Onuma Y, et al. In vivo assessment of high-risk coronary plaques at bifurcations with combined intravascular ultrasound and optical coherence tomography. JACC Cardiovasc Imaging. 2009;2:473–82.
33. Jang IK, Tearney GJ, MacNeill B, Takano M, Moselewski F, Iftima N, et al. In vivo characterization of coronary atherosclerotic plaque by use of optical coherence tomography. Circulation. 2005;111:1551–5.
34. Kume T, Akasaka T, Kawamoto T, Ogasawara Y, Watanabe N, Toyota E, et al. Assessment of coronary arterial thrombus by optical coherence tomography. Am J Cardiol. 2006;97:1713–7.
35. Stamper D, Weissman NJ, Brezinski M. Plaque characterization with optical coherence tomography. J Am Coll Cardiol. 2006;47:C69–79.
36. Ueda Y, Asakura M, Hirayama A, Komamura K, Hori M, Komada K. Intracoronary morphology of culprit lesions after reperfusion in acute myocardial infarction: serial angioscopic observations. J Am Coll Cardiol. 1996;27:606–10.
37. Jang IK, Bouma BE, Kang DH, Park SJ, Park SW, Seung KB, et al. Visualization of coronary atherosclerotic plaques in patients using optical coherence tomography: comparison with intravascular ultrasound. J Am Coll Cardiol. 2002;39:604–9.
38. Yabushita H, Bouma BE, Houser SL, Aretz HT, Jang IK, Schlendorf KH, et al. Characterization of human atherosclerosis by optical coherence tomography. Circulation. 2002;106:1640–5.
39. Keane D, Haase J, Slager CJ, Montauban van Swijndregt E, Lehmann KG, Ozaki Y, et al. Comparative validation of quantitative coronary angiography systems. Results and implications from a multicenter study using a standardized approach. Circulation. 1995;91:2174–83.
40. Ozaki Y, Yamaguchi T, Suzuki T, Nakamura M, Kitayama M, Nishikawa H, et al. Impact of cutting balloon angioplasty (CBA) prior to bare metal stenting on restenosis. Circ J. 2007;71:1–8.
41. Ozaki Y. We should use the OCT-based clinical term "acute coronary syndrome with intact fibrous cap (ACS-IFC)" rather than the pathology term "plaque erosion". J Am Coll Cardiol. 2014;63:2745.
42. Prati F, Uemura S, Souteyrand G, Virmani R, Motreff P, Di Vito L, et al. OCT-based diagnosis and management of STEMI associated with intact fibrous cap. JACC Cardiovasc Imaging. 2013;6:283–7.
43. Braunwald E. Coronary plaque erosion: recognition and management. JACC Cardiovasc Imaging. 2013;6:288–9.

Chapter 3
Dye-Staining Coronary Angioscopy and Cardioscopy

Takanobu Tomaru, Fumitaka Nakamura, Yoshiharu Fujimori, and Yasumi Uchida

Abstract Coronary angioscopy or cardioscopy using biocompatible markers is one choice for evaluation of tissues, cells, or molecules which comprise the target lesions. Angioscopy using EB as a biomarker, namely, dye-staining angioscopy, has been developed and applied for molecular imaging of the substances that constitute atherosclerotic lesions.

By dye-staining angioscopy, coronary endothelial damage can be visualized. This technique could also provide discrimination of coronary fibrin from platelets and visualization of transparent fibrin thrombi, namely, a structure that was not visible by conventional angioscopy in patients with acute coronary syndrome (ACS). Fluffy coronary luminal surface without significant stenosis nor obstructive thrombus can be observed in patients with ACS.

Following percutaneous coronary intervention, this dye-staining angioscopy could detect damaged endothelial cells on coronary stent struts in chronic phase and evaluate characterization of band and web formation on the edges of coronary stents.

Dye-staining cardioscopy enabled visualization of blood flow through the subendocardial microvessels or myocardial tissue fluid flow. This technique is useful for evaluation of the effects of coronary interventions or angiogenic therapy on coronary microcirculation.

T. Tomaru, M.D., Ph.D. (✉)
Cardiovascular Center, Toho University Medical Center Sakura Hospital, Shimoshizu 564-1, Sakura, Chiba 285-8741, Japan
e-mail: tomaru-t@sakura.med.toho-u.ac.jp

F. Nakamura, M.D.
The Third Department of Internal Medicine, Teikyo University Chiba Medical Center, Anesaki 3426-3, Ichihara, Chiba 299-0111, Japan

Y. Fujimori
Department of Internal Medicine, Suwa Central Hospital, Suwa, Japan

Y. Uchida, M.D.
Public Trust Cardiovascular Fund, Shiba 3-33-1, Minato-Ku, Tokyo 105-8574, Japan

© Springer Japan 2015
K. Mizuno, M. Takano (eds.), *Coronary Angioscopy*,
DOI 10.1007/978-4-431-55546-9_3

Keywords Dye-staining angioscopy • Dye-staining cardioscopy • Coronary thrombus • Endothelial damage

3.1 Introduction

Conventional coronary angioscopy (AS) has been proven to be more useful for evaluation of coronary plaque and thrombus than angiography. Also, cardioscopy (CS) has been proven to be more useful for the detection of intracardiac thrombi and myocardial diseases than ventriculography. However, visible light is used, both imaging modalities are limited to evaluate surface morphology and color of the target lesions, and therefore, it is beyond the scope for them to evaluate the compositions of the target lesions.

Coronary AS or CS using biocompatible markers is one choice for evaluation of tissues, cells, or molecules which comprise the target lesions.

In 1995, Uchida Y and his colleagues developed dye-staining angioscopy and applied it clinically to observation of the peripheral arteries using Evans blue (EB), which was used clinically for measurement of cardiac output and tissue permeability, as a biomarker for imaging fibrin and damaged endothelial cells [1]. They applied this imaging technique for evaluation of coronary, pulmonary, and aortic lesions in patients [2–9].

They also established dye-staining CS for examination of myocardial microcirculation using EB or fluorescein in patients [10, 11]. This article describes details of these novel imaging techniques.

3.2 Dye-Staining Coronary Angioscopy (AS)

3.2.1 Coronary AS Systems

Two AS systems were used by the present authors.

One AS system is composed of a light source (CTV-A, Olympus Corporation, Tokyo, Japan); a 5-F balloon guiding catheter with three channels, one for 0.5 mm fiberscope (AF-5, Olympus Company, Tokyo, Japan), one for 0.014 guidewire, and the remaining one for saline flush (Clinical Supply Co, Gifu, Japan); and color charge-coupled device (CCD) camera (OTV-A, Olympus Co) (Fig. 3.1a). Other AS system is composed of a light source, same as that described above, an angioscope of monorail type (VecMover, Clinical Supply Co), and a color (CCD) camera (CSVEC-10, Clinical Supply) (Fig. 3.1b).

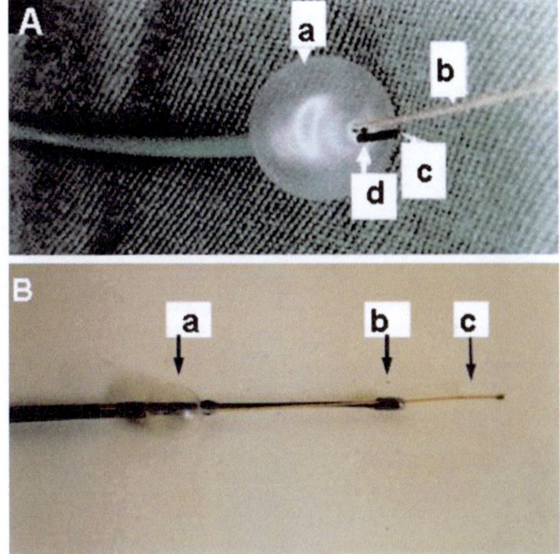

Fig. 3.1 Angioscopes for coronary use
(**a**) A fiberscope incorporated in a 5-F balloon guiding catheter with three channels *a*: Balloon. *b*: Guidewire. *c*: Fiberscope. *d*: Flush channel
(**b**) A monorail-type angioscope. *a*: Balloon. *b*: Fiberscope. *c*: Guidewire

3.2.2 Methods for Dye Staining

After coronary angiography, an angioscope was introduced into the targeted coronary artery. The balloon of the angioscope was inflated to stop the blood flow therein. The fiberscope incorporated into the angioscope was slowly advanced up to 7 cm distally to facilitate successive observations of the artery while displacing the blood by infusion of heparinized saline solution (10 IU/mL) at a rate of 2 mL/s for 10–20 s through the flush channel of the angioscope. To accurately confirm the location of the angioscope tip (and accordingly the observed portion), the angioscopic and fluoroscopic images were displayed simultaneously on a television monitor.

After observation by conventional AS, one mL of 2.5 % Evans blue (EB) solution was injected during balloon inflation into the artery through the flush channel of the angioscope to stain the damaged endothelial cells or fibrin, and then the balloon was deflated for blood flow restoration. One to 2 min later, the balloon was inflated again and the coronary luminal surface was observed by AS.

3.2.3 Imaging of Coronary Endothelial Damages Caused by Catheter Manipulation

Coronary endothelial cells protect the vascular wall against spasm and thrombus formation through release of vasodilating and antithrombotic substances. When the endothelial cells are damaged, thrombus is immediately formed on them. However, it has been difficult to visualize the damaged endothelial cells in patients in vivo.

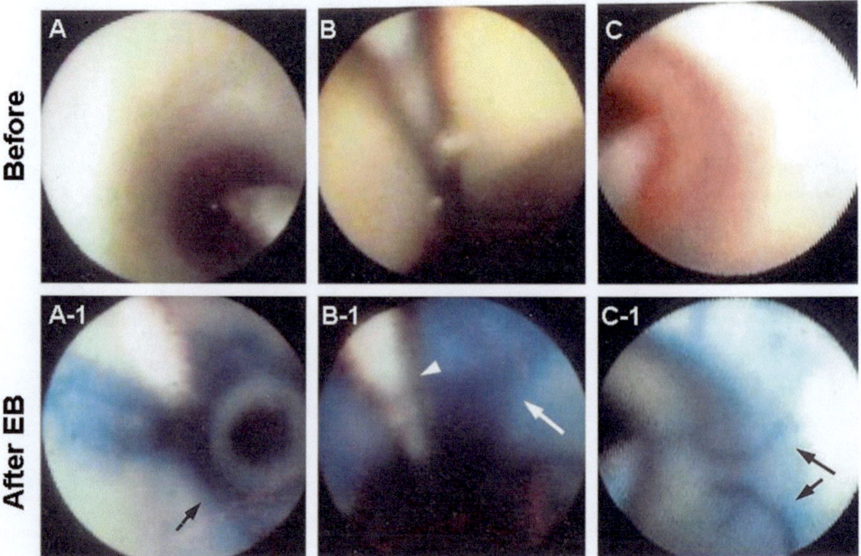

Fig. 3.2 Visualization of coronary endothelial cell damages induced by catheterization
(**a**) A conventional angioscopic image of a coronary segment after balloon inflation of a guiding catheter
(**a**-1) Dye-staining angioscopic image of the same portion. *Arrow*: Circumscribed staining with EB, indicating balloon-induced endothelial damage
(**b**) Conventional angioscopic image of a coronary segment proximal to the target lesion which had been treated by stent deployment
(**b**-1) After EB injection. The entire luminal surface was stained blue, indicating extensive endothelial cell damage (*arrow*). *Arrowhead*: Guidewire
(**c**) Conventional angioscopic image of a coronary segment after single introduction of a guidewire
(**c**-1) After EB injection. Linear endothelial cell damage caused by guidewire (*arrows*)
Cited from Ref. [3] with permission

The present authors succeeded in visualizing the damaged coronary endothelial cells. Namely, it became clear that coronary endothelial damages are caused by insertion of a catheter for percutaneous intervention, balloon inflation, and even by insertion of a guidewire (Fig. 3.2) [3, 5].

3.2.4 Discrimination of Coronary Fibrin from Platelets in Patients with Acute Coronary Syndrome (ACS)

Platelet thrombi play the key role in the genesis of ACS and it was generally considered that the white thrombus is platelet thrombus [9].

We performed dye-staining coronary AS study using EB as a marker of fibrin to examine whether white coronary thrombi in patients with ACS are composed of platelets alone. It became clear that the majority of white thrombi

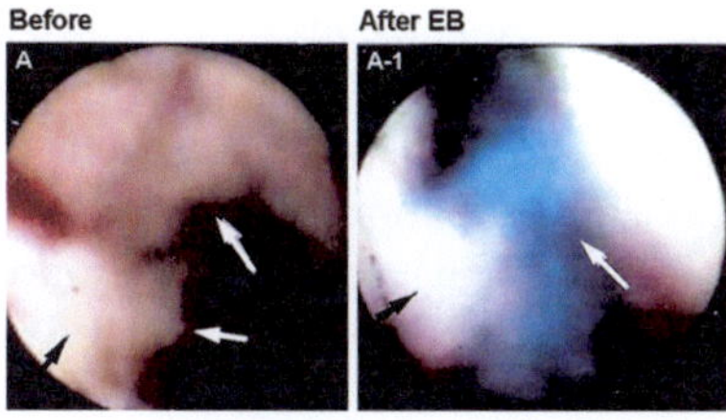

Fig. 3.3 Discrimination of fibrin from platelets in a coronary thrombus
(**a**) White coronary thrombi in a patient with acute myocardial infarction (*arrows*)
(**a**-1) After EB injection. The portions indicated by *white arrows* were stained blue, indicating presence of fibrin, but the portion indicated by a *black arrow* was not stained, indicating platelet aggregates
Cited from Ref. [10] with permission

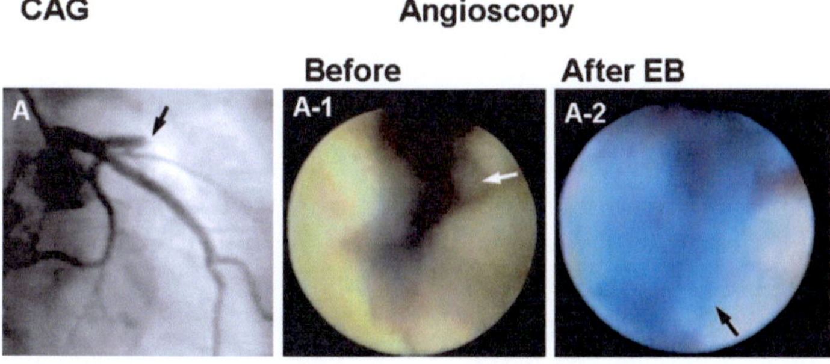

Fig. 3.4 Angiographically obstructed but angioscopically not obstructed coronary segment in a patient with acute myocardial infarction
(**a**) Coronary angiogram (CAG). Obstructed proximal segment of the left anterior descending artery (*arrow*)
(**a**-1) Conventional angioscopic image of the angiographically obstructed segment. The segment was composed of disrupted plaque but residual lumen existed (*arrow*)
(**a**-2) After EB injection. The residual lumen was stained blue, indicating that the lumen was obstructed with a transparent fibrin thrombus (*arrow*)
Cited from Ref. [12] with permission

(so-called platelet thrombi) were clearly discriminated into fibrin-rich and platelet-rich thrombi (Fig. 3.3) [3].

This imaging modality may contribute to the selection of effective primary or adjunctive thrombolytic therapy.

3.2.5 *Angiographically Obstructed but Angioscopically Not Obstructed Culprit Coronary Segment in Patients with Acute Coronary Syndrome (ACS)*

Figure 3.4 shows a patient with unstable angina (UA) in whom the left anterior descending artery was totally occluded by angiography. However, a residual lumen was observed and nothing was seen in the lumen by conventional AS. Dye-staining AS exposed a blue structure occupying the residual lumen, indicating that it was a fibrin thrombus that caused total occlusion. Transparent fibrin thrombi, namely, a structure that was not visible by conventional AS and became visible by dye-staining AS, were observed in unstable angina or non-ST elevation myocardial infarction patients but not in ST-elevation myocardial infarction patients [12].

3.2.6 Detection of Damaged Endothelial Cells on Coronary Stent Struts in Chronic Phase

Coronary in-stent thrombosis is not infrequently observed by AS even 6 months or over after stenting, despite the use of ticlopidine and aspirin. However, the mechanisms underlying this late thrombosis are not well known. Endothelial cells are highly antithrombotic. Therefore, there is a possibility that neoendothelial cells covering stent struts are damaged.

The present authors carried out angioscopic observation of the coronary segments 6 months after bare stent implantation in 44 patients. Stent struts were classified by conventional AS into subgroups: stent struts not covered by neointima (naked group), stent struts seen through the neointima (seen-through group), and those not seen through the neointima (not-seen-through group). Endothelial damages visualized by EB were observed in 13.3 % of not-seen-through group, while in 80 % of seen-through and naked groups (Fig. 3.5). The neoendothelial cells covering stent struts in the seen-through/naked group were stained blue with EB more frequently than in the not-seen-through group, indicating neoendothelial cell damage (Fig. 3.6). Neoendothelial cell damage was classified into localized damage or diffuse damage. Late stent thrombosis was observed in the latter type. In animals, late stent thrombosis was observed when the neointima thickness was within 100 μm. Neoendothelial cells may have been damaged by friction between them and the stent struts due to thin interposed neointima which might have acted as

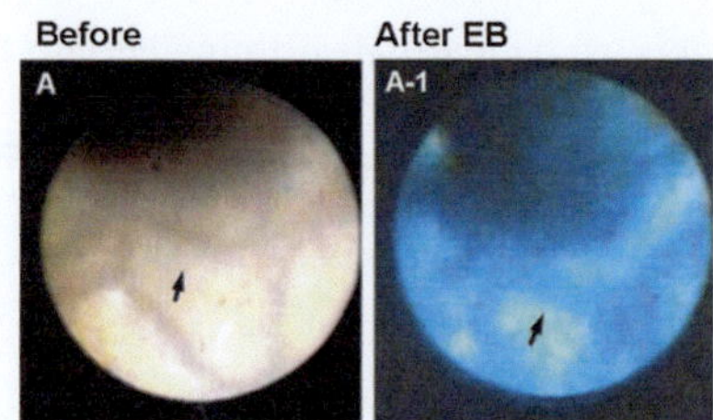

Fig. 3.5 Staining of the endothelial cells covering stent struts 6 months after stent deployment
(**a**) Stent struts were seen through at 6 months after deployment (*arrow*)
(**a**-1) After EB injection. Endothelial cells on the struts but not those in other portions were stained blue, indicating endothelial cell damage (*arrow*)
Cited from Ref. [5, 6] with permission

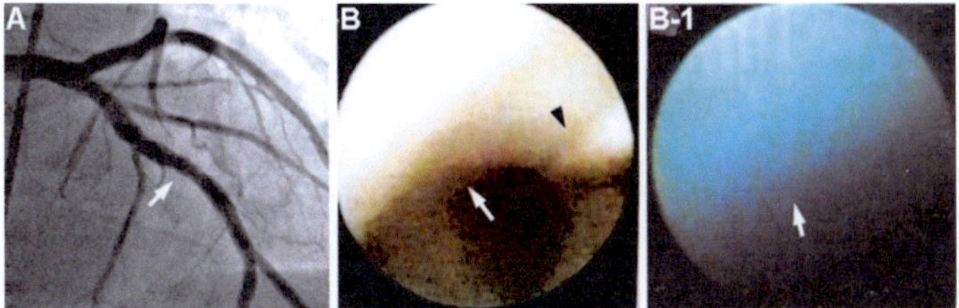

Fig. 3.6 Fluffy luminal surface of culprit non-stenotic coronary segment in a patient with acute coronary syndrome
(**a**) Coronary angiogram (CAG) of left anterior descending artery. *Arrow*: The segment where fluffy luminal surface was observed by AS
(**a**-1) Conventional angioscopy of the same segment. The luminal surface was fluffy as in the case of seagrass (*arrow*). *Arrowhead*: Guidewire
(**a**-2) After EB. The fluffy luminal surface was stained blue, suggesting presence of fibrin threads (*arrow*)
Cited from Ref. [7] with permission

a cushion, resulting in the formation of late stent thrombosis [2, 7]. These findings suggest necessity of appropriate thickening of neointima for prevention of late stent thrombosis. Similar mechanism may participate in late stent thrombosis in patients to whom drug-eluting stent was implanted.

3.2.7 Fluffy Coronary Luminal Surface Without Significant Stenosis nor Obstructive Thrombus in Patients with Acute Coronary Syndrome (ACS)

There are a considerable number of patients with ACS in whom no significant coronary obstructions are angiographically demonstrable. Hitherto, coronary spasm or accidental thrombosis was considered as underlying mechanism, however, without definite evidence. The present authors noticed that there is a certain group of patients with ACS in whom significant stenosis is not demonstrable and the suspected culprit coronary segment exhibits fluffy (or frosty glass-like) surface. In a few of these patients, a thrombus distal to the fluffy segment was detected. The fluffy surface was stained blue with EB, indicating the presence of fibrin and/or damaged endothelial cells (Fig. 3.7).

Similar changes were reproduced by mechanical damages to the artery followed by blood perfusion to produce thrombus in dogs. Fluffy surface was exposed after removal of globular thrombus. Histologically, the fluffy surface was composed of fibrin threads arising from the damaged endothelial cells and adhered by platelets. Therefore, we consider that coronary segment with frosty glass-like surface is the site of surface disruption and resultant thrombosis and frosty glass-like changes are due to residual fibrin and platelets after autolysis of the thrombus [3, 5, 8].

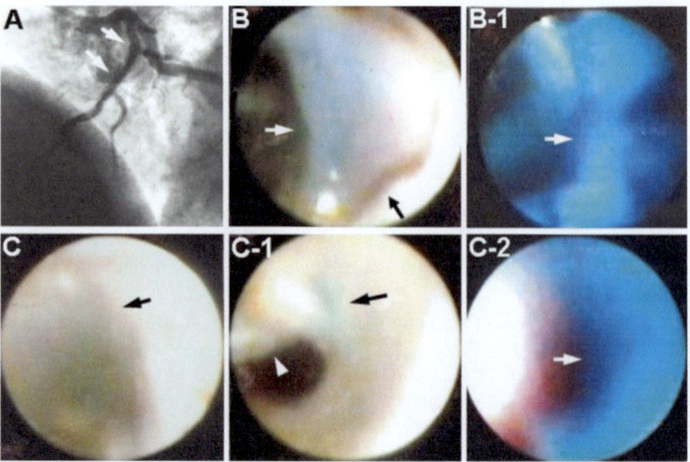

Fig. 3.7 Band-like and membranous structures on the edges of stent
(**a**) The segment of left anterior coronary artery where angioscopy was performed immediately after bare-metal stent deployment (*arrows*)
(**b**-1) Band-like structure on the proximal edge of the stent (*arrow*)
(**b**-2) The band was stained blue with EB, indicating that the band was composed of fibrin
(**b**) Membranous structure on the distal edge of the stent (*arrow*)
(**c**-1) The membranous structure was easily displaced by a guidewire (*arrow*). *Arrowhead*: Guidewire
(**c**-2) The membranous structure was stained blue with EB, indicating that the structure was composed mainly with fibrin (*arrow*)
Cited from Ref. [11] with permission

3.2.8　Characterization of Band and Web Formation on the Edges of Coronary Stents

It is a known fact that in order to treat coronary artery disease, the technique of deployment of bare-metal or drug-eluting stents into the coronary artery is widely followed. However, it is also evident that this effective therapeutic modality brings about the occurrence of several unwonted phenomena in patients, for instance, the onset of in-stent restenosis and subacute or late stent thrombosis.

In the course of conducting routine evaluations of the implanted stents through coronary AS, the authors of the present study found a frequent appearance of band-like structures connecting two or more stent struts, namely, web (W), and/or membrane-like structure connecting multiple stent struts like a curtain and obstructing the lumen, namely, membrane (M), on the edges of the implanted stents. Therefore, the incidence of this phenomenon was further investigated in the acute and chronic phases of the deployment procedure of stents in patients suffering from ACS and from effort angina pectoris. Additionally, evaluation of experiments was conducted on animals in order to obtain further clarification of the mechanisms entailed in this phenomenon.

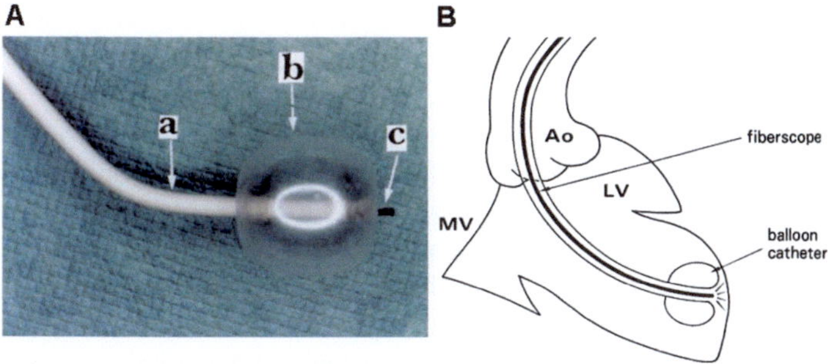

Fig. 3.8 Cardioscopy system
(**a**) Cardioscope. *a*: Balloon guiding catheter shaft. *b*: Balloon. *c*: Fiberscope
(**b**) A method to observe the left ventricular endocardial surface by the cardioscope
(**c**) *Ao* aorta, *MV* mitral valve, *LV* left ventricle

W and M were observed in patients with ACS and those with EA (80.0 % vs 18.7 %) immediately after stent deployment and also 6 months later (55.5 % vs 28.5 %). They were stained in blue with EB immediately after stent deployment but not 6 months later. In beagles, W and M were observed in 75.0 % cases at 5 h and 66.6 % cases a month later. Histological studies revealed that W and M examined 5 h after stenting were composed of fibrin whereas those examined one month later were composed of collagen fibers (Fig. 3.8) [13].

These results indicate that W and M are frequently formed on the edges of coronary stents, and they are composed of fibrin in the acute phase, whereas this fibrin was replaced by collagen fibers in chronic phase. It is conceivable that they are formed due to blood flow turbulence and affinity of stent struts to platelets/fibrin.

The findings in this study indicated that pretreatment with heparin is not sufficient for prevention of W and M formation. Therefore, prophylactic fibrinolytic therapy just before stent deployment may be necessary for prevention of this unwanted phenomenon. Slow flow phenomenon occurs in the stented coronary artery. Distal embolism and endothelial dysfunction have been proposed as the main causative mechanisms of these unwanted hemodynamic changes [14]. Also, stent edge restenosis occurs in chronic phase [15]. There is a possibility that in addition to these mechanisms, the formation of W and M on the stent edges also contributes to slow or no flow and stent edge restenosis.

3.3 Dye-Staining Cardioscopy (CS)

Structurally, the left ventricular wall of the heart comprises three myocardial layers, namely, the inner oblique, middle circular, and outer oblique myocardial layers [16]. It is the inner oblique layer that is most susceptible to ischemia [17]. Till recently, the myocardial blood flow has been evaluated by contrast echocardiography, radionuclide imaging, magnetic resonance imaging, computed tomography, and electron beam computed tomography. However, selective evaluation of the blood flow in the individual myocardial layers, especially in the inner oblique layer, namely, the subendocardial myocardium, is often difficult for these imaging modalities.

A CS system using white light as the light source and obtaining color images of the heart from the inside, namely, conventional cardioscopy [18–20], was devised by the present authors. It was applied for the differential diagnosis of myocardial and valvular diseases. This imaging modality enabled the observation of subendocardial myocardial blood flow (SMBF). However, because endocardial color was used as an indicator, the assessment of SMBF was greatly influenced by the intensity of the light source. Therefore, a more reliable method for direct imaging of SMBF was required.

As the safety of the intravascular administration of EB became evident from all these studies, intracoronary administration of this dye was performed in coronary artery disease patients to observe SMBF disturbance by CS using EB as an indicator of SMBF, namely, "dye-staining CS."

3.3.1 Cardioscopy System and Its Manipulation

The CS system was composed of a light source (CLV-A, Olympus Corporation, Tokyo), 9-F balloon guiding catheter (Clinical Supply Co, Gifu, Japan), 4.2-F fiberscope (AF 14, Olympus), and a color charge-coupled device (CCD) camera (OTV-A, Olympus) (Fig. 3.8).

The patients were pretreated with oral diazepam (10 mg) before being transferred to the catheterization laboratory. Left ventriculography was performed after administering 50 mg of intravenous lidocaine and 5000 IU heparin. A 9-F guiding balloon was then introduced into the left ventricle and the balloon was inflated with CO_2. Next, a 5-F fiberscope was advanced through the catheter so as to position the fiberscope tip at the tip of the catheter. The balloon was gently pushed against the targeted wall segment of the left ventricle, and 50–100 mL of saline solution (heparin 10 IU/mL, 37C°) was injected through the catheter at 10 mL/s to displace the blood between the balloon and the ventricular endocardial surface for observation. The anterior, apical, inferior, and lateral walls of the left ventricle were observed. The changes in the endocardial surface were recorded using a color CCD camera on a DVD recorder.

After control observation, the balloon catheter was replaced by a Judkins catheter and 1 ml of 2.5 % EB was injected into a coronary artery which irrigated the left ventricular wall segment under study. Then, the balloon catheter and fiberscope were reintroduced into the left ventricle, placing the balloon catheter tip at the same wall segment that had been previously observed, and luminal surface changes were observed again.

3.3.2 Evaluation of Subendocardial Myocardial Blood Flow (SMBF) by Dye-Staining Cardioscopy (CS) Using Evans Blue (EB) as a Biomarker

The observed portion was anteroapical segment in chest pain syndrome, the wall segment which was irrigated by the artery in which spasm was evoked by intra-coronary administration of acetylcholine in vasospastic angina, the wall segment irrigated by the stenotic artery in angina, and dys- or akinetic wall segment in old myocardial infarction.

In patients without coronary artery disease, endocardial surface was diffusely stained blue in color immediately after intracoronary injection of EB, indicating diffuse staining of subendocardial myocardium and accordingly normal SMBF in all the patients with CPS. In contrast, in patients with organic coronary artery disease due to organic coronary artery disease, patchy staining indicating patchy preservation of SMBF and no staining indicating absent SMBF were frequently observed. In addition, patchy staining was also observed in patients with VSA, a functional disease (Fig. 3.9).

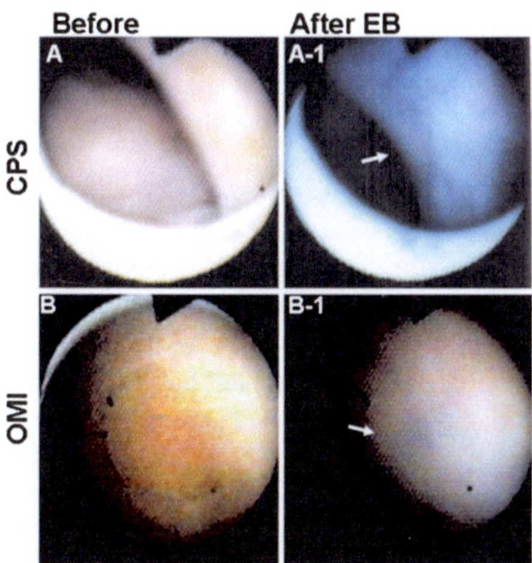

Fig. 3.9 Dye-staining cardioscopy
(**a** to **a**-1) A patient with chest pain syndrome without significant coronary stenosis
(**a**) Before EB intracoronary injection. Endocardial color was brown, indicating normal myocardial blood flow.
(**a**-1) After intracoronary EB injection. The endocardial surface was stained blue, indicating normal blood flow (*arrow*)
(**b** to **b**-1) A patient with old myocardial infarction
(**b**) The endocardial surface was white to yellowish brown
(**b**-1) After EB injection. The endocardial surface was partially stained blue, indicating partial myocardial blood flow (*arrow*)
Cited from Ref. [19] with permission

Effects of coronary stenting on SMBF were also investigated. Restoration of SMBF was confirmed by dye-staining CS in selected patients [4, 8].

3.3.3 Dye-Staining Cardioscopy Using Fluorescein as a Biomarker for Evaluation of Myocardial Tissue Fluid Flow (MTFF)

The subendocardial myocardial layer is most susceptible to ischemia. However, there is no clinically available imaging modality for selective and real-time evaluation of subendocardial myocardial microcirculation. Therefore, a fluorescent CS system which enables real-time and selective visualization of the subendocardial myocardial tissue fluid flow (MTFF) was developed by the present authors [9].

Fluorescein is a fluorescent dye and it is clinically used in the evaluation of retinal vessels [21]. When injected into the vessels, it diffuses through the microvessels of the arterial side into the interstitial spaces of the tissues and finally drains into the venous system. Therefore, if this dye in the myocardium is visualized in vivo, the real-time evaluation of myocardial microcirculation (tissue flow and accordingly regional blood flow in the microvessels) can be attained.

The present authors developed a fluorescent CS system, and using fluorescein as an indicator, the left ventricular subendocardial MTFF was evaluated in patients with coronary artery disease. Furthermore, the effects of percutaneous coronary interventions on the MTFF were evaluated.

3.3.3.1 Fluorescence Cardioscopy (FCS) System and Its Manipulation

The fluorescence cardioscopy (FCS) system was composed of a fluorescent excitation unit, angioscope, balloon guiding catheter, fluorescent emission unit, intensified CCD (ICCD) camera, camera controller, DVD recorder, and television monitor.

The fluorescent excitation unit (CLV-A, Olympus Co, Tokyo) comprised a xenon lamp and a filter disc with a band-pass filter (BP) of 470 nm for fluorescence excitation. The fluorescent emission unit (DD-2, Olympus Co, Tokyo) was composed of a dichroic membrane which cut the wavelength of light below 515 nm, a band absorption filter of 515 nm which allowed wavelength of light more than 515 nm, an intensified CCD (ICCD) camera (C3505, Hamamatsu Photonics Co, Hamamatsu), and a camera controller (C3510, Hamamatsu Photonics Co, Hamamatsu).

The cardioscope and balloon guiding catheter were the same as those used for CS using EB.

After conventional CS, the light and image guides were connected to the excitation and emission units, respectively. After setting the BP and BA filters, the light was irradiated onto the target through the BP filter and light guide. The consequently evoked autofluorescence of the target was received by the ICCD camera through the DM and BA filters.

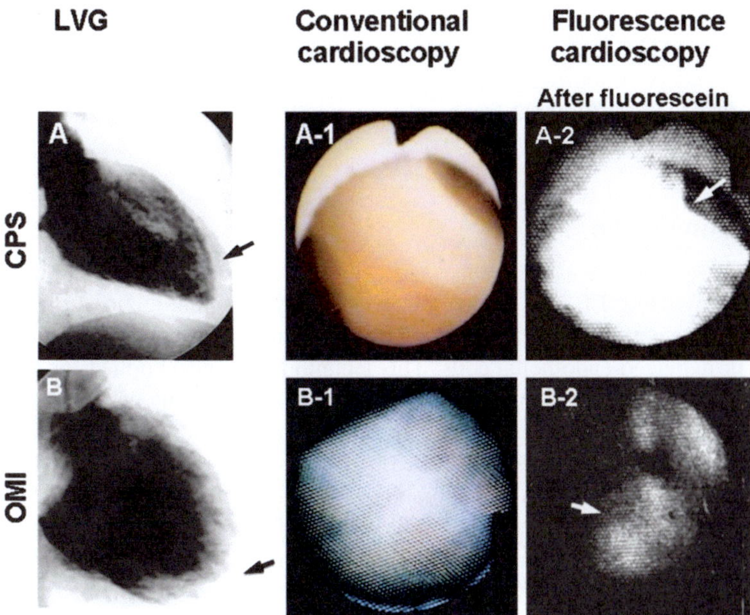

Fig. 3.10 Cardioscopy using fluorescein as a biomarker (fluorescence cardioscopy)
(**a** to **a**-2) A patient with chest pain syndrome (CPS) without demonstrable coronary stenosis
(**a**) Left ventriculogram showed normal contraction. Arrow: The portion observed by cardioscopy
(**a**-1) Conventional cardioscopy revealed normal brown color of the endocardial surface, suggesting normal myocardial blood flow
(**a**-2) After intravenous fluorescein injection. The endocardial surface exhibited strong and diffuse fluorescence, indicating normal myocardial tissue fluid flow
(**b**) Left ventriculogram of a patient with old myocardial infarction (three-vessel disease). Left ventricular contraction was severely disturbed. *Arrow*: The portion observed by cardioscopy
(**b**-1) The endocardial surface was white, indicating fibrosis and/or severe ischemia
(**b**-2) After fluorescein injection. The endocardial surface was partially stained with fluorescein, indicating severely disturbed myocardial tissue fluid flow (*arrow*)
Cited from Ref. [20] with permission

After control observation, 3 ml of 10 % fluorescein (Fluorescite®, Alcon Japan Co, Tokyo) was injected into the right femoral vein. Fluorescence images were obtained at 30 s and 1, 3, and 6 min after finishing fluorescein injection.

3.3.3.2 MTFF in Patients with Coronary Artery Disease

The fluorescence images were classified as follows: diffuse with high intensity indicating normal MTFF, diffuse but with low intensity indicating decreased MTFF, no fluorescence indicating absent MTFF, and patchy fluorescence indicating patchy preservation of MTFF. MTFF was normal in all 18 patients with chest pain syndrome; patchy, decreased, or absent MTFF in 16 of 20 patients with angina pectoris and/or old myocardial infarction due to organic coronary artery disease; and patchy MTFF in 21 of 28 patients with vasospastic angina pectoris. Ten of 20 patients underwent coronary stenting with successful angiographic results in all. However, MTFF disturbance frequently remained (Fig. 3.10) [9].

3.4 Conclusion

Angioscopy using EB as a biomarker, namely, dye-staining angioscopy, clarified hitherto unrecognized mechanisms of coronary artery disease by discriminating fibrin or damaged endothelial cells. This technique was also applied for diagnosis and treatment of aortic, pulmonary, and venous diseases. Using new biocompatible markers, this technique is now used for molecular imaging of the substances that constitute atherosclerotic lesions [22, 23].

Cardioscopy using dyes as biomarkers of blood or tissue fluid flow, namely, dye-staining cardioscopy, enabled visualization of blood flow through the subendocardial microvessels or myocardial tissue fluid flow. This technique will be useful for evaluation of the effects of coronary interventions or angiogenic therapy on coronary microcirculation.

References

1. Uchida Y, Nakamura F, Tomaru T. Observation of atherosclerotic lesions by an intravascular microscope in patients with arteriosclerosis obliterans. Am Heart J. 1995;130:1114–7.
2. Uchida Y. Recent advances in coronary angioscopy. J Cardiol. 2011;57:18–30.
3. Uchida Y. Physiological and histological basis for understanding blood stream, vascular endothelial cell damage, thrombosis, and thrombolysis. In: Uchida Y, editor. Coronary angioscopy. Armonk: Futura Publishing Ltd; 2001. p. 57–70.
4. Uchida Y. Recent advances in percutaneous cardioscopy. Curr Cardiovasc Imaging Rep. 2011;4:317–27.
5. Uchida Y, Uchida Y. Angioscopic evaluation of neointimal coverage of coronary stents. Curr Cardiovasc Imaging Rep. 2010;3:317–23.
6. Terasawa K, Fujimori Y, Morio H, Ozegawa T, Uchida Y. Evaluation of coronary endothelial damages caused by PTCA guidewire: in vivo dye staining angioscopy. J Jpn Coll Angiol. 2000;40:159–64.
7. Uchida Y, Uchida Y, Sakurai T, Kanai M, Shirai S, Oshima T, Koga A, Matsuyama A. Possible role of damaged neoendothelial cells in the genesis of coronary stent thrombus in chronic phase. Int Heart J. 2011;52:12–6.
8. Uchida Y, Uchida Y, Sakurai T, Kanai M, Shirai S, Oshima T, Koga A, Matsuyama A, Tabata T. Fluffy luminal surface of the non-stenotic culprit coronary artery in patients with acute coronary syndrome.-An angioscopic study. Circ J. 2010;75:2379–85.
9. Uchida Y, Uchida Y, Shirai S, Oshima T, Shimizu K, Tomaru T, Sakurai T, Kanai M. Angioscopic detection of pulmonary thromboemboli: with special reference to comparison with angiography, intravascular ultrasonography and computed tomography angiography. J Interven Cardiol. 2010;23:470–8.

10. Uchida Y, Uchida Y, Sakurai T, Kanai M, Sugiyama Y. Imaging of subendocardial blood flow by dye-staining cardioscopy in patients with coronary artery disease. Int Heart J. 2010;51:308–11.
11. Uchida Y, Uchida Y, Kanai M, Tomaru T, Noike F, Sakurai T. Evaluation of myocardial tissue fluid flow by fluorescence cardioscopy in patients with coronary artery disease. Int Heart J. 2010;51:153–8.
12. Uchida Y, Uchida Y, Sakurai T, Kanai M, Shirai S, Morita T. Characterization of coronary fibrin thrombus in patients with acute coronary syndrome using dye-staining angioscopy. Arterioscler Thromb Vasc Biol. 2011;31:1452–60.
13. Uchida Y, Uchida Y, Matsuyama A, Koga A, Kanai M, Sakurai T. Formation of web- and membrane-like structures on the edges of bare-metal coronary stents. Circ J. 2010;74:1830–6.
14. Airoldi F, Buriguori C, Cianflone D, Cosgrave J, Sankovic G, Godino C. Frequency of slow flow following stent implantation and effect of nitroprusside. Am J Cardiol. 2007;99:916–20.
15. Jensen LO, Maeng M, Mintz GS, Christiansen EH, Hansen KN, Galloe H. Serial intravascular ultrasound analysis of peri-stent remodeling and proximal and distal edge effects after sirolimus-eluting or paclitaxel-eluting stent implantation in patients with diabetes mellitus. Am J Cardiol. 2009;103:1083–8.
16. Bhatis S, Levi M. The pathology of congenital heart disease, vol. 1. Armonk: Futura Publishing Ltd; 1996. p. 40–1.
17. Fujita T. Myocardial anatomy. In: Human anatomy. Tokyo: Nankodo CO; 1993. p. 310.
18. Uchida Y, Nakamura F, Oshima T, Fujimori Y, Hirose J. Percutaneous fiberoptic angioscopy of the left ventricle in patients with idiopathic dilated cardiomyopathy and acute myocarditis. Am Heart J. 1990;120:677–87.
19. Uchida Y. Atlas of cardioangioscopy. Tokyo: Mrdical View Co; 1995. p. 93–161.
20. Uchida Y. Percutaneous fiberoptic angioscopy of cardiac chambers and valves. In: Zipes DP, Rowlands BJ, editors. Progress in cardiology. Philadelphia: Lea & Febiger; 1991. p. 163–91.
21. Albert DM, Jakobiec FA. Fluorescein angiography. Principles and practice of ophthalmology, vol. 2. Toronto: W.B. Saunders Co; 1994. p. 697–717.
22. Uchida Y, Maezawa Y. Molecular imaging of atherosclerotic coronary plaques by fluorescent angioscopy. In: Schaller B, editor. Molecular imaging. Rijeka: Intech; 2012. p. 247–68.
23. Uchida Y, Uchida Y, Hiruta N, Shimoyama E, Sugiyama E. Molecular imaging of native high-density lipoprotein in human coronary plaques by fluorescent angioscopy. JACC Cardiovasc Imaging. 2013;6:1015–7.

Part II
Procedure of Coronary Angioscopy

Chapter 4
Angioscopy Catheter Equipped with a Balloon for Blood Flow Attenuation

Jun-ichi Kotani

Abstract This is an angioscopy catheter equipped with a compliant balloon attached proximally to decrease blood flow in order to secure a good anterior visual field. Complete blockage of blood flow by maximally inflating the balloon is not necessary. This system is available when using regular guidewire with monorail system and can be kept in place throughout the procedure. The system can move forward or backward freely in the coronary artery and the catheter is centered with the assistance of the wire and balloon; especially in the investigation inside a coronary artery, it is very important to see the structures spatially as a cylinder.

Keywords Angioscopy • Occlusion balloon • Monorail system • Angioscopy catheter

In the early days, diagnosing diseases in humans through imaging was based on anatomy. However, when establishment tissue characterization of the target lesion was considered safe, invasive imaging gained attention and popularity. On the other hand, coronary angiography is the gold standard for assessing coronary artery disease due to atherosclerosis, but there remain some limitations, such as the inability of assessment of atherosclerosis itself, the choice of treatment, and the determination of treatment efficacy. Hence, for more detailed evaluation, invasive diagnosis that is complementary to anatomical diagnosis, based on comparisons with pathological diagnosis, has been developed. Among these, angioscopy has an established history, and its basic structure has remained almost the same [1, 2], an angioscopy catheter equipped with an occlusion balloon, and recent clinical applications are based on this system [3].

J. Kotani (⊠)
Cardiovascular Medicine, Osaka University Graduate School, 2-2 Yamada-oka,
Suita, Osaka 565-0871, Japan
e-mail: Shamallv8@aol.com

© Springer Japan 2015
K. Mizuno, M. Takano (eds.), *Coronary Angioscopy*,
DOI 10.1007/978-4-431-55546-9_4

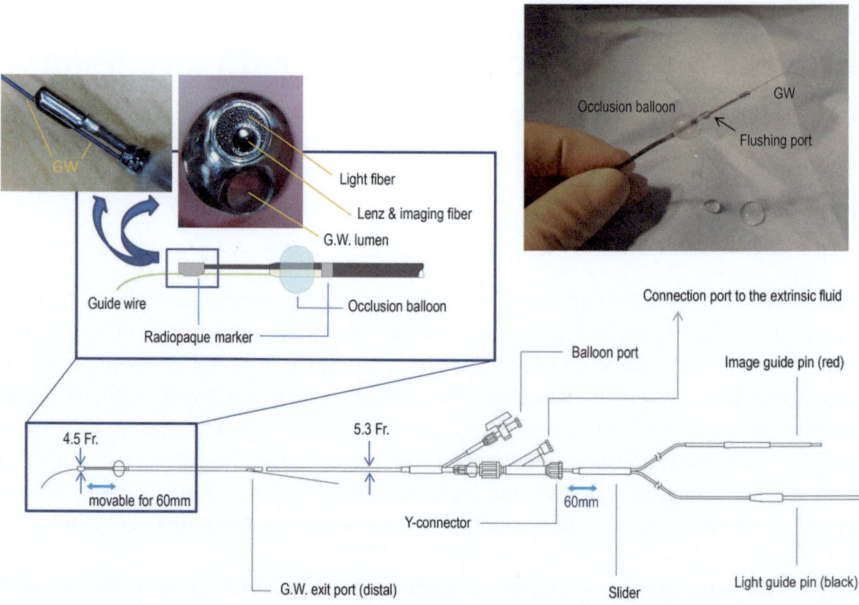

Fig. 4.1 Schema of an angioscopy catheter equipped with an occlusion balloon

4.1 Components of an Angioscopy Catheter Equipped with an Occlusion Balloon

This catheter has three characteristics. First, it is equipped with a balloon to secure a stable visual field for observation. Second, observation can be performed with a 0.014-in. guidewire in place that is compatible with standard percutaneous coronary intervention (PCI). Third, the fiber mounted on the wire (monorail system) can move forward or backward freely in the coronary artery (Fig. 4.1).

The most notable feature of this mechanism is that it contributes to a stable visual field. When evaluating the intravascular space, especially inside a stent, it is very important to see the structures spatially as a cylinder. Since a fiber without a guidewire moves linearly due to stiffness, the tip frequently comes into contact with the luminal surface and the effective visual field is restricted to the anterior direction. In addition, the fiber cannot move forward. On the other hand, a good anterior visual field is secured in this system because the catheter is centered with the assistance of the wire and balloon. Hence, the fiber can go toward a specific target site and return to it repeatedly for observation throughout the target segment. Software advancements have also been remarkable, including functions such as autofocus and white balance adjustment (Fig. 4.2).

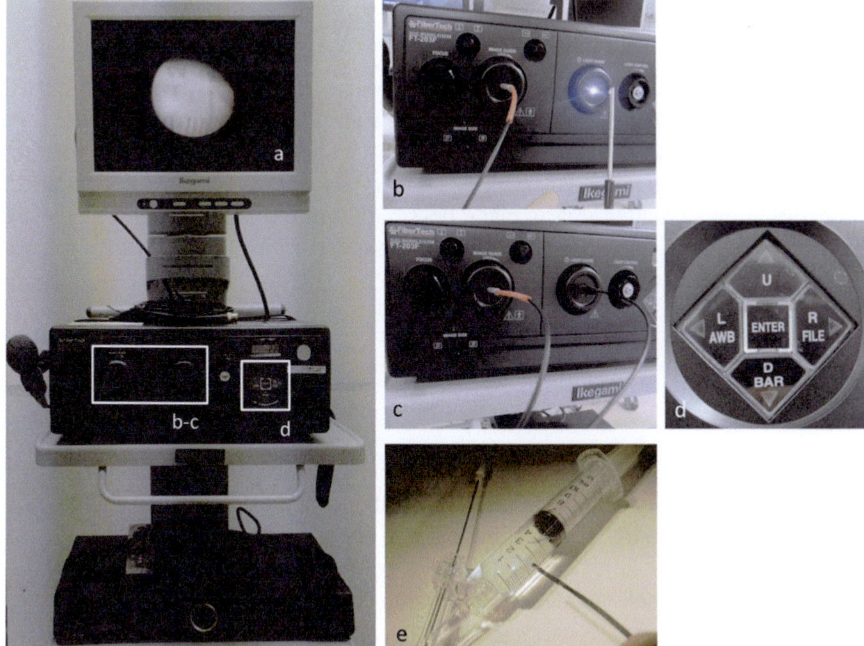

Fig. 4.2 Angioscopy system. (**a**) monitor (the monitor presents the image of panel **e**). (**b**, **c**) imaging guide (*red*) and lighting guide (*black*). (**d**) all adjustment can be done by this terminal. (**e**) autofocus adjustment

4.1.1 Occlusion Balloon and Flash Port Located on the Distal Tip

One feature of this catheter, as indicated by its name, is the presence of a compliant balloon attached proximally to decrease blood flow in order to secure a good anterior visual field. Complete blockage of blood flow by maximally inflating the balloon is not necessary. In clinical use, lactated Ringer's or low molecular weight dextran-L is flashed from the head in order to prevent retrograde blood flow coming from the anterior direction or side branches due to collateral circulation. Hence, a small degree of residual antegrade blood flow does not create a problem. Inflating the balloon may not be necessary during the observation of small vessels. For these reasons, the method of inflating the equipped balloon using CO_2 gas, while checking the monitor after flashing, has been widely adopted, replacing the traditional method of inflating the balloon with a diluted contrast agent under fluoroscopic guidance. While an inflated balloon cannot be checked with this method, the advantage is that inflation time can be shortened and an air vacuum is not required.

4.1.2   Monorail System

Observation with this catheter can be carried out with a 0.014-in. guidewire used for PCI in the coronary artery, which is also common for other imaging devices. Furthermore, using a proximally located slider, the tip of the fiber can move forward and backward on the guidewire with its support. By blocking off blood flow once, observation in a broader area is made possible. Furthermore, since the guidewire becomes a supporting device, the fiber can pass closer to the center of the inner cavity, contributing to a wider visual field.

4.2   Operation

Because each unit is integrated, operation after insertion is straightforward. However, despite the various functions mentioned above, understanding the role of each part and making thorough preparations prior to insertion are vital. Since this system must be connected to an exterior equipment, cooperation and communication with healthcare professionals such as clinical engineers are important.

4.2.1   System Outline

This system is comprised of (1) a fiber catheter, (2) a light source system main unit, (3) a computer and hard disc, and (4) a monitor. The fiber catheter has been described above. This system has compatibility with angioscopy of non-balloon occlusion type (Chap. 5).

4.2.2   Preparation of the Catheter

As with catheters in general, remove the catheter from the packaging and place it in the holder filled with water to prevent it from drying out. Wipe off any dust on the terminals connected to the light source with dry gauze, and avoid getting the connecting terminals wet. The distal part of the catheter has several holes; each of them is a lumen through which the guidewire, balloon, fluid for flashing, or the optical fiber or lens can pass.

The proximal portion of the catheter is separated into a balloon port with a two-way stopcock and a slider attached to a Y connector. Attach the slider, which moves the fiber forward or backward relative to the Y connector, and attach the intravenous circuit for flashing to the side tube. These parts, in addition to the Y connector, must be connected to the exterior equipment. The tip of the slider branches into two connection terminals (red, imaging guide; black, lighting guide). Connect a three-way stopcock with an intravenous circuit so that pressure can be externally applied. Completely extract any air from the intravenous circuit, and then connect it to the Y connector. After connecting it to the Y connector, move the slider forward and backward to completely extract any air bubbles from inside of the Y connector. Flash repeatedly in order to extract any bubbles from the inside of the catheter. After confirming that all air bubbles are completely removed, position the slider 1 mm distal to the tip of the slider so that it cannot move or come closer. Gently screw the Y connector to fasten it in place. If the slider cannot move or come closer when the catheter is inserted in the patient, not only will the slider not move, but it may also become unexpectedly ejected due to a kickback caused by forceful movement of the slider, which is dangerous. Before insertion, inflate the balloon in water once to check its integrity. When inflating a balloon with contrast agent, thoroughly extract any air. When using a viscous contrast agent, exercise care since it may take more time to deflate; extracting air from inside the system may not occur smoothly.

4.2.3 Connection to External Equipment

Connect the imaging guide and lighting guide to the main unit's light source. Check the monitor to make sure there is no dust on the tips of the terminals or damage to the fiber. Next, adjust the white balance. Simply push the adjustment button with the head of the catheter pointing in the direction of the white board with DIC-F27 or RAL9010 for Europe (at a distance of 1–2 mm away from the fixed white board to mimic the actual relative distance between the fiber and the vascular wall inside the body). This step is important to avoid halation within the vessel (Fig. 4.3).

In order to reduce the risk of complications, the composition of the infusion solution used for flashing is important. Blood is replaced with the infusion solution during observation. Use of heparinized saline may cause a prolonged QT interval, arrhythmia, and bleeding. To avoid these problems, use infusion solutions that are mainly comprised of extracellular fluid, such as lactated Ringer's or low molecular weight dextran-L.

4.2.4 Catheter Manipulation

X-ray is required during catheter manipulation. Procedures for inserting a system into the aortic root are the same as the standard procedures for a catheter for angioplasty. However, the following should be kept in mind before inserting a catheter into the coronary artery.

Fig. 4.3 White balance adjustment (focus and color balance are automatically adjusted by this procedure). *(1)* Move the head of the fiber close to fixed pure white panel (DIC-F24 or RAL9010). *(2)* Maintain conditions and push the adjustment button for 2–3 s. *(3)* Confirm that adjustment is complete on the monitor

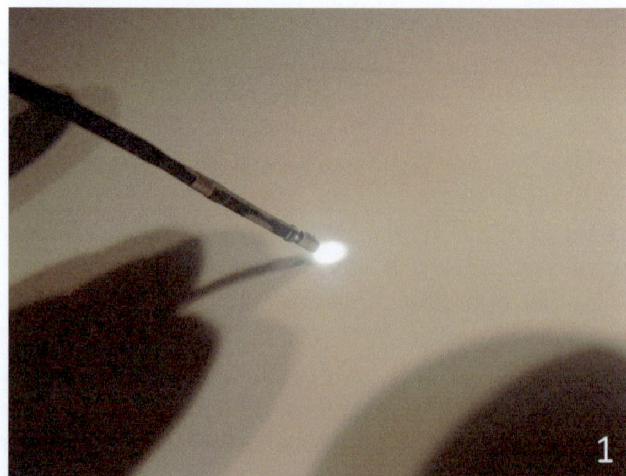

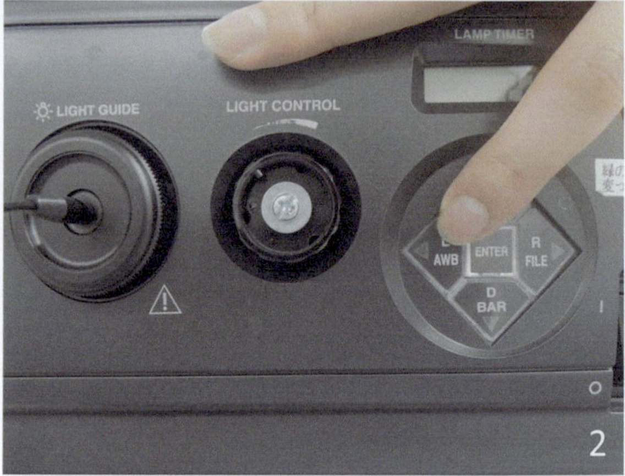

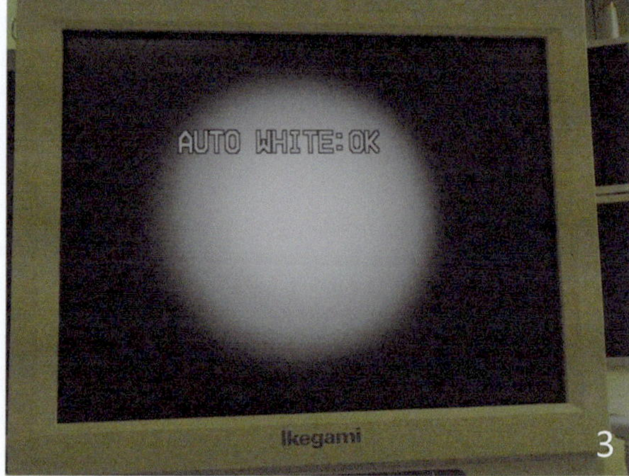

4.2.4.1 Inserting a Catheter into the Coronary Artery

As explained in the section on structure, the tip of this catheter is made of metal and has a complex structure. Compared to the coronary stent delivery system, it is slightly more bulky and rigid. As a result, if the catheter is forcefully pushed forward, there is a greater risk of damage to the vessel wall. However, the structure used to slide the tip can improve conformability, and there is no need for strong backup support of a guide catheter. Maintaining a straight line between the ostium and the proximal segment of the coronary artery coaxially is important when inserting the catheter. If the catheter becomes stuck, move the slider forward and position the tip distally (to change the stiffness of the distal part of the system) before moving the entire catheter forward again. Forward movement may help to advance the catheter by "buddy effect".

4.2.4.2 Coronary Artery Observation

After confirming that the radio-opaque part of the catheter attached to the balloon is positioned inside the coronary artery, perform fluid flashing from the head and inflate the balloon. Slowly inflate the balloon until the anterior visual field is secured (Fig. 4.4). At the same time, start electrocardiographic monitoring, and watch it closely. Normally, one moves the slider forward slowly and observes the coronary artery in the proximal to distal direction. Of course, with this system the same site can be repeatedly observed by pulling on the slider. The slider alignment distance is 60 mm. At that point, if ischemic sign appears, immediately stop moving the slider and flashing, and deflate the occlusion balloon. If you reinflate the balloon and restart the flashing after the ischemia has been resolved, observation can be continued at the same location. When the tip of the fiber does not move forward

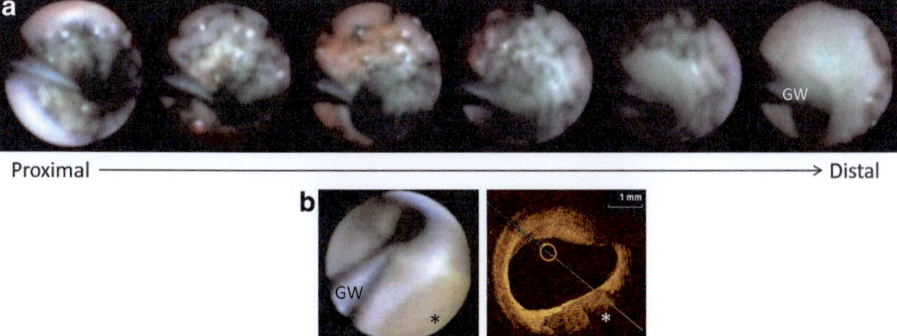

Fig. 4.4 Representative cases. (**a**) circumferential image of 3.0×20 mm stent is provided by the system with occluded balloon equipped angioscopy (Proximal-LAD, immediately after stent implantation). (**b**) Comparative images between angioscopy (*left*) and optical coherence tomography (*right*). *, calcium image; *GW*, guidewire

due to a bend in the coronary artery, do not forcibly move the slider. Rather, change the bias of the entire catheter or the guidewire, and then see if it moves smoothly. Changing the rigidity of the guidewire or using the buddy wire technique may also be effective.

4.2.5 Recording and Storage of Media

As with frequency-domain optical coherence tomography (FD-OCT), start recording once removal of blood from the vessel has been confirmed. Recording images with voice announcement and recording the initial part of catheter manipulation in cine-film mode are useful for off-line analysis.

References

1. Mizuno K, Arai T, Satomura K, Shibuya T, Arakawa K, Okamoto Y, Miyamoto A, Kurita A, Kikuchi M, Nakamura H, et al. New percutaneous transluminal coronary angioscope. J Am Coll Cardiol. 1989;13:363–8.
2. Nanto S, Ohara T, Mishima M, Hirayama A, Komamura K, Matsumura Y, Kodama K. Coronary angioscopy: a monorail angioscope with movable guide wire. Am J Card Imaging. 1991;1:1–5.
3. Uchida Y. Coronary angioscopy. 1st ed. New York: Futura Publishing Company, Inc.; 2001.

Chapter 5
System and Procedure of Nonocclusion Type of Angioscopy

Tadateru Takayama

Abstract Nonocclusion type of angioscopy was developed in Japan. The design of the device is relatively simple, consisting of a probe catheter and fiber catheter. Low molecular weight dextran is injected through the outer probe, removing red blood cells from the vessel wall in order to create a clear field of view for observing the lesion. This paper will describe the procedural requirements to undertake nonocclusion type of angioscopy.

Keywords Nonocclusion type of angioscopy • Procedure • Intravascular imaging

5.1 Introduction

Angioscopy visualizes atherosclerotic lesions in vivo, with yellow plaque indicating lipid-rich plaque and high vulnerability [1–10]. Nonocclusion type of angioscopy has been used to assess plaque morphology in patients with acute coronary syndrome and plaque stabilization or regression by statin treatment in a number of clinical trials [11–13]. Recently, some reports have evaluated neointimal coverage and thrombus formation after drug-eluting stent implantation by angioscopy [14–17].

The type of angioscopy system (Fig. 5.1a) comprises of a light source and a CCD camera. There are two types of angioscopy systems, which are distinguished according to the use of an occlusion balloon. Both balloon occlusion and nonocclusion types of catheters are commercially available in Japan. In particular, the unique feature of the nonocclusion type of angioscopic procedure is that the lumen of the vascular can be observed without requiring a blood occlusion, minimizing myocardial ischemia compared to a balloon occlusion type.

Although angioscopy is a commercially available and FDA-approved optical imaging technology that has been available for many years, its use in the United

T. Takayama, M.D., Ph.D. (✉)
Division of Cardiology, Department of Medicine, Nihon University School of Medicine, 30-1 Ohyaguchi-kamicho, Itabashi-ku, Tokyo 173-8610, Japan
e-mail: takayama.tadateru@nihon-u.ac.jp

© Springer Japan 2015
K. Mizuno, M. Takano (eds.), *Coronary Angioscopy*,
DOI 10.1007/978-4-431-55546-9_5

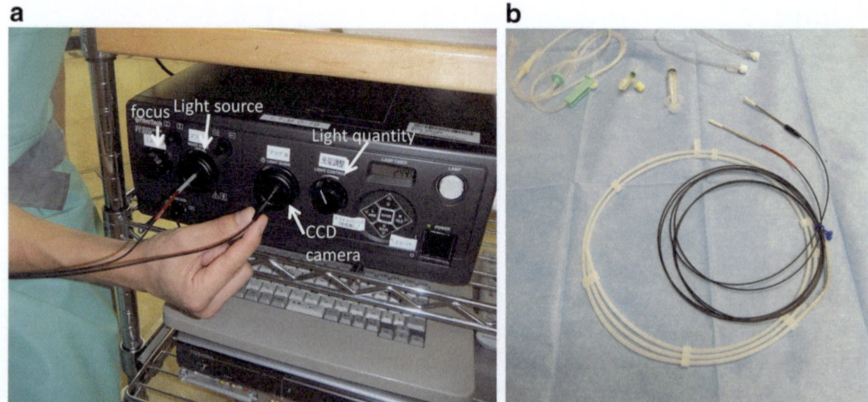

Fig. 5.1 Fiber catheter of nonocclusion type of angioscopy and imaging system. (**a**) This device has a built-in a light source and a CCD camera. (**b**) This catheter is 6,000 pixels. This probing catheter consists of inner catheter and outer catheter. A tube and a T-shaped stopcock for the connection with dextran are required. 5 ml syringes for flashbulbs are also necessary

States has been largely restricted to research applications rather than clinical practice. Limitations of the technology include the requirement to clear the coronary lumen of blood by the infusion of saline, the large catheter diameter that limits the evaluation of distal segments, the inability to pass significant lesions, and the difficulties associated with accurate interpretation of the images, which therefore mandate expertise [18, 19]. Balloon occlusion-induced myocardial ischemia and the complicated procedure arising from the use of an occlusion type angioscopy may be a concern in the United States.

Nonocclusion type of angioscopy was developed in Japan in order to eliminate the risk associated with the balloon occlusion device, with approval obtained from the Ministry of Health, Labor and Welfare. The design of the device is relatively simple, consisting of a probe catheter and fiber catheter. Low molecular weight dextran is injected through the outer probe, removing red blood cells from the vessel wall in order to create a clear field of view for observing the lesion. This paper will describe the procedural requirements to undertake nonocclusion type of angioscopy.

5.2 Nonocclusion Type of Angioscopy System

A description of the angioscopy device and catheter is outlined in Fig. 5.1a, b. The physician operates the fiber and probe catheters, while a 2nd operator flushes low molecular weight dextran through the manifold.

5.3 Preparation of Nonocclusion Type of Angioscopy

1. Preparation of nonocclusion type of angioscopy (VISIBLE Fiber (FT-203F; Fiber Tech Co. Ltd., Tokyo, Japan), a fiber imaging system, and a console (Inter-tec Medicals Co. Ltd., Osaka, Japan) is as follows: both the inner and outer probing catheter are flushed with heparin and assembled.
2. The 2nd operator assembles the manifold, ensuring that no air is introduced with the low molecular weight dextran. A 5 ml syringe is also attached (Fig. 5.2).
3. A 0.014-in. guidewire is inserted through the probing catheter, introduced via a guiding catheter (>6Fr) for coronary angioplasty and advanced to lesion location, while viewing fluoroscopic images on the monitor (Fig. 5.3).
4. Then, the inner catheter and guidewire are removed, and the 5 ml syringe is connected while confirming presence of reverse blood flow and that no air has been introduced. The fiber catheter is then inserted.

5.4 Preparation for the Probing Catheter

The probing catheter requires rinsing with saline solution. The outer and inner catheters are then separated and rinsed using a 10 ml syringe which is also effective in removing residual air. The probe catheter is rinsed in a tray (it is important to ensure that the catheter does not dry out). The catheter should be carefully rinsed

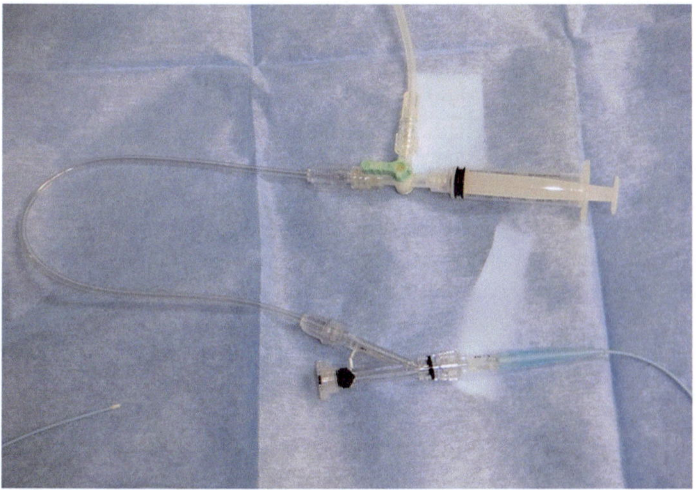

Fig. 5.2 System of nonocclusion type of angioscopy (probing catheter and flushing system). This shows the connection method with the syringe for Y-connector and flashbulbs

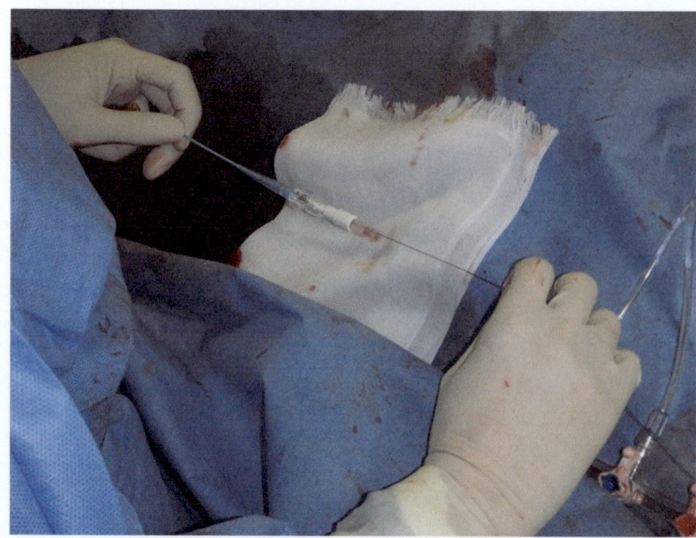

Fig. 5.3 Advancing probing catheter on the guidewire. 0.014-in. guidewire is inserted through the probing catheter, introduced via a guiding catheter and advanced to lesion location, while viewing fluoroscopic images on a fluoroscopic monitor

to ensure that no residual air remains (residual air bubbles in the tip of the probing catheter will result in interference of the field of imaging). The inner catheter is placed within the outer catheter while immersed in saline solution. As the catheter is relatively thin, the use of a small tray may affect the ability to insert the catheter effectively, and excessive force may result in damage to the catheter. The catheter is easily inserted in a straight position, and should resistance be encountered, it may be effective to pre-insert the guidewire in the inner catheter prior to insertion into the outer catheter (Fig. 5.4). If there is residual air inside the catheter, air bubbles or ST elevation on the electrocardiograph is observed during the procedure; a 20–30 ml syringe of saline solution should be used to repetitively flush the coronary arteries and wash out any air post procedure. When the probing catheter in the angioscopy catheter set cannot cross over severe stenosis, an aspiration catheter (>7Fr) for thrombectomy can be used instead of the original probing catheter.

5.5 Focus Alignment of Angioscopy

In order to align the focus of the angioscopy catheter, the tip should be placed close to a dry gauze in order to confirm the imaging. The image should be focused to align either the 2×2 or 3×3 markers (Fig. 5.5). The focusing dial should be adjusted carefully and the focus confirmed. Following repetitive use, the tip should be cleaned with damp gauze and the focus readjusted. When protein becomes attached

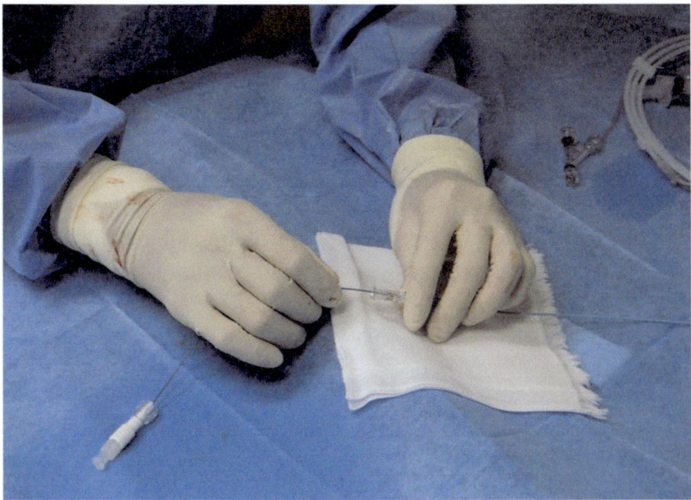

Fig. 5.4 Inserting inner catheter to outer probing catheter. Outer probing catheter should be as straight as possible while inserting the inner probing catheter. The inner catheter is placed within the outer catheter while immersed in saline solution

Fig. 5.5 Focus alignment of angioscopy. The image should be focused to align either the 2x2 or 3x3 markers

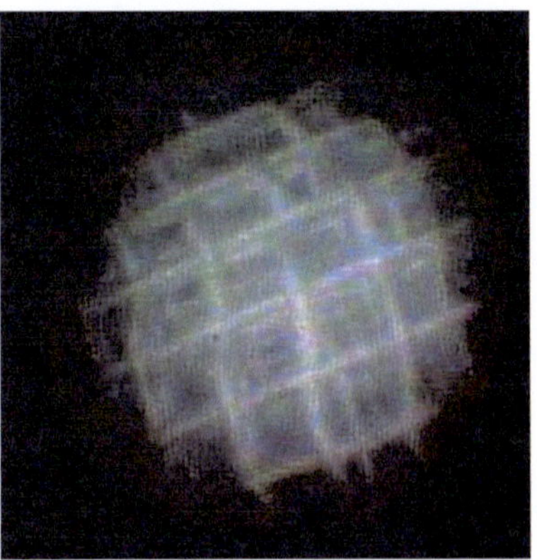

to the tip, the image may become unfocused. When large particles are observed on the image, it may be resultant from particles contained within the connection rather than the catheter tip. The connection should be wiped with either gauze or cotton swab or the "white balance" button reset.

5.6 Insertion of the Fiber Catheter into the Probing Catheter

Similar to other catheters, the fiber catheter is easily damaged under excessive bending. When the fiber is broken, sufficient light is unable to reach the catheter tip. When product is not in use, it is recommended to place a cover over the fiber when stored. The probing catheter is inserted beyond the target location. Care should be given that the guiding catheter does not become disengaged when the probing catheter is inserted into tortuous vasculature (the guiding catheter should ideally be coaxially positioned). It might be impossible to advance the fiber catheter when the guiding catheter is bent. When the catheter is placed in position, the inner catheter and guidewire are removed (quickly removing product may result in the introduction of air). Use a 2.5 ml syringe to remove any residual air, and confirm the backflow of blood. When reverse blood flow is not observed, the catheter may have become wedged in a smaller vessel diameter, and under minimal negative pressure, the catheter should be pulled slightly proximal. Not correcting this issue may result in an ST elevation.

5.7   Care During Insertion

The 2nd operator should introduce low molecular dextran removing residual air with the Y-connector connected. The fiber catheter is then inserted though probing catheter. Further flushing of dextran should be performed again with the catheter inserted at a 40–50 cm depth to ensure removal of all residual air. Finally, the fiber catheter is further inserted just prior to the tip of the guide catheter. If the guiding catheter tip is positioned at a bend, some resistance may be incurred during insertion. If the fiber catheter is within the guiding catheter, it can be advanced further even under some resistance. If the guiding catheter is excessively bent, the guiding catheter positioning should be corrected. Insertion resistance will be increased if the probing catheter is also placed in a bent position. A fluoroscopic marker is located at the tip, and the catheter should be advanced 1 cm at a time. The catheter should be inserted as straight as possible to avoid damage to the catheter. Excessive force may result in the fiber catheter breaking.

When image recording is commenced, it can be difficult to determine the vessel location and whether target location is pre- or posttreatment. All significant lesion locations should be recorded on cine angiography while imaging, noting details such as the position of the catheter and the grade of the plaque.

5.8   Careful Consideration During Imaging

It is important that the lead physician be aware of the positioning of both probing catheter tip and fiber catheter when pulling the probing catheter back. The image in Fig. 5.6a is the correct positioning.

When the fiber catheter is positioned far from the tip of probing catheter, the observational range is small, and the whole image is dark as in Fig. 5.6b. The image is improved by reducing the distance between catheters. In addition, if blood removal was inadequate by appropriate dextran flushing due to strong blood flow,

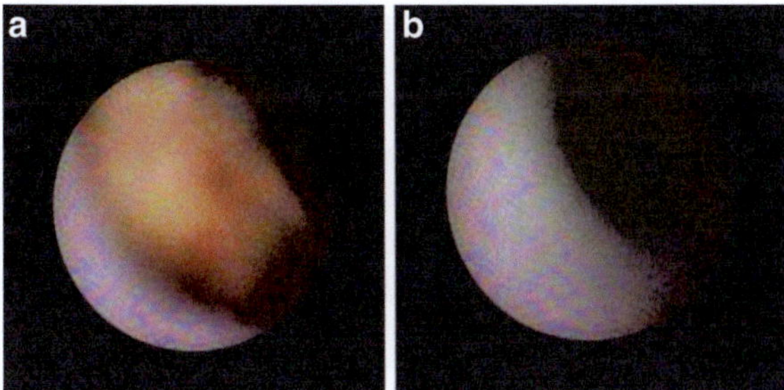

Fig. 5.6 The positioning of fiber catheter in probing catheter. (**a**) The fiber catheter placed at correct position from the tip of probing catheter. Yellow plaque clearly evident. (**b**) When the fiber catheter is far from the tip of the probing catheter, the observational range is small, and the whole image is dark. The image is improved by reducing the distance to the tip of the catheter. In addition, if blood removal was not adequately performed by appropriate dextran flushing because of strong blood flow, the image might be improved by increasing the light quantity without bringing the catheter closer to the tip

the image might be improved by increasing light quantity without reducing the distance between catheters. As flushing may cause a slight offset, it is important to correct the positioning. There is a 1–2 s delay between pullback and the image, making it difficult to determine accurate positioning if retracted too quickly. Further, it is important that the fiber catheter is not retracted before the probing catheter as this may result in injury to the vessel.

5.9 Complication with Procedure of Angioscopy

The general complications of this nonocclusion type of angioscopy are similar to the imaging modality in other blood vessels, for example, catheter-induced spasm, intimal injury, deformation of stent, etc., and there are no specific complications. However, it is important that we do not push it forcibly when the probing catheter cannot reach for the target lesion because of resistance with a severe stenosis, calcification, bending vessel, and the stent edge when we advance probing catheter in the vessel.

5.10 Future Prospects

The inability to see through blood flow because of its opaque nature and the resulting need to remove blood from the visual field using dextran-flushing technique remain the primary obstacles to the widespread and routine use of nonocclusion type of angioscopy to evaluate the luminal wall.

At present, certain angioscopic techniques may possibly recognize the presence of coronary artery calcification, but assessment/quantification of coronary artery calcification is not a current application of this evolving technique.

However, angioscopy is able to observe vulnerable plaque and arteriosclerotic change, as well as identify the presence of thrombus, currently not feasible with an IVUS or OCT system. It is considered that the use of this device will become more prevalent, although the advancement of hardware of the nonocclusion type of angioscopy system is a requirement moving forward.

References

1. Spears JR, Marais HJ, Serur J, Pomerantzeff O, Geyer RP, Sipzener RS, Weintraub R, Thurer R, Paulin S, Gerstin R, Grossman W. In vivo coronary angioscopy. J Am Coll Cardiol. 1983;1:1311–14.
2. Sherman CT, Litvack F, Grundfest W, Lee M, Hickey A, Chaux A, Kass R, Blanche C, Matloff J, Morgenstern L, et al. Coronary angioscopy in patients with unstable angina pectoris. N Engl J Med. 1986;315:913–19.
3. Uchida Y, Tomaru T, Nakamura F, Furuse A, Fujimori Y, Hasegawa K. Percutaneous coronary angioscopy in patients with ischemic heart disease. Am Heart J. 1987;114:1216–22.
4. Mizuno K, Arai T, Satomura K, Shibuya T, Arakawa K, Okamoto Y, Miyamoto A, Kurita A, Kikuchi M, Nakamura H, et al. New percutaneous transluminal coronary angioscope. J Am Coll Cardiol. 1989;13:363–8.
5. Siegel RJ, Ariani M, Fishbein MC, Chae JS, Park JC, Maurer G, Forrester JS. Histopathologic validation of angioscopy and intravascular ultrasound. Circulation. 1991;84:109–17.
6. White CJ, Ramee SR, Collins TJ, Mesa JE, Jain A. Percutaneous angioscopy of saphenous vein coronary bypass grafts. J Am Coll Cardiol. 1993;21:1181–5.
7. Mizuno K, Miyamoto A, Satomura K, Kurita A, Arai T, Sakurada M, Yanagida S, Nakamura H. Angioscopic coronary macromorphology in patients with acute coronary disorders. Lancet. 1991;337:809–12.
8. Ueda Y, Asakura M, Hirayama A, Komamura K, Hori M, Kodama K. Intracoronary morphology of culprit lesions after reperfusion in acute myocardial infarction: serial angioscopic observations. J Am Coll Cardiol. 1996;27:606–10.
9. Mizote I, Ueda Y, Ohtani T, Shimizu M, Takeda Y, Oka T, Tsujimoto M, Hirayama A, Hori M, Kodama K. Distal protection improved reperfusion and reduced left ventricular dysfunction in patients with acute myocardial infarction who had angioscopically defined ruptured plaque. Circulation. 2005;112:1001–7.
10. Ueda Y, Asakura M, Yamaguchi O, Hirayama A, Hori M, Kodama K. The healing process of infarct-related plaques: insights from 18 months of serial angioscopic follow-up. J Am Coll Cardiol. 2001;38:1916–22.
11. Hirayama A, Saito S, Ueda Y, Takayama T, Honye J, Komatsu S, Yamaguchi O, Li Y, Yajima J, Nanto S, Takazawa K, Kodama K. Qualitative and quantitative changes in coronary plaque associated with atorvastatin therapy. Circ J. 2009;73(4):718–25.
12. Hirayama A, Saito S, Ueda Y, Takayama T, Honye J, Komatsu S, Yamaguchi O, Li Y, Yajima J, Nanto S, Takazawa K, Kodama K. Plaque-stabilizing effect of atorvastatin is stronger for plaques evaluated as more unstable by angioscopy and intravenous ultrasound. Circ J. 2011;75(6):1448–54.
13. Kodama K, Komatsu S, Ueda Y, Takayama T, Yajima J, Nanto S, Matsuoka H, Saito S. Hirayama A Stabilization and regression of coronary plaques treated with pitavastatin proven by angioscopy and intravascular ultrasound–the TOGETHAR trial. Circ J. 2010;74(9):1922–8.

14. Kotani J, Awata M, Nanto S, Uematsu M, Oshima F, Minamiguchi H, Mintz GS, Nagata S. Incomplete neointimal coverage of sirolimus-eluting stents: angioscopic findings. J Am Coll Cardiol. 2006;47(10):2108–11.
15. Oyabu J, Ueda Y, Ogasawara N, Okada K, Hirayama A, Kodama K. Angioscopic evaluation of neointima coverage: sirolimus drug-eluting stent versus bare metal stent. Am Heart J. 2006;152(6):1168–74.
16. Awata M, Kotani J, Uematsu M, Morozumi T, Watanabe T, Onishi T, Iida O, Sera F, Nanto S, Hori M, Nagata S. Serial angioscopic evidence of incomplete neointimal coverage after sirolimus-eluting stent implantation: comparison with bare-metal stents. Circulation. 2007;116(8):910–16.
17. Takayama T, Hiro T, Akabane M, Kawano T, Ichikawa M, Kanai T, Fukamachi D, Haruta H, Saito S, Hirayama A. Degree of neointimal coverage is not related to prevalence of in-stent thrombosis in drug-eluting stents: a coronary angioscopic study. Int J Cardiol. 2012;156(2):224–6.
18. Suter MJ, Nadkarni SK, Weisz G, Tanaka A, Jaffer FA, Bouma BE, Tearney GJ. Intravascular optical imaging technology for investigating the coronary artery. JACC Cardiovasc Imaging. 2011;4(9):1022–39.
19. Fujii K, Hao H, Ohyanagi M, Masuyama T. Intracoronary imaging for detecting vulnerable plaque. Circ J. 2013;77(3):588–95.

Chapter 6
Classification of Plaque and Thrombus

Kyoichi Mizuno

Abstract The composition of plaque and thrombus can be determined from their appearance. Plaque is classified into yellow and white according to color and smooth or complex according to shape. Complex plaque is subdivided to three categories: ulceration (erosion), intimal flap, and intimal cleft. Yellow plaque seems to have thin fibrous cap or superficial or diffuse lipid deposition with or without lipid core. Tiny calcium particle, macrophage foam cells, or degenerated collagen fiber may glisten yellow. White plaque is histologically composed of dense collagen fiber (fibrous) or thick fibrous or calcified cap covered with lipid and macrophage foam cell-free endothelia with lipid pool below. Yellow plaque is likely to be vulnerable, whereas white plaque seems to be stable.

Thrombus is classified into red and white according to color and mural and luminal according to shape. White thrombus is platelet rich; on one hand, red thrombus contains an abundance of fibrin mixed with erythrocytes and platelets. This pathological presentation may explain why the thrombolysis treatment using tPA is less effective in patients with unstable angina or non-ST elevation myocardial infarction.

Keywords Yellow plaque • White plaque • Red thrombus • White thrombus

6.1 Characteristics of Angioscopy

Angioscopy provides a full-color, three-dimensional perspective image of intra-coronary artery surface morphology [1, 2]. Color discrimination in angioscopy makes it relatively easy to distinguish between yellow and white plaque [3–9]. Angioscopy can also distinguish a thrombus and a plaque even if a clot is very small. Furthermore, the composition of plaque and thrombus can be determined from their appearance [10, 11]. The three-dimensional perspective and high resolution of angioscopy can disclose luminal changes in minute plaque rupture, ulceration,

K. Mizuno (⊠)
Mitsukoshi Health and Welfare Foundation, Nippon Medical School, 1-24-1 Nishi-shinjuku, Shinjuku-ku, Tokyo 160-0023, Japan
e-mail: mizunokyoichi@gmail.com

© Springer Japan 2015
K. Mizuno, M. Takano (eds.), *Coronary Angioscopy*,
DOI 10.1007/978-4-431-55546-9_6

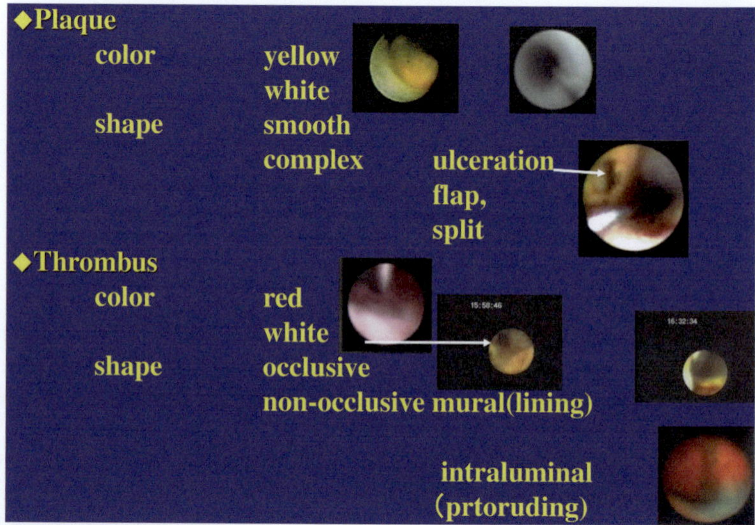

Fig. 6.1 Classification of coronary angioscopic findings. Plaque is classified into yellow and white according to the color and smooth or complex according to the shape. Thrombus is classified into red and white according to the color and mural or transluminal according to their shapes

or intimal flap. Angioscopy provides information about the macromorphology of coronary artery disease that previous was available only during autopsy.

6.2   Classification of Plaque

Plaque is classified into yellow and white according to color and smooth or complex according to shape (Fig. 6.1). Complex plaque is subdivided to three categories: ulceration (erosion), intimal flap, and intimal cleft. This classification is based on morphologic appearance and cleft orientation. Ulceration is defined as a crater-like lesion suggesting gap in the intima (Fig. 6.2). Clinically, ulceration is usually called plaque rupture. Erosion and plaque rupture may be difficult to classify by angioscopy [12, 13]. Other diagnostic modalities such as OCT can help distinguish two conditions. Detailed definition of erosion is described in another chapter. Intimal flaps are defined as a small, thin, disrupted fragment floating in the lumen. Intimal split is defined as sharp cleft in the inner lumen. We use this term only after PTCA. Figure 6.2 is an example of angioscopic findings of normal artery, plaque, and thrombus.

Normal artery appears angioscopically smooth in contour and has a uniform glistering white.

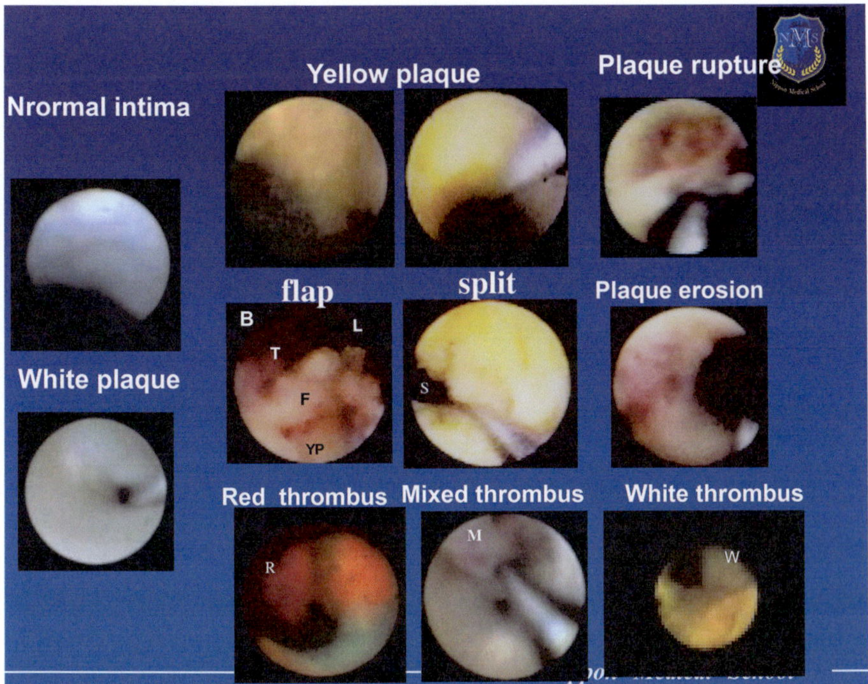

Fig. 6.2 Angioscopic examples of normal coronary (normal intima), plaque, and thrombus. *T* thrombus, *F* flap, *L* lumen, *YP* yellow plaque, *R* red thrombus, *M* mixed thrombus, *W* white thrombus

6.2.1 Yellow Plaque and White Plaque

Many studies including our previous study [14] showed that yellow plaque is more common in patients with acute coronary syndromes such as acute myocardial infarction or unstable angina; conversely, white plaque was seen in patients with stable coronary syndromes such as stable angina or old myocardial infarction. Yellow plaque is likely to be vulnerable, and white plaque seemed to be stable.

6.2.2 Comparison of Plaque Color and Pathological Findings

6.2.2.1 Autopsy Study

Lipid Pool (Lipid Core) Beneath Fibrous Cap

One hundred ninety-eight coronary segments were evaluated by angioscopy, and then 46 yellow plaque lesions and 61 white plaque lesions of atheroma (lipid pool beneath fibrous cap) were excised and prepared for pathological examination [15].

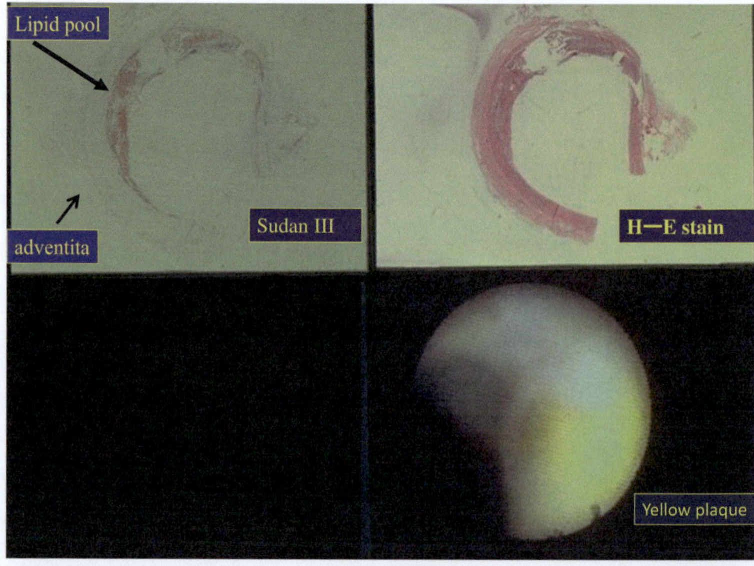

Fig. 6.3 Comparison of yellow plaque and pathological finding. Angioscopy shows yellow plaque (*right lower panel*). Hematoxylin-eosin stain at the same segment of yellow plaque (*right upper panel*). Sudan III stain shows lipid pool (*pink*) with thin fibrous cap (*left upper panel*)

Fig. 6.4 Comparison of the thickness of the fibrous cap between yellow plaque group and white plaque group. The thickness of the fibrous cap is significantly thinner in the yellow plaque group than in the white plaque group (Isoda et al. [15])

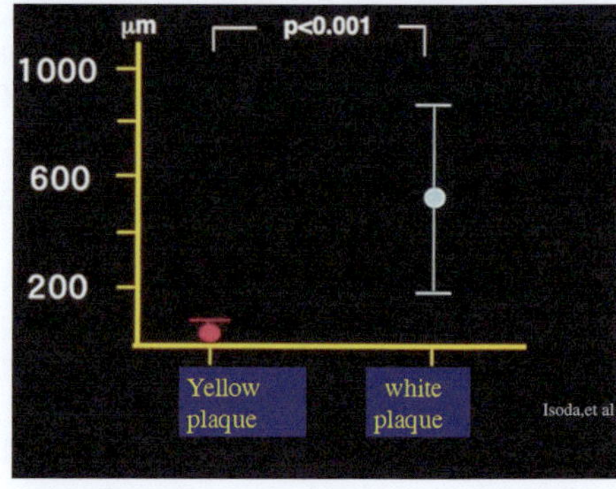

Yellow plaque has thin fibrous cap (Fig. 6.3). The thickness of fibrous cap was 58 ± 18 μm (35–90 μm) in yellow plaque group and 648 ± 356 μm (190–1,731 μm) in white plaque group. The thickness of fibrous cap was significantly thinner in the yellow plaque group than in the white plaque group (Fig. 6.4). White plaque has thick fibrous cap (Fig. 6.5).

Comparison of the stenosis and the plaque area between yellow and white plaque group showed both stenosis and plaque were significantly higher in the white plaque group than in the yellow plaque group. Comparison of the lipid core area and the lipid core (pool) size relative to overall plaque size between yellow plaque group and white plaque group is shown in Fig. 6.6. The lipid core (pool) area was not significant between two groups, but the lipid core (pool) size relative to plaque size

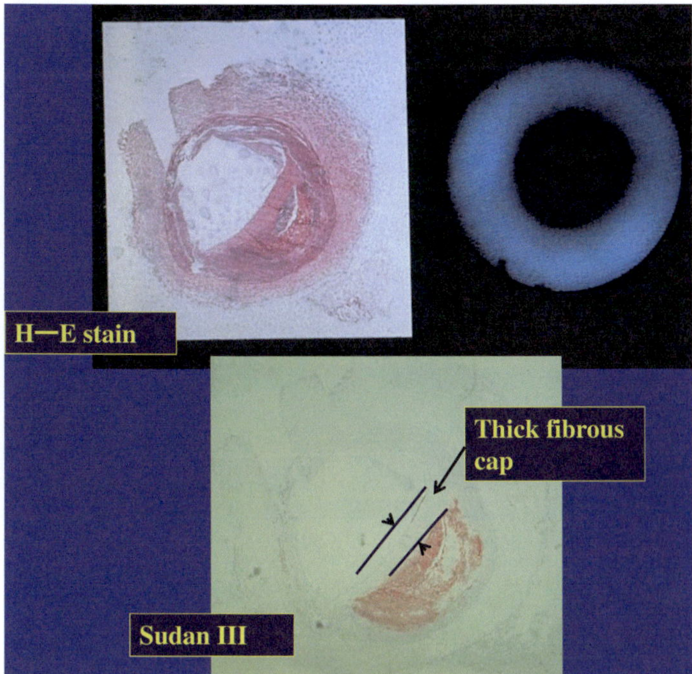

Fig. 6.5 Comparison of white plaque and pathological findings. Angioscopy shows white plaque (*right upper panel*). Hematoxylin-eosin stain at the same segment of white plaque (*left upper panel*). Sudan III stain shows lipid pool with thick fibrous cap (*lower panel*)

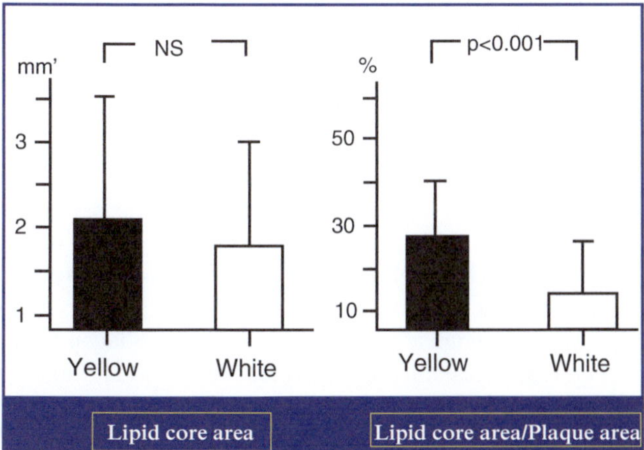

Fig. 6.6 Comparison of the stenosis and the plaque area between yellow and white plaque group. The lipid core (pool) area was not significant between two groups, but the lipid core (pool) size relative to plaque size was significantly higher in the yellow plaque group than in the white plaque group (Isoda et al. [15])

Fig. 6.7 Diffuse lipid deposition with macrophage foam cell. Yellow plaque (Y) exists in the artery (*left panel*). Angioscopy revealed yellow plaque (*right upper panel*). A large amount of inflammation cells such as probably macrophage with diffuse lipid deposition is seen (*right lower panel*)

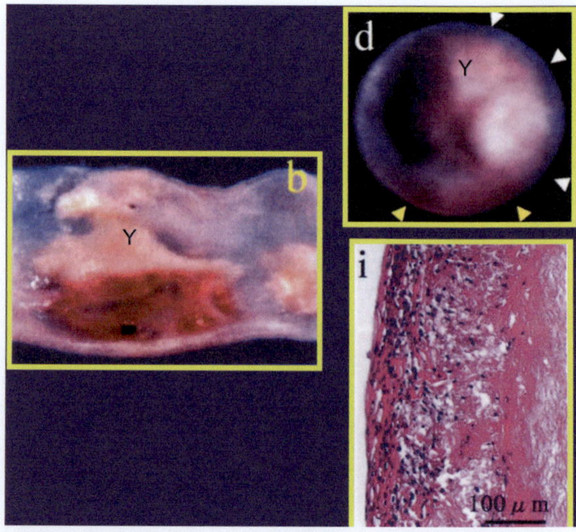

Table 6.1 Classification of plaque according to color

Yellow plaque	Thin fibrous cap superficial or diffuse lipid deposition
Glistening yellow plaque	Tiny calcium particle, macrophage foam cells, or degenerated collagen fiber
White plaque	Dense collagen fiber (fibrous) or calcified cap covered with lipid-free and macrophage foam cell-free endothelia with lipid pool

was significantly higher in the yellow plaque group than in the white plaque group. Yellow plaque reflects thin fibrous cap rather than size of lipid pool [16].

Superficial or Diffuse Lipid Deposition with or Without Lipid Core

Superficial or diffuse lipid deposition in intima is diagnosed as yellow plaque by angioscopy (Fig. 6.7). In this lipid deposition, tiny calcium particle, macrophage foam cells, or degenerated collagen fiber may glisten yellow plaque(glistening yellow plaque) [17, 18]. High yellow color intensity region may not necessarily represent thin-cap fibroatheroma.

White plaque was histologically composed of dense collagen fiber (fibrous) or thick fibrous (Fig. 6.5) or calcified cap covered with lipid and macrophage foam cell-free endothelia with lipid pool below (Table 6.1).

6.2.2.2 Directional Coronary Atherectomy Study

Yellow plaque color was closely related to degenerated plaque or atheroma. Gray white lesion represented fibrous plaque without degeneration in 64 % and with degeneration in 36 %. Fibrous cap could not be clarified by directional coronary atherectomy [19].

6.2.3 Quantitative Evaluation of Angioscopy

It is hypothesized that yellow color is due to visualization of reflected light from the lipid-rich yellow color through a thin fibrous cap. Thus, quantification of yellow color saturation (intensity) may estimate plaque cap thickness and identification vulnerable plaque [20] (Fig. 6.8). High yellow color saturation (intensity) is associated with lipid core underneath thin fibrous cap (Fig. 6.9) [21].

6.2.4 Comparison of Angioscopic Plaque Color and Optical Coherent Tomography

Optical coherence tomography (OCT) has the excellent capability to measure fibrous cap thickness covering a lipid plaque. There was an inverse relationship between color intensity {white (grade 0), light yellow (grade 1), yellow (grade 2), dark yellow (grade 2)} and fibrous cap thickness [22, 23] (Fig. 6.10). Plaque color intensity of coronary angioscopy was determined by the fibrous cap thickness. Yellow plaque of higher color grade might have thinner fibrous cap.

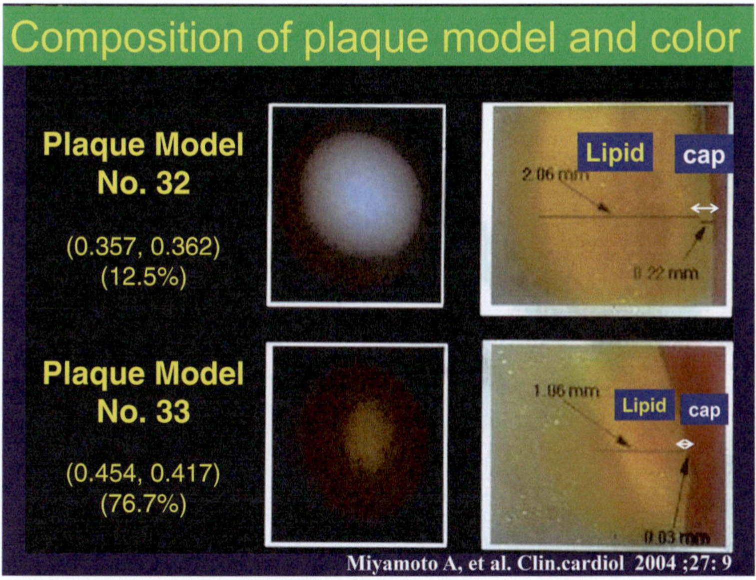

Fig. 6.8 Angioscopic images of plaque model and histology. Angioscopic image with low yellow saturation (12.5 %) and corresponding cross section of plaque with cap thickness (220 μm) (*top*). Angioscopic image with high yellow saturation (76.7 %) and corresponding histology with thin cap thickness (30 μm) (Miyamoto et al. [20])

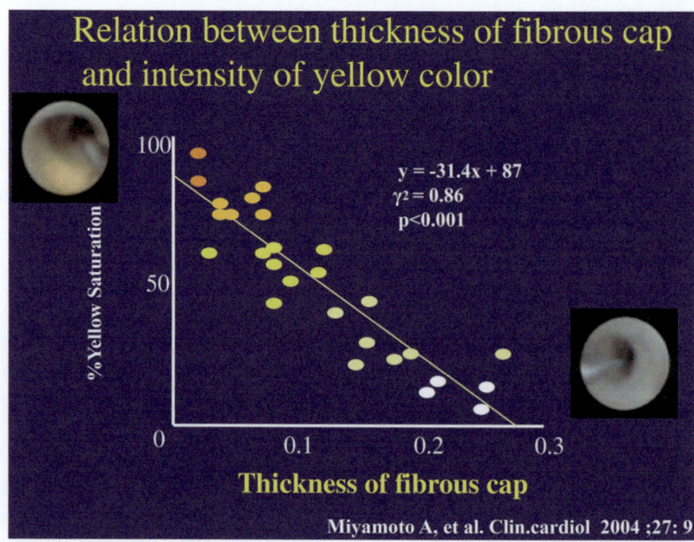

Fig. 6.9 Relationship between the percent yellow saturation and cap thickness in the lipid-rich plaque model. The percent yellow saturation had a strong inverse linear correlation with cap thickness (Miyamoto et al. [20])

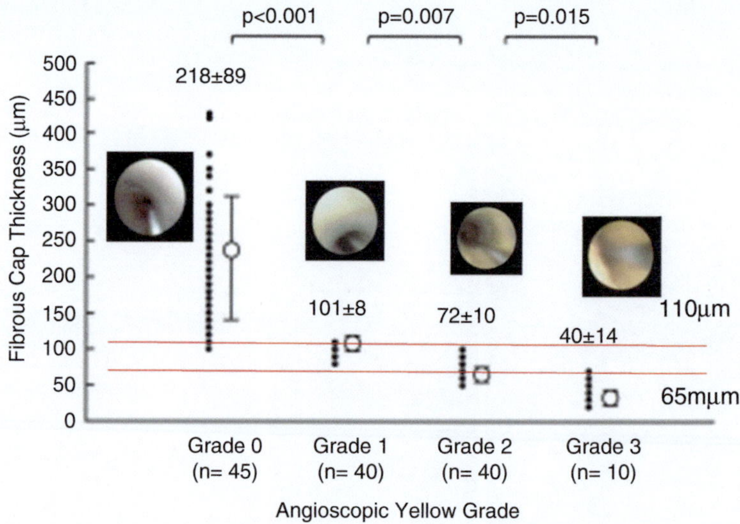

Fig. 6.10 Relationship between the angioscopic yellow grade and the fibrous cap thickness. Measured by optical coherence tomography (OCT). The fibrous cap thickness by OCT decreased significantly as yellow grade by angioscopy rose (Takano et al. [22])

6.3   Classification of Thrombus

Thrombus is defined as a red and/or white solid material adhering to the intima or protruding into the inner lumen despite flushing with clear liquid such as normal saline. Thrombus is classified as red and white according to color and mural and luminal according to shape (Figs. 6.1 and 6.2).

A serial observation of coronary thrombus produced by copper coil in canine coronary showed that white component of thrombus and fibrin-like material was existed around the copper coil in a few minutes after coil insertion. Thereafter, thin mixed thrombotic white and red components formed around the copper coil and grow in size. Thrombus finally obstructed the coronary lumen.

The thrombus taken from the copper coil is mixed white and red type (Fig. 6.11). White-type thrombus is larger than red-type thrombus. Microscopic examination of thrombus revealed platelet aggregate and fibrin network with red blood cell coagulation (Fig. 6.11). White thrombus is platelet rich, whereas red thrombus contains an abundance of fibrin mixed with erythrocytes and platelets [24].

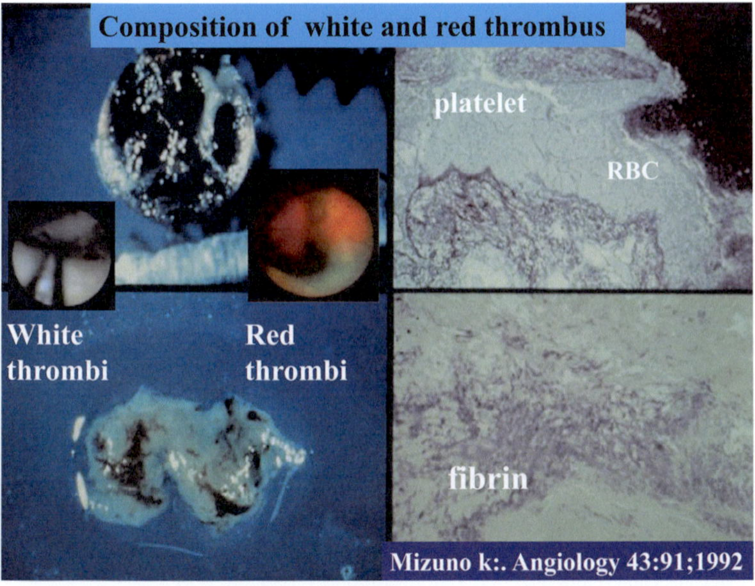

Fig. 6.11 Macroscopic and microscopic examination of coronary thrombus made by copper coil insertion into canine coronary artery. Antegrade view of coronary thrombus in copper coil (*left upper panel*). The thrombus taken from the copper coil is mixed white and red type. White-type thrombus is larger than red-type thrombus (*left lower panel*). Microscopic examination of thrombus revealed platelet aggregate and fibrin network with red blood cell coagulation. White thrombus is platelet rich, whereas red thrombus contains an abundance of fibrin mixed with erythrocytes and platelets (*right upper panel*)

Angioscopic study has reported the significantly higher prevalence of red thrombus in patients with acute myocardial infarction; on the other hand, white thrombus was observed in patients with unstable angina and non-ST segment elevation myocardial infarction [25]. Occlusive thrombi occurred frequently in patients with acute myocardial infarction but were not seen in patients with unstable angina. The color differences of thrombus may be observed via angioscopy among patients with varying acute coronary syndromes. Differences in color probably reflect differences in the composition of thrombus, which are perhaps related in part to the age of thrombus or the presence and absence of blood flow in the coronary artery. Red thrombus tends to form under the condition of stasis (as in an occluded vessel); white thrombus tend to form the blood flow has not been completely interrupted. White thrombus was found to be older than red thrombus and had a tight fibrin network [26] and large amount platelets.

Platelets release plasminogen activator inhibitor and induce cross-link of fibrin. This pathological presentation may explain why the thrombosis treatment using tPA is less effective in patients with unstable angina or non-ST elevation myocardial infarction.

References

1. Mizuno K, Arai T, Satomura K, Shibuya T, Arakawa K, Okamoto Y, et al. New percutaneous transluminal coronary angioscope. J Am Coll Cardiol. 1989;13:363–8.
2. Sherman CT, Litbac F, Grundfest W, et al. Coronary angioscopy in patients with unstable angina. New Engl J Med. 1986;325:913–19.
3. Mizuno K. Angioscopic examination of the coronary arteries: what have we learned? Heart Dis Stroke. 1992;1:320–4.
4. Mizuno K, Nakamura H. Percutaneous coronary angioscopy: present role and future direction. Ann Med. 1993;25:12.
5. Mizuno K. Clinical application of angioscopy. Asian Med J. 1996;39:300–6.
6. Mizuno K, Sakai S, Okuni M. Development and clinical feasibility of percutaneous coronary angioscope. J Nippon Med Sch. 1999;66:7–14.
7. Mizuno K, Sakai S, Yokoyama S, Ohba T, Uemura R, Seimiya Y, Takano M, Tanabe J, Tomimura M, Imaizumi T, Ma SM, Inami S, Okamatsu K, Hata N. Percutaneous transluminal angioscopy during coronary intervention. Diagn Ther Endosc. 2000;7:1520.
8. Mizuno K. Coronary angioscopy. In: Rosch J, Lanzer P, editors. Vascular diagnostic. Berlin/Heidrberg/New York: Springer; 1994. p. 498–508.
9. Mizuno K, Wang Z, Inami S, Takano M, Yasutake M, Asai K, Takano H. Coronary angioscopy: current topics and future direction. Cardiovasc Interv Ther. 2011;26:89–97.
10. Heuer PD, Foley DP, Hillege JM, Lablanche JM, Duke PB, Franzen D, Morice MC, Serra A, Scheerder IK, Serruys PW, Lie KI. The 'Ermenonville' classification of observation at coronary angioscopy – evaluation of intra-and inter-observer agreement. Eur Heart J. 1994;15:815–22.
11. Siegel RJ, Ariani M, Fishbein MC, Chae JS, Park JC, Maurer G, Forrester JS. Histopathologic validation of angioscopy and intravascular ultrasound. Circulation. 1991;84:109–17.
12. Kubo T, Imanishi T, Takarada S, Kuroi A, Ueno S, Yamano T, Tanimoto T, Matsuo Y, Masho T, Kitabata H, Tsuda K, Tomobuchi Y, Akasaka Y. Assessment of culprit lesion morphology in acute myocardial infarction: ability of optical coherence tomography compared with intravascular ultrasound and coronary angioscopy. J Am Coll Cardiol. 2007;50:933–9.

13. Ozaki Y, Okumura M, Ismail TF. Coronary CT angioscopic characteristics of culprit lesions in acute coronary syndromes not related to plaque rupture as defined by optical coherence tomography and angioscopy. Eur Heart J. 2011;32:2814–23.
14. Mizuno K, Miyamoto A, Satomura K, Kurita A, Arai T, Yanagida S, et al. Angioscopic coronary macromorphology in patients with acute coronary disorders. Lancet. 1991;337:809–12.
15. Isoda K, Satomura K, Ohsuzu F. Pathological characterization of yellow and white plaques under angioscopy. Int J Angiol. 2001;10:183–7.
16. Kawasaki M, Tkatsu H, Noda Y, Sano K, Ito Y, Hayakawa K, Tuchiya K, Arai M, Nishigaki K, Takemura G, Minatoguchi S, Fujiwara T, Fujiwara H. In vivo quantitative tissue characterization of human coronary arterial plaques by use of integrated backscatter intravascular ultrasound and comparison with angioscopic findings. Circulation. 2002;105:2487–92.
17. Uchida Y, Nakamura F, Tomaru T, Morita T, Oshima T, Sakai T, et al. Prediction of acute coronary syndromes by percutaneous coronary angioscopy in patients with stable angina. Am Heart J. 1995;130:195–203.
18. Uchida Y, Uchida Y, Hituta N. Histological characteristics of glistening yellow coronary plaques seen on angioscopy-with special reference of vulnerable plaques. Circ J. 2011;75:1913–19.
19. Thieme T, Wernecke KD, Meyer R, Brandenstein E, Habedank D, Hinz A, et al. Angioscopic evaluation of atherosclerotic plaques: validation by histomorphologic analysis and association with stable and unstable coronary syndromes. J Am Coll Cardiol. 1996;28:1–6.
20. Miyamoto A, Prieto AR, Friedl SE, Lin FC, Muller JE, Nesto RW, et al. Atheromatous plaque cap thickness can be determined by quantitative color analysis during angioscopy: implications for identifying the vulnerable plaque. Clin Cardiol. 2004;27:9–15.
21. Ishibashi F, Mizuno K, Kawamura A, Singh PP, Nesto RW, Waxman S. High yellow color intensity by angioscopy with quantitative colorimetry to identify high-risk features in culprit lesions of patients with acute coronary syndromes. Am J Cardiol. 2007;100:1207–11.
22. Takano M, Jang IK, Inami S, Yamamoto M, Murakami D, Okamatsu K, et al. In vivo comparison of optical coherence tomography and angioscopy for the evaluation of coronary plaque characteristics. Am J Cardiol. 2008;101:471–6.
23. Kubo T, Imanishi T, Takarada S, Kuroi A, Ueno S, Yamano T, et al. Implication of plaque color classification for assessing plaque vulnerability: a coronary angioscopy and optical coherence tomography investigation. J Am Coll Cardiol Interv. 2008;1:74–80.
24. Miuzuno K, Miyamoto A, Isojima K, Kurita A, Senoo A, Arai T, et al. A serial observation of coronary thrombi in vivo by a new percutaneous trans coronary angioscopy. Angiology. 1992;43:91–9.
25. Mizuno K, Satomura K, Miyamoto A, Arakawa K, Shibuya T, Arai T, et al. Angioscopic evaluation of coronary-artery thrombi in acute coronary syndromes. N Engl J Med. 1992;326:287–91.
26. Uchida Y, Masuo M, Tomaru T, Kato A, Sugimoto T. Fiberoptic observation of thrombosis and thrombolysis in isolated human coronary arteries. Am Heart J. 1986;112:691–6.

Chapter 7
Vulnerable Plaque

Masanori Kawasaki

Abstract The pathogenesis of acute coronary syndromes (ACSs) is not fully understood because it is multifactorial and complex. Coronary plaques prone to fissure have been identified as "vulnerable plaques." These plaques have thin fibrous caps with active inflammation, large lipid cores, and endothelial denudation with superficial platelet aggregation. The frequency of ruptured plaques causing ACS has been estimated to be approximately 1–5 %/year. Angioscopy applies fiber-optic technology to directly visualize the luminal surface and is able to characterize plaque composition on the basis of luminal appearance. Therefore, angioscopy can partly identify features of vulnerable plaques. The grade of yellow color as defined by angioscopy is correlated with the fibrous cap thickness. There are a large number of clinical studies that have investigated the pathogenesis of ACS using angioscopy.

Keywords Angioscopy • Vulnerable plaque • Acute coronary syndrome • Imaging

7.1 History of Vulnerable Plaque

In 1966, Friedman et al. demonstrated communication of a preexisting intramural atheromatous abscess with the occluding thrombus in 39 of 40 autopsied coronary arteries in patients with acute myocardial infarction [1]. They also demonstrated that such communications were accomplished by destruction of the portion of the arterial wall that separated the necrotic mass from luminal blood. The destruction was preceded by or associated with an infiltration of the vessel wall by lipid-containing macrophages extending from remnants of tissue encompassing the abscess. They concluded that the communication between lumen and atheromatous abscess preceded and was responsible for the formation of the thrombus [1]. In 1978, Horie et al. examined serial section of coronary arteries in 108 necropsies and demonstrated that plaque rupture into the vessel lumen may precede and cause

M. Kawasaki (✉)
Department of Cardiology, Gifu University Graduate School of Medicine, 1-1 Yanagido, Gifu 501-1194, Japan
e-mail: masanori@ya2.so-net.ne.jp

© Springer Japan 2015
K. Mizuno, M. Takano (eds.), *Coronary Angioscopy*,
DOI 10.1007/978-4-431-55546-9_7

thrombus formation, resulting in acute myocardial infarction in a pathological study [2]. In 1992, Mizuno et al. performed an angioscopic study in vivo and demonstrated that disruption or erosion of vulnerable plaques followed by thrombosis was the most frequent cause of acute coronary syndrome (ACS) [3].

As insights into this process have evolved, the relevant terminology has been continually updated. In the 1980s, Falk and Davies and Thomas used "plaque disruption" synonymously with "plaque rupture" [4, 5]. Later, Muller and colleagues used "vulnerable" to describe rupture-prone plaques as the underlying cause of most clinical coronary events [6, 7]. Falk introduced the concept of plaque rupture [8]. Rupture of the plaque surface, often with thrombosis superimposed, occurs frequently during the evolution of coronary atherosclerotic lesions [8]. It is probably the most important mechanism underlying the sudden, rapid plaque progression responsible for ACS. The risk of plaque rupture depends on plaque type (composition) rather than plaque size (volume), because only plaques rich in soft extracellular lipids are vulnerable (rupture prone) [4]. The stability of atherosclerotic plaques is related to histological composition and the thickness of fibrous caps. Therefore, recognition of the tissue characteristics of coronary plaques is important to understand and prevent ACS. Accurate in vivo identification of the tissue characteristics of coronary plaques may allow the identification of vulnerable plaques before the development of ACS.

7.2 Features of Vulnerable Plaque

According to a previous pathological and clinical review [9], the following major criteria are necessary for the detection of vulnerable plaque: (1) active inflammation with extensive macrophage accumulation, (2) thin fibrous cap with a large lipid core (thin-cap fibroatheroma, TCFA) (Fig. 7.1), (3) endothelial denudation with superficial platelet aggregation, (4) fissured/injured plaque, and (5) severe stenosis. The minor criteria for detection of vulnerable plaque include the following: (1) superficial calcified nodules, (2) yellow color (on angioscopy), (3) intraplaque hemorrhage, (4) endothelial dysfunction, and (5) expansive (positive) remodeling [9].

7.3 Frequency of Vulnerable Plaque and Acute Coronary Syndrome

Since all vulnerable plaques do not always cause ACS, it is important to determine the incidence of ACS due to vulnerable plaque. Ohtani et al. followed patients for 4.8 years after angioscopy and found that respective incidence of ACS was 2.2- and 3.8-fold higher in patients with ≥ 2 and ≥ 5 yellow plaques per vessel, compared

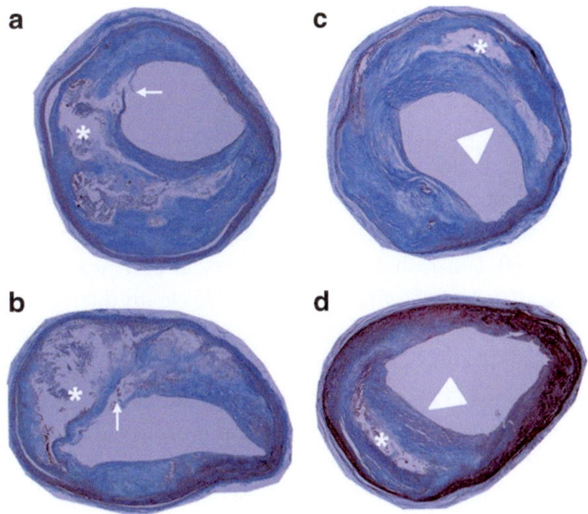

Fig. 7.1 Pathological images of coronary plaques. (**a**, **b**) Vulnerable plaques with thin fibrous cap (*arrow*) and large lipid core (*). (**c**, **d**) Stable plaques with relatively thick fibrous cap (*arrowhead*) and small lipid core (*)

with those who had ≤1 yellow plaque per vessel [10]. On the basis of angioscopy, plaque is defined as a nonmobile, elevated, and/or protruding structure that can be clearly demarcated from the adjacent vessel wall. Coronary plaques are divided into yellow or nonyellow plaques (white plaque) according to the surface color. Ueda et al. estimated that vulnerable plaques may cause ACS at a rate of approximately 0.3–1.0 %/year [11]. Taking into consideration the estimated frequency of vulnerable plaque to ruptured/disrupted plaque, the frequency of ruptured plaques causing ACS may be approximately 1–5 %/year [11]. Another prospective angioscopic study that was conducted in the non-statin era reported that yellow plaques caused ACS at a rate of 5.9 %/ year, whereas white plaques caused ACS at a rate of 2.1 %/year [12].

In patients who died of plaque rupture, additional lesion sites remote from the culprit plaque show TCFAs in 70 % of cases. On the other hand, TCFAs are less frequent (30 %) in cases where death is attributed to fibrocalcific plaques with flow-limiting stenosis, regardless of whether there is myocardial infarction or plaque erosion [13].

All vulnerable plaques are not likely to progress to rupture. Therefore, it is important to consider the results of a pathological study in which the coronary arteries were sectioned serially from the coronary ostium to a distal intramyocardial location. In this study, mean luminal narrowing was the least in lesions with TCFAs (59.6 %), intermediate in lesions with hemorrhage into a plaque (68.8 %), and greatest in acute plaque ruptures (73.3 %) or healed plaque ruptures (72.8 %) [14]. Approximately 50 % of the TCFAs occur in the proximal portions of the major coronary arteries (left anterior descending > left circumflex > right coronary artery), with another one third in the midportion and the remaining few in the distal portion [14]. The number of vulnerable plaques correlated with both high total cholesterol and the total cholesterol/high-density lipoprotein cholesterol ratio [15].

7.4 Plaque Erosion as Vulnerable Plaque

Plaque rupture/disruption refers to a lesion consisting of a necrotic core with an overlying thin ruptured fibrous cap that leads to luminal thrombosis because of contact of flowing blood with a highly thrombogenic necrotic core [16]. On the other hand, plaque erosion shows a luminal thrombus with an underlying base rich in smooth muscle cells and proteoglycans with mild inflammation [17]. Erosion of proteoglycan-rich and smooth muscle cell-rich plaques lacking a superficial lipid core is one of the findings in sudden death due to coronary thrombosis. Compared with plaque ruptures, these lesions are more often seen in younger individuals and women, have less luminal narrowing and less calcification, and fewer macrophages and T cells [17]. Kolodgie et al. postulated that the lack of significant inflammation at the site of erosion raises the possibility that erosion represents chronic injury rather than true atherogenesis. The abundance of a proteoglycan and hyaluronan matrix suggests their potential role in the development of thrombosis [18]. Although erosion can be detected by angioscopy and optical coherence tomography (OCT) [19, 20], the exact type of images that indicate pre-stage erosion has not yet been determined. Angheloiu et al. observed superficial foam cells in erosion-prone plaques by intrinsic fluorescence spectroscopy and diffuse reflectance spectroscopy in an autopsy study [21].

7.5 Vulnerable Plaques Detected by Angioscopy

Angioscopy applies fiber-optic technology to directly visualize the luminal surface and is able to characterize plaque composition on the basis of luminal appearance and to distinguish between white and red thrombus [22]. Endoluminal irregularities such as ulceration, fissures, erosions, and tears also can be seen using angioscopy. Therefore, among the major criteria of vulnerable plaques that are mentioned above, endothelial denudation with superficial platelet aggregation and fissured/injured plaque are the features that can be detected by angioscopy. Furthermore, among the minor criteria, superficial calcified nodules, yellow color (on angioscopy), and intraplaque hemorrhage are the features that can be detected by angioscopy. Takano et al. compared angioscopic findings with the results of OCT [23]. Angioscopic findings were semiquantitatively classified based on the surface color as 0, white; 1, light yellow; 2, medium yellow; and 3, dark yellow. They demonstrated that there was an inverse relationship between yellow grade and the fibrous cap thickness (grade 0, 218 ± 89 μm; grade 1, 101 ± 8 μm; grade 2, 72 ± 10 μm; grade 3, 40 ± 14 μm). Angioscopic yellow plaques can be identified as lipid plaques with high sensitivity (98 %) and specificity (96 %) based on the fibrous cap thickness measured at 110 μm [24]. Therefore, another major criterion for vulnerable plaque (thin fibrous cap with a large lipid core) can be indirectly detected

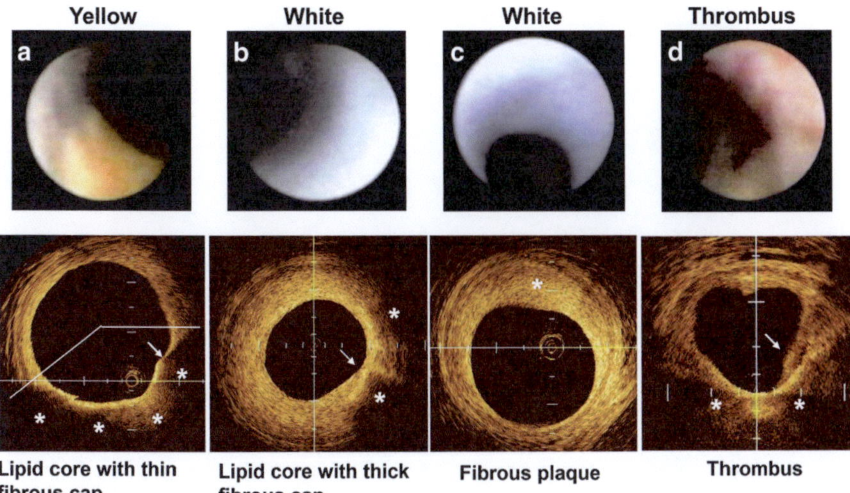

Fig. 7.2 (Courtesy of Dr. Takano M and Prof. Mizuno K). Corresponding angioscopic images and optical coherence tomography (OCT). *Upper*: angioscopic images. *Lower*: OCT. (**a**) A dark yellow plaque (yellow grade 3) is presented as a lipid plaque (*) with a thin fibrous cap (*white arrow*). The minimal thickness of the fibrous cap is 20 μm. The arc of lipid was measured as an angle between the two straight lines that joined the center of lumen to both ends of the lipid area. (**b**) A white plaque (yellow grade 0) contains lipid core (*) under a fibrous cap. The fibrous plaque thickness at the thinnest part (*white arrow*) is 130 μm. (**c**) A white plaque (yellow grade 0) that is diagnosed as a fibrous plaque (*) by OCT. (**D**) A red thrombus on a yellow plaque is observed by angioscopy. Protruding thrombus (*white arrow*) overlying thin-cap lipid plaque (*) is recognized by OCT

by angioscopy (Fig. 7.2). Regarding detecting vulnerable plaques, MacNeill et al. showed macrophage infiltration in coronary plaques in vivo using OCT and elucidated the relationships between increased macrophage infiltration and the incidence of ACS (Fig. 7.3) [25]. Virmani et al. reported that a thin cap <65 μm is a more specific precursor of plaque rupture [26]. However, Tanaka et al. demonstrated by OCT study that some plaque rupture may occur in thick fibrous cap depending on exertion levels (Fig. 7.4) [27].

Uchida et al. employed another classification of yellow color on angioscopic images [28]. They divided yellow plaques into glistening yellow plaques and non-glistening yellow plaques. A glistening yellow plaque is a plaque exhibiting yellow fluorescence-like color with a glistening portion usually located in the area of the plaque center. Yellow fluorescence-like color is a yellow color closely resembling the reflected light by yellow fluorescent paint. Collagen fiber density in fibrous caps in glistening yellow plaques was smaller than that in white or non-glistening plaques, indicating that glistening yellow plaques were histologically vulnerable plaques [24].

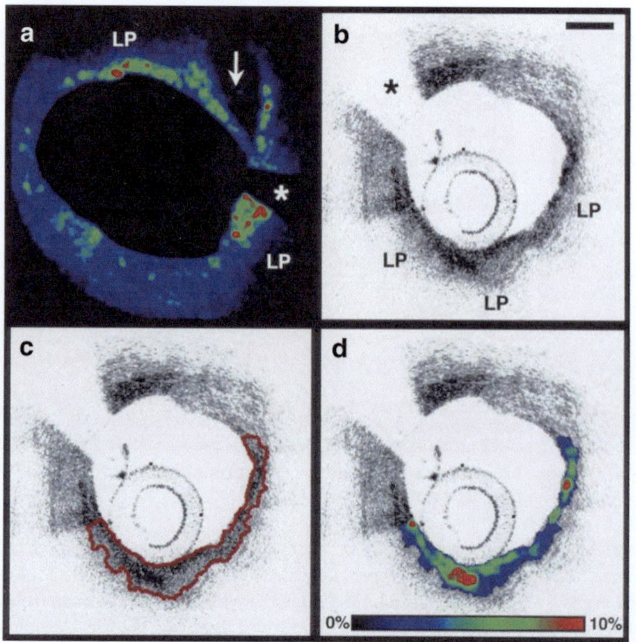

Fig. 7.3 Fibrous cap segmentation and macrophage density images for lipid-rich plaques. (**a**) A normalized standard deviation (NSD) image. (**b**) Optical coherence image of a lipid pool (LP). *: guide wire shadow artifact. (**c**) Outline (*red*) of the segmented fibrous cap of the OCT image depicted in *panel b*. (**d**) NSD image superimposed over a standard intensity image shows locations corresponding to increased macrophage density. The color scale bar represents the color mapping of the NSD parameter (Ref. [25])

7.6 Mechanical Stress as a Vulnerability of Coronary Plaques

When plaques eventually start to intrude into the lumen, shear stress in the area surrounding the plaque changes substantially, increasing tensile stress at the plaque shoulders leading to fissuring and thrombosis [28]. This elevated shear stress has been proposed to cause mechanically induced rupture of the cap [29]. Local biologic effects induced by high shear stress can destabilize the cap, particularly on its upstream side, and turn it into a rupture-prone, vulnerable plaque [28]. Therefore, mechanical stress that influences plaque vulnerability is an important factor as well as the plaque tissue characteristics [30]. Shear stress induces important biologic effects in endothelial cells that can affect the crucial balance between cap-reinforcing matrix synthesis by synthetic smooth muscle cells and matrix breakdown by metalloproteinases, which are produced by macrophages [31]. In humans, outward vascular remodeling seems to be increased proximal to a coronary stenosis, compared with the impaired outward remodeling seen distally [32].

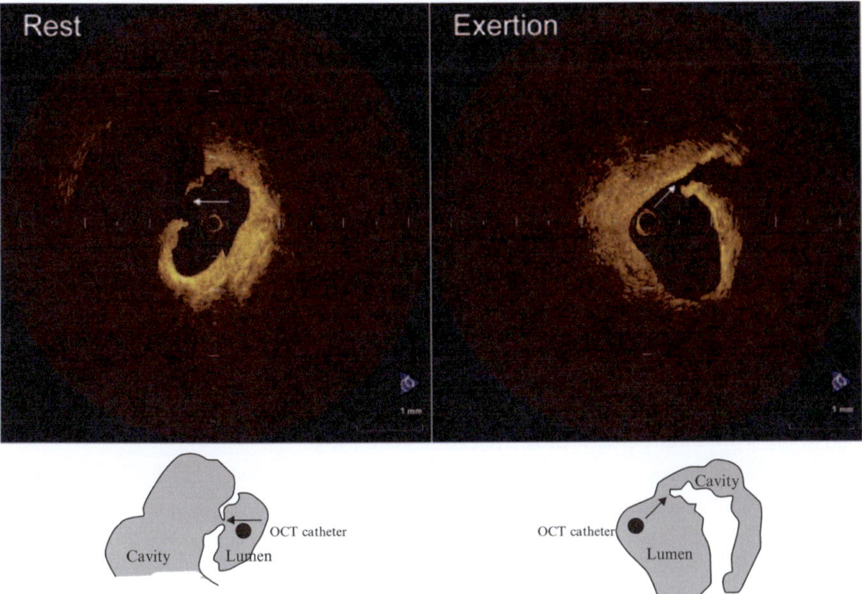

Fig. 7.4 Representative cases of plaque rupture occurring at rest or with exertion. *Left*: plaque rupture that occurred at rest. Fibrous cap was broken at the midportion, and a thin fibrous cap could be observed. *Right*: plaque rupture that occurred during heavy farm work. Thick fibrous cap was broken at the shoulder of plaque (Ref. [27])

Preliminary calculations that were made by applying computational fluid dynamics coupled with solid deformation mechanics to a symmetric lesion model showed that a relatively small (20 mmHg) pressure drop can induce $\geq$10 kPa axial tensile stress in a 75-μm thick cap. Given that the average minimum cap thickness in one previous study was 5.6 μm in patients who died after exertion [33], a peak tensile stress of 134 kPa would load the cap as predicted by the model. This far exceeds the fracture stresses in the lowest tertile reported for caps covering lipid pools in human aortic tissue samples (75 kPa for non-ulcerated plaques and 20 kPa for ulcerated plaques) [34]. This finding might explain why plaque rupture at the midcap (75 %) was the most frequent cause of death (68 %) in the exertion group [33]. In contrast, plaque rupture accounted for only 23 % of the subjects who died at rest and mostly occurred at the plaque shoulders (65 %) [33]; thus, a blood pressure surge might have been a more likely trigger in this group. Fukumoto et al. demonstrated that localized high shear stress might be a trigger for fibrous cap rupture, although the absolute value of shear stress is not sufficient to directly provoke mechanical destruction of the fibrous cap using computational color mapping of the distributions of the streamline, blood pressure, and shear stress [35].

7.7 Recent Investigations on Vulnerable Plaques

The ability of environmental, physical, or emotional stressors to trigger myocardial infarction has been attributed to a surge in sympathetic nervous system activity and catecholamine release that leads to increases in heart rate, blood pressure, and cardiac work as well as local vasoconstriction at the site of vulnerable plaques, thereby precipitating plaque rupture [36]. There is an intriguing working hypothesis that shifts in environmental factors, including local saturation of cholesterol, temperature, pH, and hydration status, could alone or in various combinations lead to cholesterol crystallization with sudden and forceful volume expansion causing plaque fissure and thrombosis [36, 37]. However, this hypothesis needs to be confirmed in larger studies. Intraplaque hemorrhage can enhance this mechanism by triggering the crystallization of free cholesterol from erythrocyte membranes and causing abrupt enlargement of the necrotic core [38].

Hyperglycemia is an important factor in cardiovascular damage, working through different mechanisms such as the activation of the protein kinase C, polyol or hexosamine pathways, and the production of advanced glycation end products [39]. Moreover, hyperinsulinemia has been established as an important factor associated with the occurrence of new cardiovascular events in patients with a first myocardial infarction [40]. The common mechanisms that contribute to insulin resistance and endothelial dysfunction also include glucotoxicity, lipotoxicity, and inflammation, which are associated with oxidative stress and increase the risk of cardiovascular events [41].

References

1. Friedman M, Van den Bovenkamp GJ. The pathogenesis of a coronary thrombus. Am J Pathol. 1966;48:19–44.
2. Horie T, Sekiguchi M, Hirosawa K. Coronary thrombosis in pathogenesis of acute myocardial infarction. Histopathological study of coronary arteries in 108 necropsied cases using serial section. Br Heart J. 1978;40:153–61.
3. Mizuno K, Satomura K, Miyamoto A, Arakawa K, Shibuya T, Arai T, Kurita A, Nakamura H, Ambrose JA. Angioscopic evaluation of coronary artery thrombi in acute coronary syndromes. N Engl J Med. 1992;326:287–91.
4. Falk E. Plaque rupture with severe pre-existing stenosis precipitating coronary thrombosis: characteristics of coronary atherosclerotic plaques underlying fatal occlusive thrombi. Br Heart J. 1983;50:127–34.
5. Davies MJ, Thomas AC. Plaque fissuring: the cause of acute myocardial infarction, sudden ischaemic death, and crescendo angina. Br Heart J. 1985;53:363–73.
6. Muller J, Tofler G, Stone P. Circadian variation and triggers of onset of acute cardiovascular disease. Circulation. 1989;79:733–43.
7. Muller JE, Abela GS, Nesto RW, Tofler GH. Triggers, acute risk factors and vulnerable plaques: the lexicon of a new frontier. J Am Coll Cardiol. 1994;23:809–13.
8. Falk E. Why do plaques rupture? Circulation. 1992;86(6 Suppl):III30–42.

9. Naghavi M, Libby P, Falk E, Casscells SW, Litovsky S, Rumberger J, Badimon JJ, Stefanadis C, Moreno P, Pasterkamp G, Fayad Z, Stone PH, Waxman S, Raggi P, Madjid M, Zarrabi A, Burke A, Yuan C, Fitzgerald PJ, Siscovick DS, de Korte CL, Aikawa M, Juhani Airaksinen KE, Assmann G, Becker CR, Chesebro JH, Farb A, Galis ZS, Jackson C, Jang IK, Koenig W, Lodder RA, March K, Demirovic J, Navab M, Priori SG, Rekhter MD, Bahr R, Grundy SM, Mehran R, Colombo A, Boerwinkle E, Ballantyne C, Insull Jr W, Schwartz RS, Vogel R, Serruys PW, Hansson GK, Faxon DP, Kaul S, Drexler H, Greenland P, Muller JE, Virmani R, Ridker PM, Zipes DP, Shah PK, Willerson JT. From vulnerable plaque to vulnerable patient: a call for new definitions and risk assessment strategies: Part I. Circulation. 2003;108:1664–72.
10. Ohtani T, Ueda Y, Mizote I, Oyabu J, Okada K, Hirayama A, Kodama K. Number of yellow plaques detected in a coronary artery is associated with future risk of acute coronary syndrome: detection of vulnerable patients by angioscopy. J Am Coll Cardiol. 2006;47:2194–200.
11. Ueda Y, Ogasawara N, Matsuo K, Hirotani S, Kashiwase K, Hirata A, Nishio M, Nemoto T, Wada M, Masumura Y, Kashiyama T, Konishi S, Nakanishi H, Kobayashi Y, Akazawa Y, Kodama K. Acute coronary syndrome: insight from angioscopy. Circ J. 2010;74:411–17.
12. Uchida Y, Nakamura F, Tomaru T, Morita T, Oshima T, Sasaki T, Morizuki S, Hirose J. Prediction of acute coronary syndromes by percutaneous coronary angioscopy in patients with stable angina. Am Heart J. 1995;130:195–203.
13. Finn AV, Nakano M, Narula J, Kolodgie FD, Virmani R. Concept of vulnerable/unstable plaque. Arterioscler Thromb Vasc Biol. 2010;30:1282–92.
14. Kolodgie FD, Burke AP, Farb A, Gold HK, Yuan J, Narula J, Finn AV, Virmani R. The thin-cap fibroatheroma: a type of vulnerable plaque: the major precursor lesion to acute coronary syndromes. Curr Opin Cardiol. 2001;16:285–92.
15. Burke AP, Farb A, Malcom GT, Liang YH, Smialek J, Virmani R. Coronary risk factors and plaque morphology in men with coronary disease who died suddenly. N Engl J Med. 1997;336:1276–82.
16. Grønholdt ML, Dalager-Pedersen S, Falk E. Coronary atherosclerosis: determinants of plaque rupture. Eur Heart J. 1998;19(Suppl C):C24–9.
17. Farb A, Burke AP, Tang AL, Liang TY, Mannan P, Smialek J, Virmani R. Coronary plaque erosion without rupture into a lipid core. A frequent cause of coronary thrombosis in sudden coronary death. Circulation. 1996;93:1354–63.
18. Kolodgie FD, Burke AP, Wight TN, Virmani R. The accumulation of specific types of proteoglycans in eroded plaques: a role in coronary thrombosis in the absence of rupture. Curr Opin Lipidol. 2004;15:575–82.
19. Mizukoshi M, Imanishi T, Tanaka A, Kubo T, Liu Y, Takarada S, Kitabata H, Tanimoto T, Komukai K, Ishibashi K, Akasaka T. Clinical classification and plaque morphology determined by optical coherence tomography in unstable angina pectoris. Am J Cardiol. 2010;106:323–8.
20. Ozaki Y, Okumura M, Ismail TF, Motoyama S, Naruse H, Hattori K, Kawai H, Sarai M, Takagi Y, Ishii J, Anno H, Virmani R, Serruys PW, Narula J. Coronary CT angiographic characteristics of culprit lesions in acute coronary syndromes not related to plaque rupture as defined by optical coherence tomography and angioscopy. Eur Heart J. 2011;32:2814–23.
21. Angheloiu GO, Arendt JT, Müller MG, Haka AS, Georgakoudi I, Motz JT, Scepanovic OR, Kuban BD, Myles J, Miller F, Podrez EA, Fitzmaurice M, Kramer JR, Feld MS. Intrinsic fluorescence and diffuse reflectance spectroscopy identify superficial foam cells in coronary plaques prone to erosion. Arterioscler Thromb Vasc Biol. 2006;26:1594–600.
22. Suh WM, Seto AH, Margey RJ, Cruz-Gonzalez I, Jang IK. Intravascular detection of the vulnerable plaque. Circ Cardiovasc Imaging. 2011;4:169–78.
23. Takano M, Jang IK, Inami S, Yamamoto M, Murakami D, Okamatsu K, Seimiya K, Ohba T, Mizuno K. In vivo comparison of optical coherence tomography and angioscopy for the evaluation of coronary plaque characteristics. Am J Cardiol. 2008;101:471–6.
24. Uchida Y, Uchida Y, Hiruta N. Histological characteristics of glistening yellow coronary plaques seen on angioscopy. -With special reference to vulnerable plaques-. Circ J. 2011;75:1913–19.

25. MacNeill BD, Jang IK, Bouma BE, Iftimia N, Takano M, Yabushita H, Shishkov M, Kauffman CR, Houser SL, Aretz HT, DeJoseph D, Halpern EF, Tearney GJ. Focal and multi-focal plaque macrophage distributions in patients with acute and stable presentations of coronary artery disease. J Am Coll Cardiol. 2004;44:972–9.
26. Virmani R, Burke AP, Kolodgie FD, Farb A. Pathology of the thin-cap fibroatheroma: a type of vulnerable plaque. J Interv Cardiol. 2003;16:267–72.
27. Tanaka A, Imanishi T, Kitabata H, Kubo T, Takarada S, Tanimoto T, Kuroi A, Tsujioka H, Ikejima H, Ueno S, Kataiwa H, Okouchi K, Kashiwaghi M, Matsumoto H, Takemoto K, Nakamura N, Hirata K, Mizukoshi M, Akasaka T. Morphology of exertion-triggered plaque rupture in patients with acute coronary syndrome: an optical coherence tomography study. Circulation. 2008;118:2368–73.
28. Wentzel JJ, Gijsen FJ, Stergiopulos N, Serruys PW, Slager CJ, Krams R. Shear stress, vascular remodeling and neointimal formation. J Biomech. 2003;36:681–8.
29. Gertz SD, Roberts WC. Hemodynamic shear force in rupture of coronary arterial atherosclerotic plaques. Am J Cardiol. 1990;66:1368–72.
30. Chatzizisis YS, Coskun AU, Jonas M, Edelman ER, Feldman CL, Stone PH. Role of endothelial shear stress in the natural history of coronary atherosclerosis and vascular remodeling: molecular, cellular, and vascular behavior. J Am Coll Cardiol. 2007;49:2379–93.
31. Libby P. Molecular bases of the acute coronary syndromes. Circulation. 1995;91:2844–50.
32. Ward MR, Jeremias A, Huegel H, Fitzgerald PJ, Yeung AC. Accentuated remodeling on the upstream side of atherosclerotic lesions. Am J Cardiol. 2000;85:523–6.
33. Burke AP, Farb A, Malcom GT, Liang Y, Smialek JE, Virmani R. Plaque rupture and sudden death related to exertion in men with coronary artery disease. JAMA. 1999;281:921–6.
34. Burleigh MC, Briggs AD, Lendon CL, Davies MJ, Born GV, Richardson PD. Collagen types I and III, collagen content, GAGs and mechanical strength of human atherosclerotic plaque caps: span-wise variations. Atherosclerosis. 1992;96:71–81.
35. Fukumoto Y, Hiro T, Fujii T, Hashimoto G, Fujimura T, Yamada J, Okamura T, Matsuzaki M. Localized elevation of shear stress is related to coronary plaque rupture: a 3-dimensional intravascular ultrasound study with in-vivo color mapping of shear stress distribution. J Am Coll Cardiol. 2008;51:645–50.
36. Crea F, Giovanna L. Pathogenesis of acute coronary syndrome. J Am Coll Cardiol. 2013;61:1–11.
37. Abela GS, Aziz K, Vedre A, Pathak DR, Talbott JD, Dejong J. Effect of cholesterol crystals on plaques and intima in arteries of patients with acute coronary and cerebrovascular syndromes. Am J Cardiol. 2009;103:959–68.
38. Tziakas DN, Kaski JC, Chalikias GK, Romero C, Fredericks S, Tentes IK, Kortsaris AX, Hatseras DI, Holt DW. Total cholesterol content of erythrocyte membranes is increased in patients with acute coronary syndrome: a new marker of clinical instability? J Am Coll Cardiol. 2007;49:2081–9.
39. Fiorentino TV, Prioletta A, Zuo P, Folli F. Hyperglycemia-induced oxidative stress and its role in diabetes mellitus related cardiovascular diseases. Curr Pharm Des. 2013;19:5695–703.
40. García RG, Rincón MY, Arenas WD, Silva SY, Reyes LM, Ruiz SL, Ramirez F, Camacho PA, Luengas C, Saaibi JF, Balestrini S, Morillo C, López-Jaramillo P. Hyperinsulinemia is a predictor of new cardiovascular events in Colombian patients with a first myocardial infarction. Int J Cardiol. 2011;148:85–90.
41. Kim JA, Montagnani M, Koh KK, Quon MJ. Reciprocal relationships between insulin resistance and endothelial dysfunction: molecular and pathophysiological mechanisms. Circulation. 2006;113:1888–904.

Chapter 8
Plaque Erosion

Shigenobu Inami

Abstract Acute coronary syndrome results from the intimal injury of an epicardial coronary artery. Plaque erosion is intimal injury which does not exhibit plaque rupture.

Pathological studies have shown that plaque erosion often develops on intimal thickening or a fibroatheroma, with few lipid core and calcification. The exposed intima at the eroded site is predominantly comprised of vascular smooth muscle cells and proteoglycans. Plaque erosions are more often observed in younger individuals and smokers compared with plaque ruptures.

There have been few angioscopic investigations of plaque erosion. Because the injured intima hides behind a thrombus, the plaque morphology is often overlooked by angioscopy. The combination of angioscopy and an intravascular imaging device visualizing cross-sectional images of an artery is thought to be helpful for identifying plaque erosion. A recent study using both angioscopy and intravascular ultrasound demonstrated that the morphologies of culprit lesions are associated with the clinical features of the patients with acute myocardial infarction. Identifying the morphology of intimal injury may help to determine the optimal management of acute coronary syndrome.

Keywords Intima • Erosion • Acute coronary syndrome

8.1 What Is Plaque Erosion?

Acute coronary syndrome (ACS) is caused by the formation or presence of a thrombus in an epicardial coronary artery. The formation of a thrombus results from intimal injury, which has a variety of morphologies. Pathological studies have shown that plaque rupture is the main morphology observed in the culprit lesions of ACS patients. Plaque rupture is defined as a perforation of a fibrous cap overlying a lipid core. Plaque rupture is not observed in approximately one-fourth

S. Inami, M.D. (✉)
Department of Cardiology, International University of Health and Welfare, Sioya Hospital, 77, Tomita, Yaita City, Tochigi 329-2145, Japan
e-mail: sigenobu@iuhw.ac.jp

© Springer Japan 2015
K. Mizuno, M. Takano (eds.), *Coronary Angioscopy*,
DOI 10.1007/978-4-431-55546-9_8

of the patients with acute events. Plaque erosion is an intimal injury which does not exhibit plaque rupture. The ruptured site is characterized by a thin fibrous cap, large lipid core, and numerous activated inflammatory cells. On one hand, erosion often develops on intimal thickening or a fibroatheroma with few lipid core and calcification. The exposed intima at the eroded site is predominantly comprised of vascular smooth muscle cells and proteoglycans [1]. According to pathological studies, plaque erosions are more often observed in younger individuals and smokers compared with plaque ruptures [2, 3].

8.2   Angioscopic Findings of Plaque Erosion

Angioscopy can visualize the luminal surface of the intima and thrombus. The injured intima hides behind the intraluminal and mural thrombus, so the plaque morphology is often overlooked. Just after the thrombus has disappeared or decreased in size, the injured intima becomes visible. Typically, plaque erosion is diagnosed if there is only reddening and a rough surface, with no evidence of trans-cap ruptures, such as a dissection, cleft, or depressed ulceration (Fig. 8.1). Kubo et al. analyzed the culprit lesions in patients with myocardial infarction by optical coherence tomography (OCT), angioscopy, and intravascular ultrasound (IVUS). There was a significant difference in the incidence of plaque erosion diagnosed by these intravascular imaging devices (23 %, 3 %, and 0 % by OCT, angioscopy, and IVUS, respectively; $p = 0.003$). The difference in the incidence of erosion was significant between OCT and CAS ($p = 0.026$) or between OCT and IVUS ($p = 0.005$), but not between CAS and IVUS ($p = 0.500$) [4]. The combination of angioscopy and an intravascular imaging device visualizing the cross-sectional images of an artery is thought to be helpful in identifying plaque erosion (Fig. 8.2). Ozaki et al. assessed coronary CT angiographic characteristics of culprit lesions in acute coronary syndromes not related to plaque rupture as defined by optical coherence tomography and angioscopy. CT angiography revealed that a low-attenuation plaque, positive remodeling, and spotty calcification were significantly less common in the ACS not related to plaque rupture than ACS related to plaque rupture, but similar to stable angina [5].

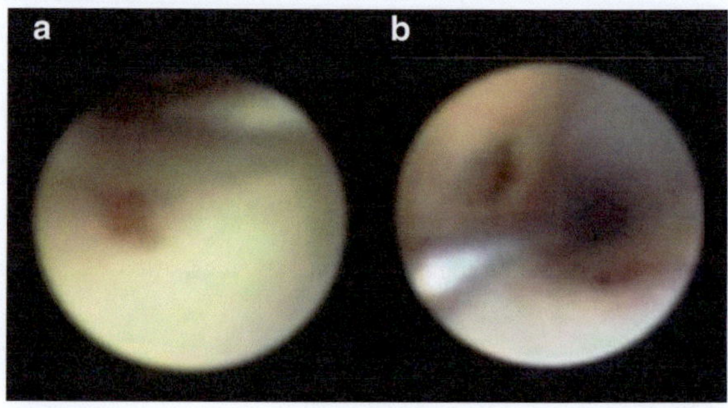

Fig. 8.1 Angioscopic finding of plaque erosion and rupture. (**a**) Plaque erosion, only reddening with no evidence of trans-cap ruptures, (**b**) plaque rupture, perforation of a fibrous cap overlying lipid core

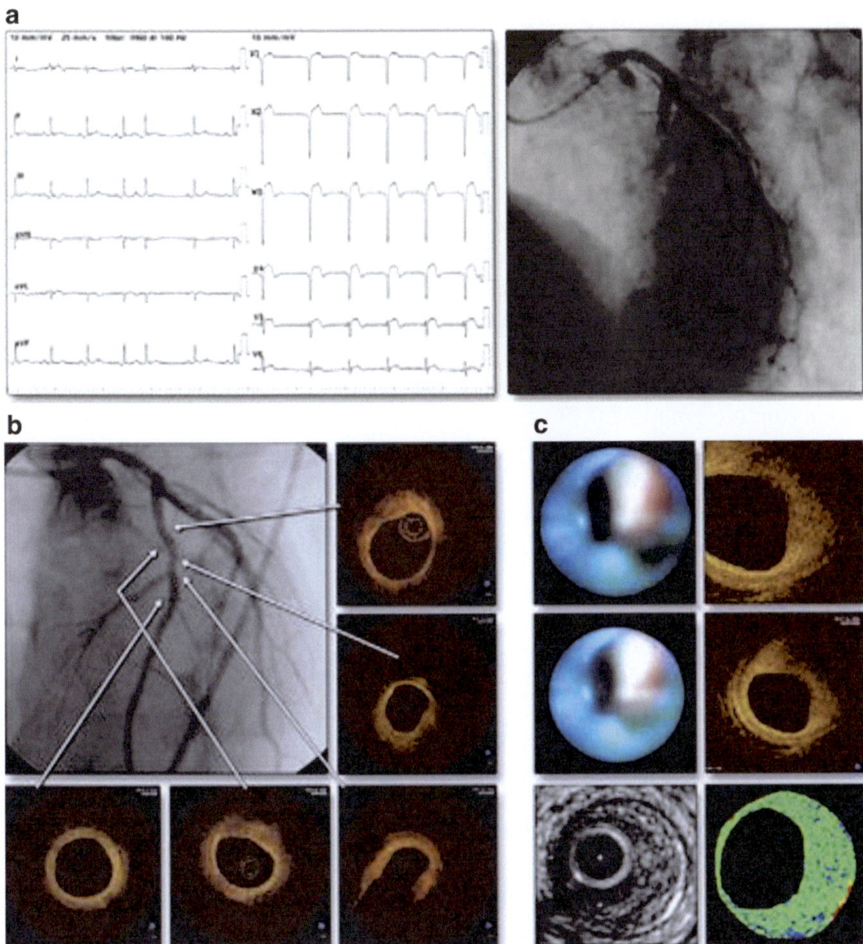

Fig. 8.2 Coronary angiography and intravascular imaging in patient with ST-segment elevation myocardial infarction not related to plaque rupture. (**a**) An electrocardiogram revealed ST-segment elevation in precordial leads. Coronary angiography showed total occlusion of the proximal segment of left anterior descending coronary artery. (**b**) Coronary angiography and OCT after thrombolysis demonstrated no significant stenosis and no perforation of fibrous cap. (**c**) Coronary angioscopy showed faint red thrombus formation through the blue coronary angioscopy guide catheter, whereas OCT did not show a typical red thrombus with a high backscattering protrusion mass with signal-free shadowing, but some signal reduction was observed from 12 to 3 o'clock positions. Intravascular ultrasound and integrated backscatter intravascular ultrasound demonstrated predominantly a fibrous plaque (*green*) and negligible lipid-rich component (*blue*) (From Prati F et al. [6])

8.3 Clinical Implications of Plaque Erosions Observed by Angioscopy

Angioscopy, which shows gross pathological findings in vivo, has the potential to clarify the differences in the pathogenic mechanisms between an erosion and rupture. Hayashi et al. examined the relationship between the morphologies of culprit lesions and the clinical features of the patients with acute myocardial infarction using coronary angioscopy and intravascular ultrasound [7]. These studies were performed immediately before percutaneous coronary intervention was undertaken. They found that the patients with eroded plaque lesions had smaller infarctions than those with ruptured plaque lesions. Furthermore, distal embolization was less frequent in the erosion group compared with the rupture group (rupture group 37.0 % vs. erosion group 0.0 %; $P = 0.0026$). These results also suggest that the morphology of the intimal injury may help to determine the optimal management of ACS. The mechanical stress caused by coronary spasm is suspected to contribute to the formation of erosion. The angioscopic findings of coronary spasm are discussed in detail in the next section.

8.4 Summary

There have been few angioscopic investigations of plaque erosion. Because a thrombus attaches to the injured intima, the morphology of the intima is often overlooked by angioscopy. The combination of angioscopy and an intravascular imaging device visualizing the cross-sectional images of the artery is thought to be helpful in identifying a plaque erosion. Identifying the morphology of the intimal injury may help to determine the optimal management of ACS.

References

1. Virmani R, Kolodgie FD, Burke AP, Farb A, Schwartz SM. Lessons from sudden coronary death: a comprehensive morphological classification scheme for atherosclerotic lesions. Arterioscler Thromb Vasc Biol. 2000;20:1262–75. doi:10.1161/01.ATV.20.5.1262.
2. Burke AP, Farb A, Malcom GT, Liang YH, Smialek J, Virmani R. Coronary risk factors and plaque morphology in men with coronary disease who died suddenly. N Engl J Med. 1997;336:1276–82. doi:10.1056/NEJM199705013361802.
3. Farb A, Burke AP, Tang AL, Liang TY, Mannan P, Smialek J, Virmani R. Coronary plaque erosion without rupture into a lipid core. A frequent cause of coronary thrombosis in sudden coronary death. Circulation. 1996;93:1354–63. doi:10.1161/01.CIR.93.7.1354.
4. Kubo T, Imanishi T, Takarada S, Kuroi A, Ueno S, Yamano T, Tanimoto T, Matsuo Y, Masho T, Kitabata H, Tsuda K, Tomobuchi Y, Akasaka T. Assessment of culprit lesion morphology in acute myocardial infarction: ability of optical coherence tomography compared with intravascular ultrasound and coronary angioscopy. J Am Coll Cardiol. 2007;50:933–9. doi:10.1016/j.jacc.2007.04.082.

5. Ozaki Y, Okumura M, Ismail TF, Motoyama S, Naruse H, Hattori K, Kawai H, Sarai M, Takagi Y, Ishii J, Anno H, Virmani R, Serruys PW, Narula J. Coronary CT angiographic characteristics of culprit lesions in acute coronary syndromes not related to plaque rupture as defined by optical coherence tomography and angioscopy. Eur Heart J. 2011;32:2814–23. doi:10.1093/eurheartj/ehr189. Epub 2011 June 30.
6. Prati F, Uemura S, Souteyrand G, Virmani R, Motreff P, Di Vito L, Biondi-Zoccai G, Halperin J, Fuster V, Ozaki Y, Narula J. OCT-based diagnosis and management of STEMI associated with intact fibrous cap. JACC Cardiovasc Imaging. 2013;6:283–7. doi:10.1016/j.jcmg.2012.12.007.
7. Hayashi T, Kiyoshima T, Matsuura M, Ueno M, Kobayashi N, Yabushita H, Kurooka A, Taniguchi M, Miyataka M, Kimura A, Ishikawa K. Plaque erosion in the culprit lesion is prone to develop a smaller myocardial infarction size compared with plaque rupture. Am Heart J. 2005;149:284–90. doi:10.1016/j.ahj.2004.06.020.

Chapter 9
Angioscopy and Coronary Endothelial Function

Yoshiaki Mitsutake and Takafumi Ueno

Abstract The endothelium plays a critical role in regulating vascular homeostasis. Damage of endothelial cells is an initial step in atherosclerosis, and endothelial dysfunction is a predictor of long-term atherosclerotic disease progression and future cardiovascular events. Recently, endothelial dysfunction associated with drug-eluting stent has been reported.

This section will focus on the relationship between coronary endothelial function and morphological findings by intravascular imaging modalities.

Keywords Neointimal coverage • Drug-eluting stent • Endothelial function • Spasm

9.1 Introduction

The vascular endothelium is the monolayer of endothelial cells lining the lumen of the vascular beds and envelopes the circulating blood. The endothelium plays a critical role in vascular tone through the release of several autocrine and paracrine substances [1]. In addition, a healthy endothelium affects inhibition of platelet aggregation and adhesion, monocyte and leukocyte adhesion, smooth muscle cell proliferation, and thrombosis [2]. Damage of endothelial cells is an initial step in atherosclerosis and is an important manifestation of ischemic heart disease process. Coronary endothelial dysfunction plays a pivotal role in not only coronary spasm [3] but also acute coronary syndrome and sudden cardiac death [4, 5]. Increasing evidence suggests that coronary endothelial dysfunction is a predictor of long-term atherosclerotic disease progression and future cardiovascular events [6, 7].

Y. Mitsutake • T. Ueno (✉)
Division of Cardiovascular Medicine, Kurume University School of Medicine, 67 Asahi-machi, Kurume 830-0011, Japan
e-mail: takueno@med.kurume-u.ac.jp

© Springer Japan 2015
K. Mizuno, M. Takano (eds.), *Coronary Angioscopy*,
DOI 10.1007/978-4-431-55546-9_9

9.2 Assessment of Endothelial Function

In the clinical setting, endothelial function is often assessed as a vascular response to pharmacological or physiological stimuli, e.g., acetylcholine (Ach), adenosine, ergonovine, bradykinin, serotonin, and blood flow (shear stress) [8]. Nowadays, intracoronary infusion of Ach could be considered as the golden standard method for coronary endothelial function testing in patients. Under healthy endothelial conditions, Ach causes vasodilation by inducing the release of a nitric oxide (NO). In contrast, if endothelial dysfunction exists, paradoxical vasoconstrictive response to Ach is observed because of a disturbed NO release and a direct effect on vascular smooth muscle cells [9, 10].

9.2.1 Endothelial Function and Intravascular Imaging Modalities

Some studies have investigated morphological findings at the endothelium-dependent vasoconstriction site using intravascular imaging modalities in human coronary arteries. Etsuda et al. revealed that even coronary vasoconstriction sites were angiographically normal; those sites had intimal injuries (hemorrhage, flap, thrombus, or ulcer) by angioscopy [11]. Likewise, Yamagishi et al. showed atheroma by intravascular ultrasound (IVUS) was present at vasoconstriction sites, even in the absence of angiographically significant coronary disease [12]. Zeiher et al. and Miyao et al. demonstrated that intimal thickening had a relationship with the vasoconstrictive response to Ach [13, 14]. Furthermore, Morikawa et al. examined the morphological characteristics of coronary arteries with coronary spasm using optical coherence tomography (OCT) and revealed OCT findings at the vasoconstrictive segments were homogeneous and diffuse thickening of the intimal layer without lipid and/or calcium accumulation [15]. Similarly, Tsujita et al. showed the intima in spastic coronary arteries was diffusely thickened, and a major component of the intima thickening was a fibrous tissue in virtual histology IVUS [16]. In contrast, Lavi et al. demonstrated that coronary endothelial dysfunction was associated with necrotic cores by virtual histology IVUS [17]. Some studies have failed to identify morphological features of vessel wall with endothelial dysfunction [18–20]. Thus, the relation between morphological findings by intravascular imaging modalities and endothelial dysfunction might be still a matter of debate.

9.3 Endothelial Function and Drug-Eluting Stents

Drug-eluting stent (DES) has significantly reduced in-stent restenosis and targets lesion revascularization after percutaneous coronary intervention (PCI), as compared with bare-metal stent (BMS) [21]. Despite these beneficial effects of

DES, the use of first-generation DES, sirolimus-eluting stent (SES) (Cypher™, Cordis Corporation, Florida), and paclitaxel-eluting stent (PES) (Taxus™, Boston Scientific Corporation, Massachusetts) could be associated with the risk of late stent thrombosis (LST) [22]. Several clinical studies revealed coronary endothelial dysfunction at segments adjacent to the SES and PES [23–27]. Although the mechanisms of LST have not been fully elucidated, recent human autopsy studies suggested that the most powerful histological predictor of LST is impaired re-endothelialization after DES implantation [28, 29].

9.3.1 Endothelial Dysfunction and Delayed Arterial Healing in First-Generation DES

Several coronary angioscopic observational data revealed poor neointimal coverage and thrombus formation at the first-generation DES implanted site [27, 30–33]. Delayed arterial healing after DES implantation is considered the most important morphometric predictor of LST as well as impaired re-endothelialization [28, 29]. We examined endothelial function and intra-stent condition by angioscopy in patients with stable angina at 9 months after SES and PES implantation. Our study demonstrated that the degree of coronary endothelial dysfunction was similar between the SES and PES (Fig. 9.1), and endothelial dysfunction distal to the stent was greater in the poor stent strut coverage compared with the good coverage (Figs. 9.2, 9.3, and 9.4) [27]. Moreover, we found that poor strut coverage was associated with thrombus formation (Fig. 9.5), and the presence of in-stent thrombus and the degree of neointimal stent strut coverage were the independent factors of endothelial dysfunction distal to the first-generation DES [27]. Therefore, our results suggested evaluation intra-stent condition by angioscopy may be a surrogate for endothelial function with first-generation DES.

9.3.2 Possible Mechanisms of Endothelial Dysfunction with First-Generation DES

Previous studies have reported some potential mechanisms of abnormal endothelial function with DES. Re-endothelialization is nearly completed after BMS implantation [34], but not after DES implantation [28, 29]. Accordingly, reduced NO production attributable to delayed re-endothelialization and/or endothelial dysfunction at the stented site could be associated with endothelial dysfunction at areas adjacent to the DES. Sahler LG, et al. showed that antiproliferative drugs may have locally diffused through the vaso vasorum to the non-stented distal segments, leading to impaired endothelial function distal to the DES [35]. Pendyala LK, et al. reported polymer incompatibility and potentiation of superoxide activity may be

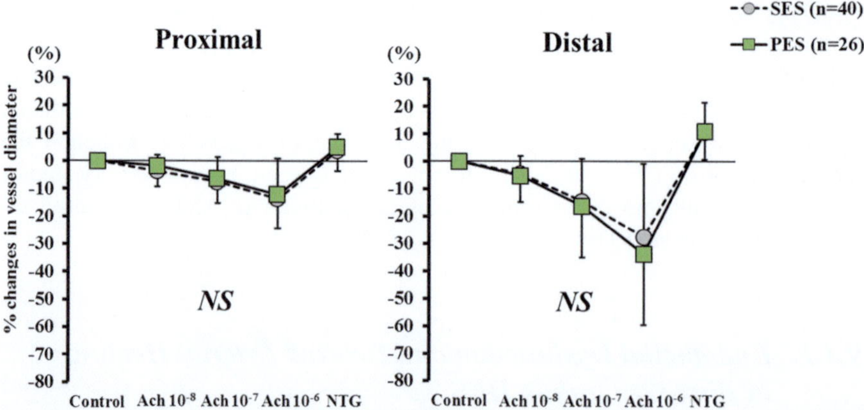

Fig. 9.1 Changes in vessel diameter in response to Ach and NTG infusion expressed as percentage of changes versus the baseline diameter in comparison between the SES and the PES. *Ach* acetylcholine, *NTG* nitroglycerin, *SES* sirolimus-eluting stent, *PES* paclitaxel-eluting stent

LAD, SES

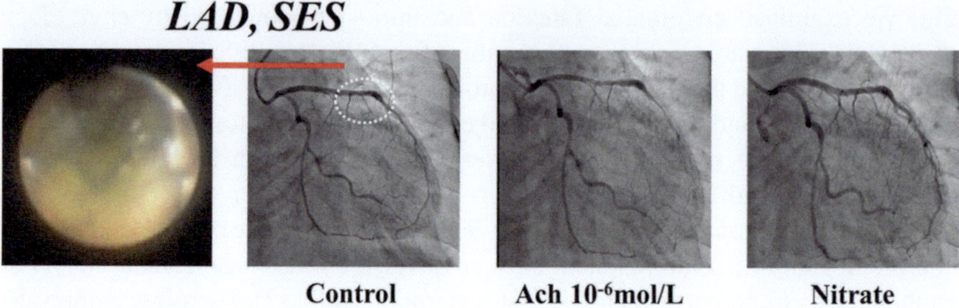

Fig. 9.2 A representative case with SES. In this case, SES was implanted in the LAD. At 9 months follow-up, restenosis was not found. Severe vasoconstriction to Ach distal to the stent was observed, while vasodilation to NTG was preserved. In angioscopic evaluation, poor neointimal coverage and yellow plaque between the strut were observed in the SES. *SES* sirolimus-eluting stent, *LAD* left anterior descending artery, *NTG* nitroglycerin

a culprit of endothelial dysfunction with PES [36]. We have previously reported that thrombi release several vasoactive substances which are shed into the distal site and would impair distal endothelial function in the canine model of acute coronary syndromes [37, 38] and endothelial dysfunction distal to the stent is strongly associated with existence of thrombus inside the first-generation DES implantation in the clinical setting [27]. Thus, poor re-endothelialization and thrombus at the stent site might work together to aggravate endothelial function adjacent to the first-generation DES.

LAD, PES

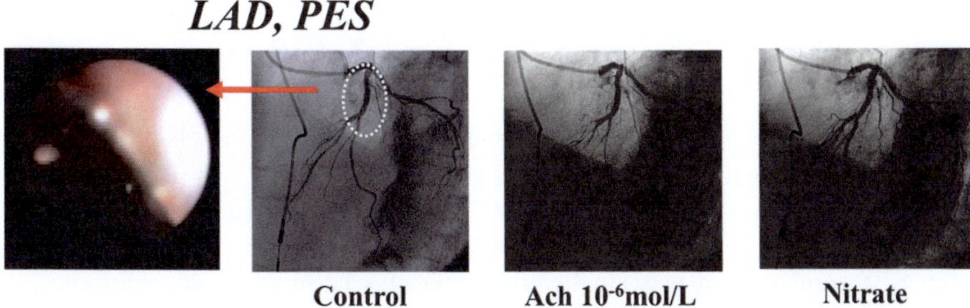

Fig. 9.3 A representative case with PES. PES was implanted in the LAD. At 9 months follow-up, severe vasoconstriction to Ach distal to the stent was observed, while vasodilation to NTG was preserved. The poor neointimal coverage and red thrombus formation were observed in the PES by angioscopy. *PES* paclitaxel-eluting stent, *LAD* left anterior descending artery, *NTG* nitroglycerin

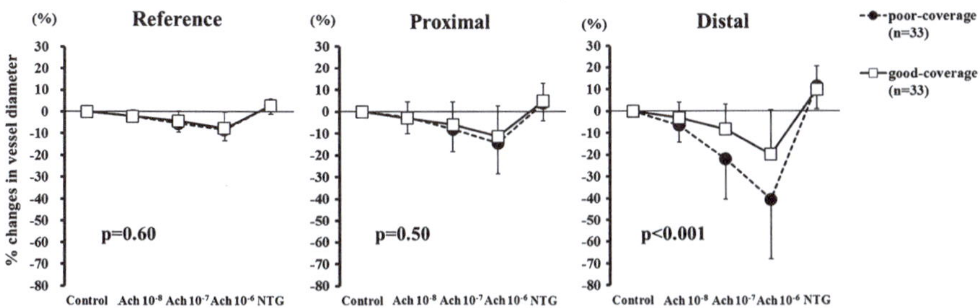

Fig. 9.4 Changes in vessel diameter in response to Ach and NTG infusion expressed as percentage of changes versus the baseline diameter in comparison between the poor-coverage group and the good-coverage group. *p* values indicate difference between the poor-coverage group and the good-coverage group. *Ach* acetylcholine, *NTG* nitroglycerin

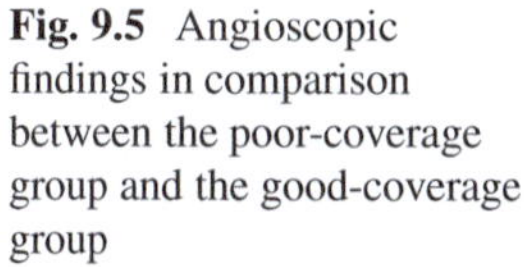

Fig. 9.5 Angioscopic findings in comparison between the poor-coverage group and the good-coverage group

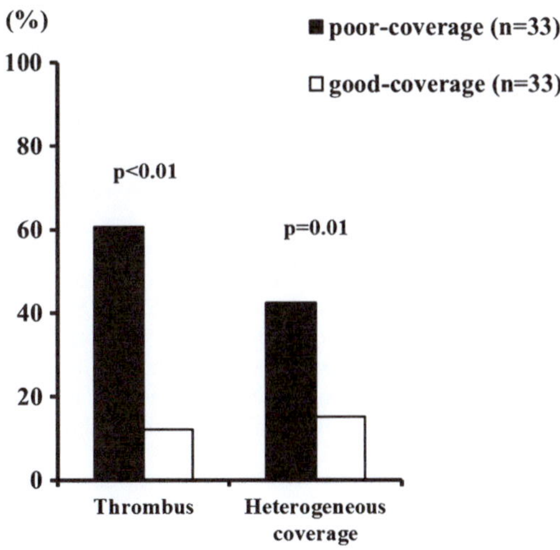

9.3.3 Endothelial Dysfunction and Delayed Healing with First-Generation DES Persist for a Long-Term?

Some angioscopic studies revealed delayed arterial healing associated with first-generation DES is still observed at 2–5 years after PCI [31, 33]. However, there are few investigations that evaluated how long endothelial dysfunction persists after DES implantation. Kitahara et al. showed endothelial dysfunction at >12 months after SES implantation was smaller than that at <12 months [26]. However, in their study, only low-dose Ach infusion was used, and additionally serial change in endothelial function was not examined. We examined serial changes in endothelial function and intra-stent condition by angioscopy in comparison between 9 months and over 24 months after PES implantation. In that study, endothelial dysfunction distal to the PES and delayed healing improved slightly as time passed; however, those findings were still observed over 24 months after stent implantation (Figs. 9.6, 9.7, and 9.8) [39]. Thus, the restoration of coronary endothelial function and arterial healing associated with first-generation DES might be significantly delayed.

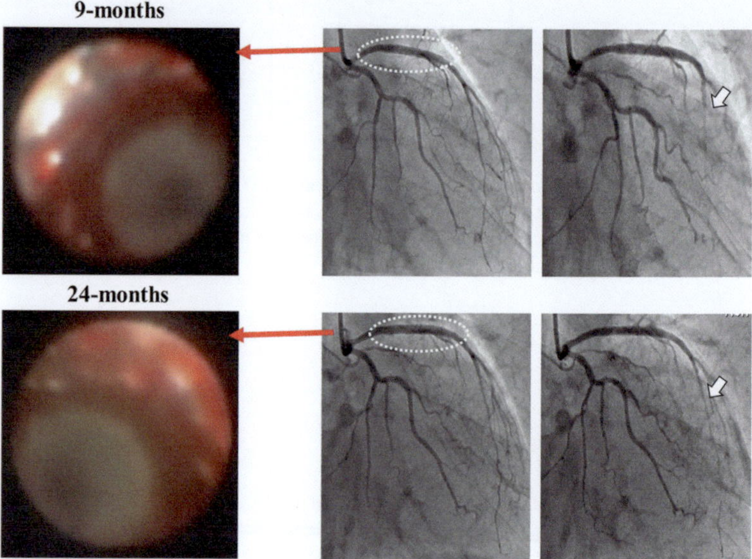

Fig. 9.6 A representative case with PES (2). In this case, PES was implanted in the LAD. At 9 months follow-up, restenosis was not found. Severe vasoconstriction to Ach distal to the stent was observed. At 24 months follow-up, vasoconstriction to Ach was still observed at the distal segment to the stent. In angioscopic evaluation, the maximum neointimal coverage site was grade 3 coverage. In contrast, many uncovered struts and red thrombus were found at both 9 and 24 months follow-up, similarly in the minimum neointimal coverage site. *PES* paclitaxel-eluting stent, *LAD* left anterior descending artery

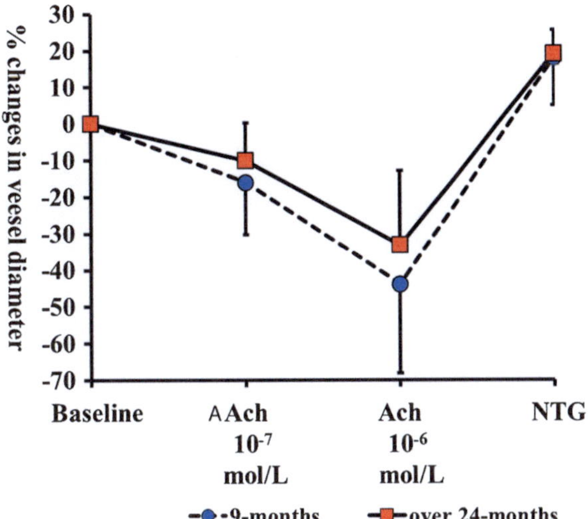

Fig. 9.7 Changes in vascular response to Ach and NTG distal to PES in comparison between 9 months and over 24 months. *Ach* acetylcholine, *NTG* nitroglycerin, *PES* paclitaxel-eluting stent

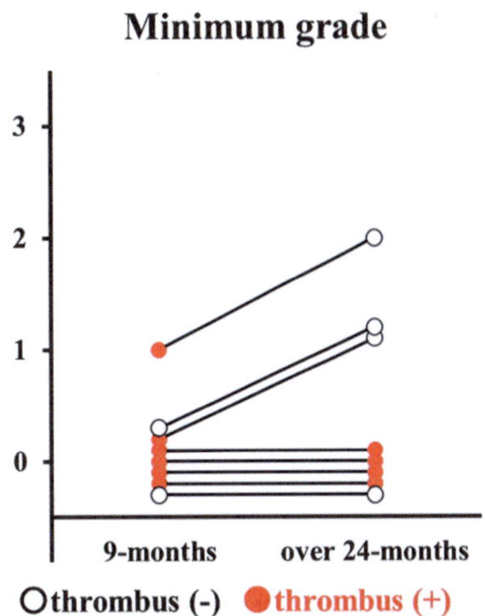

Fig. 9.8 Angioscopic findings at minimum coverage site in PES in comparison between 9 months and over 24 months

9.3.4 Endothelial Function and Arterial Healing in Newer-Generation DES

Several newer-generation DESs have been developed with different drugs, polymers, drug release kinetics, and stent designs. Zotarolimus-eluting stent (ZES) (Endeavor[TM], Medtronic Inc., Santa Rosa, California) and everolimus-eluting stent (EES) (Xience[TM], Abbott Vascular, Santa Clara, California) are newly developed DES. Both ZES and EES showed better outcomes compared with first-generation DES in real-world patients [40, 41].

LAD, EES

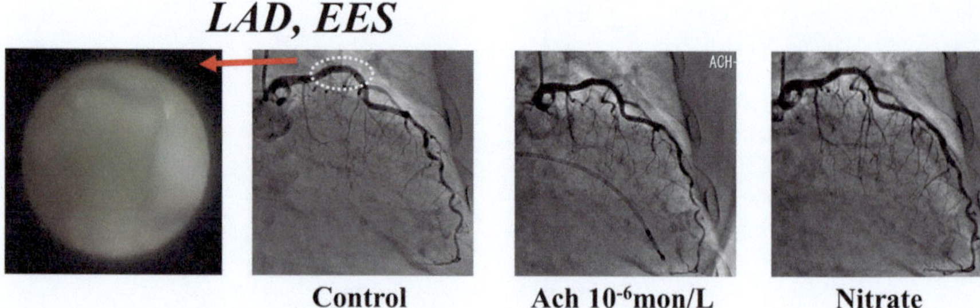

Fig. 9.9 A representative case with EES. EES was implanted in the LAD. At 9 months follow- up, vascular response to Ach was very small, and vasodilation to NTG was preserved. In angioscopic observation, relatively good neointimal coverage was observed, and there was no thrombus in the EES. *EES* everolimus-eluting stent, *LAD* left anterior descending artery, *NTG* nitroglycerin

LAD, ZES

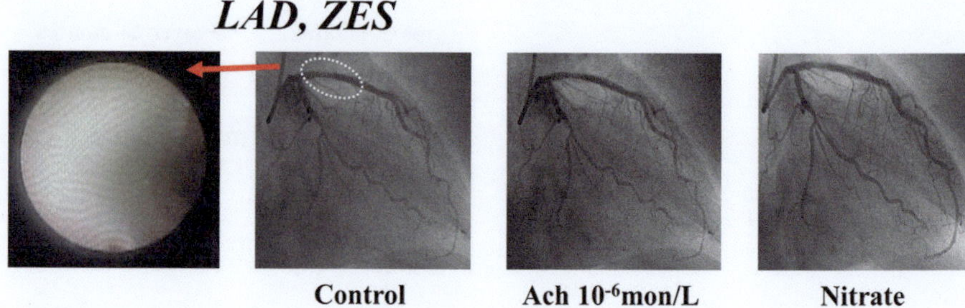

Fig. 9.10 A representative case with ZES. EES was implanted in the LAD. At 9 months follow-up, vascular response to Ach and NTG was preserved. In angioscopic observation, complete neointimal coverage was obtained, and there was no thrombus in the ZES. *ZES* zotarolimus-eluting stent, *LAD* left anterior descending artery, *NTG* nitroglycerin

In our study, ZES and EES demonstrated better endothelial function and arterial healing than first-generation DES at 9 months after PCI (Figs. 9.8, 9.9, 9.10, 9.11, and 9.12) [42], similar to other reports [43–46].

9.4 Conclusion

To evaluate endothelial function using intravascular imaging modalities in human coronary arteries would be challenging. However, in patients with DES, assessment of intra-stent condition by imaging modalities, especially angioscopy which enables to visually inspect the macroscopic pathology, could be a surrogate for endothelial function with DES.

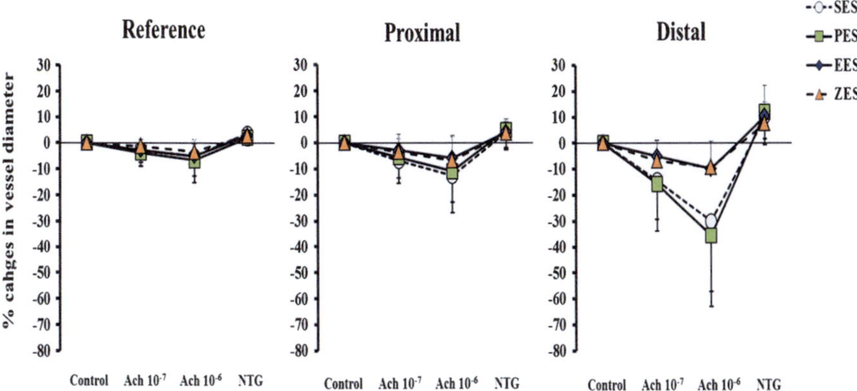

Fig. 9.11 Changes in vessel diameter in response to Ach and NTG infusion expressed as percentage of changes versus the baseline diameter in comparison between the first-generation DES and the second-generation DES. *Ach* acetylcholine, *NTG* nitroglycerin, *DES* drug-eluting stent, *SES* sirolimus-eluting stent, *PES* paclitaxel-eluting stent, *EES* everolimus-eluting stent, *ZES* zotarolimus-eluting stent

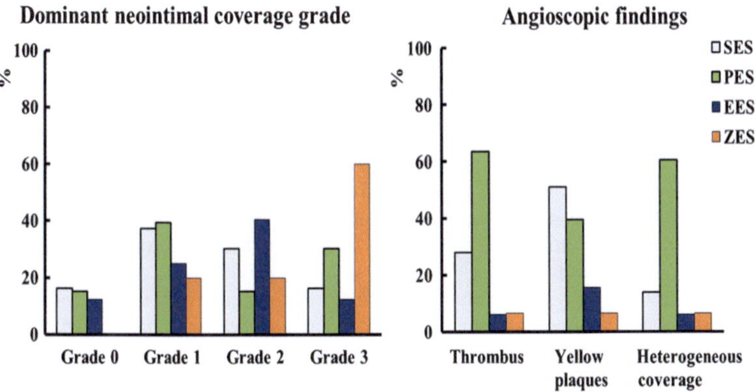

Fig. 9.12 Angioscopic findings in comparison between the first-generation DES and the second-generation DES. *DES* drug-eluting stent, *SES* sirolimus-eluting stent, *PES* paclitaxel-eluting stent, *EES* everolimus-eluting stent, *ZES* zotarolimus-eluting stent

References

1. Moncada S, Higgs A. The L-arginine-NO pathway. N Engl J Med. 1993;329:2002–12.
2. Vane JR, Anggard EE, Botting RM. Regulatory functions of the vascular endothelium. N Engl J Med. 1990;323:27–36.
3. Kugiyama K, Yasue H, Okumura K, et al. Nitric oxide activity is deficient in spasm arteries of patients with coronary spastic angina. Circulation. 1996;94:266–71.
4. Naghavi M, Libby P, Falk E, et al. From vulnerable plaque to vulnerable patient: a call for new definitions and risk assessment strategies: Part I. Circulation. 2003;108:1664–72.

5. Naghavi M, Libby P, Falk E, et al. From vulnerable plaque to vulnerable patient: a call for new definitions and risk assessment strategies: Part II. Circulation. 2003;108:1772–8.
6. Schächinger V, Britten MB, Zeiher AM. Prognostic impact of coronary vasodilator dysfunction on adverse long-term outcome of coronary heart disease. Circulation. 2000;101:1899–906.
7. Widlansky ME, Gokce N, Keaney Jr JF, et al. The clinical implications of endothelial dysfunction. J Am Coll Cardiol. 2003;42:1149–60.
8. Anderson TJ. Assessment and treatment of endothelial dysfunction in humans. J Am Coll Cardiol. 1999;34:631–8.
9. Ludmer PL, Selwyn AP, Shook TL, et al. Paradoxical vasoconstriction induced by acetylcholine in atherosclerotic coronary arteries. N Engl J Med. 1986;315:1046–51.
10. Quyyumi AA, Dakak N, Andrews NP, et al. Nitric oxide activity in the human coronary circulation. Impact of risk factors for coronary atherosclerosis. J Clin Invest. 1995;95:1747–55.
11. Etsuda H, Mizuno K, Arakawa K, et al. Angioscopy in variant angina: coronary artery spasm and intimal injury. Lancet. 1993;342:1322–4.
12. Yamagishi M, Miyatake K, Tamai J, et al. Intravascular ultrasound detection of atherosclerosis at the site of focal vasospasm in angiographically normal or minimally narrowed coronary segments. J Am Coll Cardiol. 1994;23:352–7.
13. Zeiher AM, Schächlinger V, Hohnloser SH, et al. Coronary atherosclerotic wall thickening and vascular reactivity in humans. Elevated high-density lipoprotein levels ameliorate abnormal vasoconstriction in early atherosclerosis. Circulation. 1994;89:2525–32.
14. Miyao Y, Kugiyama K, Kawano H, et al. Diffuse intimal thickening of coronary arteries in patients with coronary spastic angina. J Am Coll Cardiol. 2000;36:423–7.
15. Morikawa Y, Uemura S, Ishigami K, et al. Morphological features of coronary arteries in patients with coronary spastic angina: assessment with intracoronary optical coherence tomography. Int J Cardiol. 2011;146:334–40.
16. Tsujita K, Sakamoto K, Kojima S, et al. Coronary plaque component in patients with vasospastic angina: a virtual histology intravascular ultrasound study. Int J Cardiol. 2013;168:2411–15.
17. Lavi S, Bae JH, Rihal CS, et al. Segmental coronary endothelial dysfunction in patients with minimal atherosclerosis is associated with necrotic core plaques. Heart. 2009;95:1525–30.
18. Nishimura RA, Lerman A, Chesebro JH, et al. Epicardial vasomotor responses to acetylcholine are not predicted by coronary atherosclerosis as assessed by intracoronary ultrasound. J Am Coll Cardiol. 1995;26:41–9.
19. Reddy KG, Nair RN, Sheehan HM, et al. Evidence that selective endothelial dysfunction may occur in the absence of angiographic or ultrasound atherosclerosis in patients with risk factors for atherosclerosis. J Am Coll Cardiol. 1994;23:833–43.
20. Manfrini O, Cenko E, Verna E, et al. Endothelial dysfunction versus early atherosclerosis: a study with high resolution imaging. Int J Cardiol. 2013;168:1714–16.
21. Stetter C, Wandel S, Allemann S, et al. Outcomes associated with drug-eluting and bare-metal stents: a collaborative network meta-analysis. Lancet. 2007;370:937–48.
22. McFadden EP, Stabile E, Regar E, et al. Late thrombosis in drug-eluting coronary stents after discontinuation of antiplatelet therapy. Lancet. 2004;364:1519–21.
23. Hofma SH, van der Giessen WJ, van Dalen BM, et al. Indication of long-term endothelial dysfunction after sirolimus-eluting stent implantation. Eur Heart J. 2006;27:166–70.
24. Shin DI, Kim PJ, Seung KB, et al. Drug-eluting stent implantation could be associated with long-term coronary endothelial dysfunction. Int Heart J. 2007;48:553–67.
25. Kim JW, Suh SY, Choi CU, et al. Six-month comparison of coronary endothelial dysfunction associated with sirolimus-eluting stent versus paclitaxel-eluting stent. J Am Coll Cardiol Intv. 2008;1:65–71.
26. Kitahara H, Fujimoto Y, Ishikawa K, et al. Recovery of endothelial function after sirolimus-eluting stent implantation: a pilot study. Angiology. 2013;64:211–15.
27. Mitsutake Y, Ueno T, Yokoyama S, et al. Coronary endothelial dysfunction distal to stent of first-generation drug-eluting stents. JACC Cardiovasc Interv. 2012;5:966–73.

28. Joner M, Finn AV, Farb A, et al. Pathology of drug-eluting stents in humans: delayed healing and late thrombotic risk. J Am Coll Cardiol. 2006;48:193–202.
29. Finn AV, Joner M, Nakazawa G, et al. Pathological correlates of late drug-eluting stent thrombosis: strut coverage as a marker of endothelialization. Circulation. 2007;115:2435–41.
30. Kotani J, Awata M, Nanto S, et al. Incomplete neointimal coverage of sirolimus-eluting stents: angioscopic findings. J Am Coll Cardiol. 2006;47:2108–11.
31. Awata M, Kotani J, Uematsu M, et al. Serial angioscopic evidence of incomplete neointimal coverage after sirolimus-eluting stent implantation: comparison with bare-metal stents. Circulation. 2007;116:910–16.
32. Awata M, Nanto S, Uematsu M, et al. Heterogeneous arterial healing in patients following paclitaxel-eluting stent implantation: comparison with sirolimus-eluting stents. J Am Coll Cardiol Intv. 2009;2:453–8.
33. Yamamoto M, Takano M, Murakami D, et al. The possibility of delayed arterial healing 5 years after implantation of sirolimus-eluting stents: serial observations by coronary angioscopy. Am Heart J. 2011;161:1200–6.
34. Grewe PH, Deneke T, Machraoui A, et al. Acute and chronic tissue response to coronary stent implantation: pathologic findings in human specimen. J Am Coll Cardiol. 2000;35:157–63.
35. Sahler LG, Davis D, Saad WE, et al. Comparison of vasa vasorum after intravascular stent placement with sirolimus drug-eluting and bare metal stent. J Med Imaging Radiat Oncol. 2008;52:570–5.
36. Pendyala LK, Li J, Shinke T, et al. Endothelium-dependent vasomotor dysfunction in pig coronary arteries with Paclitaxel-eluting stents is associated with inflammation and oxidative stress. JACC Cardiovasc Interv. 2009;2:253–62.
37. Ikeda H, Koga Y, Oda T, et al. Free oxygen radicals contribute to platelet aggregation and cyclic flow variations in stenosed and endothelium-injured canine coronary arteries. J Am Coll Cardiol. 1994;24:1749–56.
38. Eguchi H, Ikeda H, Murohara T, et al. Endothelial injuries of coronary arteries distal to thrombotic sites: role of adhesive interaction between endothelial P-selectin and leukocyte sialyl lewis X. Circ Res. 1999;84:525–35.
39. Mitsutake Y, Ueno T, Yokoyama S, et al. Coronary endothelial dysfunction and delayed arterial healing persist over 24 months after paclitaxel-eluting stent implantation. 17th Transcatheter Cariovascular Therapeutics Asia Pacific Seoul, Korea, April 2012
40. Kandzari DE, Leon MB, Meredith I, et al. Final 5-year outcomes from the Endeavor zotarolimus-eluting stent clinical trial program: comparison of safety and efficacy with first-generation drug-eluting and bare-metal stents. JACC Cardiovasc Interv. 2013;6:504–12.
41. Kedhi E, Joesoef KS, McFadden E, et al. Second-generation everolimus-eluting and paclitaxel-eluting stents in real-life practice (COMPARE): a randomised trial. Lancet. 2010;375:201–9.
42. Mitsutake Y, Ueno T, Yokoyama S, et al. Second-generation drug-eluting stents demonstrate better vascular function and healing than first-generation drug-eluting stents. EuroPCR 2012, Paris, France, May 2012
43. Awata M, Nanto S, Uematsu M, et al. Angioscopic comparison of neointimal coverage between zotarolimus- and sirolimus-eluting stents. J Am Coll Cardiol. 2008;52:789–90.
44. Kim JW, Seo HS, Park JH, et al. A prospective, randomized, 6-month comparison of the coronary vasomotor response associated with a zotarolimus- versus a sirolimus-eluting stent: differential recovery of coronary endothelial dysfunction. J Am Coll Cardiol. 2009;53:1653–9.
45. Hamilos M, Ribichini F, Ostojic MC, et al. Coronary vasomotion one year after drug-eluting stent implantation: comparison of everolimus-eluting and Paclitaxel-eluting coronary stents. J Cardiovasc Transl Res. 2014;7:406–12.
46. Sawada T, Shinke T, Otake H, et al. Comparisons of detailed arterial healing response at seven months following implantation of an everolimus- or sirolimus-eluting stent in patients with ST-segment elevation myocardial infarction. Int J Cardiol. 2013;168:960–6.

Chapter 10
Acute Coronary Syndrome vs. Stable Angina Pectoris: Angioscopic Point of View

Masafumi Ueno and Shunichi Miyazaki

Abstract Coronary artery disease (CAD) has two broad categories of clinical syndromes such as acute coronary syndrome (ACS) and stable angina pectoris (SAP). ACS is well recognized to be a significant contributor to both morbidity and mortality in worldwide, and it is pivotal to understand the mechanisms of ACS in order to predict the occurrence of ACS using a combination of novel imaging modalities and noninvasive biomarkers. Currently, several imaging modalities are investigated to detect vulnerable plaques. In particular, coronary angioscopy can evaluate the luminal surface by direct visualization and plays an important role to elucidate morphological interaction between the plaque and thrombus. In this review, we will focus on the differences in angioscopic findings of plaque morphology, such as plaque color and presence of thrombus in patients with ACS and those with SAP.

Keywords Acute coronary syndrome • Stable angina pectoris • Vulnerable plaque • Plaque rupture • Erosion • Plaque color • Thrombus

10.1   Introduction

The prognosis of patients with stable angina pectoris (SAP) is generally good with an incidence of death or nonfatal myocardial infarction (MI) not exceeding 2 % per year [1]. On the other hand, patients with an acute coronary syndrome (ACS) without ST elevation have much worse prognosis with a 10–15 % incidence of death or nonfatal MI within 1 year after admission [2]. Despite a similar anatomical background, there are different pathophysiologic mechanisms between ACS and SAP. ACS is a clinical syndrome characterized by acute change of ischemic symptom. Plaque disruption, platelet activation, and flow-limiting thrombus formation are recognized as key events in the pathogenesis of ACS [3]. In contrast, such changes do not occur in SAP patients. Because angiography can only provide

M. Ueno, M.D. • S. Miyazaki, M.D. (☒)
Division of Cardiology, Department of Internal Medicine, Faculty of Medicine, Kinki University, 377-2 Ohnohigashi Osakasayama, Osaka 589-8511, Japan
e-mail: smiyazak@med.kindai.ac.jp

© Springer Japan 2015
K. Mizuno, M. Takano (eds.), *Coronary Angioscopy*,
DOI 10.1007/978-4-431-55546-9_10

a two-dimensional silhouette of the lumen, it is not suitable to identify plaque vulnerability. Therefore, the challenge for the future is to identify vulnerable plaques prone to disrupt before thrombotic complications occur. There are several imaging techniques that could detect local plaque vulnerability leading to an ACS [4]. Of these, only coronary angioscopy can provide detailed information of the luminal surface of a plaque, such as color, thrombus, or disruption. In the present review, we will focus on the angioscopic characteristics of ACS and SAP.

10.2 Characteristics of the Current Intravascular Imaging Modalities

Intravascular imaging devices can show detailed plaque composition that cannot be detected by angiography, and these findings are thought to play an important role in order to predict future cardiac events such as ACS. Each imaging device has its own advantages and disadvantages (Table 10.1) [4, 5].

Several studies have demonstrated differences in plaque components between ACS and SAP patients using different intravascular imaging devices. When comparing ACS and SAP using intravascular ultrasound imaging (IVUS), patients with ACS have more frequently positive remodeling and noncalcified attenuated plaque in the culprit lesion than in those with SAP [6, 7]. According to optical coherence tomography (OCT) findings, thrombi and plaque disruption and thin-cap fibroatheroma are frequently found within the culprit lesions of ACS patients [8]. In addition to these findings, several studies evaluated surface morphology between lesions in ACS and SAP patients using angioscopy.

Table 10.1 Advantages and disadvantages of the different intravascular imaging devices

Devices	Advantages	Disadvantages
Angioscopy	Good surface visualization (color, thrombus)	Effect of blood noise
	High resolution (10–50 μm)	Unable to visualize the entire circumference
	Forward viewing	Unable to observe deep tissue
		Difficult to quantify
IVUS	Quantification of plaque, wall thickness, and lumen size	Unable to distinguish thrombi from plaque components
	Tissue characterization	Low resolution (80–120 μm)
	Remodeling assessment	
OCT	High resolution (10–20 μm)	Effect of blood noise
	Small-diameter catheters	Limited depth of penetration (1.5–2 mm)
	Fast data acquisition	
	Can detect endothelization, thin cap, and lipid pool	

The angioscopy system is classified into an occlusion balloon type (monorail on guidewire system) or a non-occlusion one (bare fiber system). Angioscopic examination using balloon occlusion type (FULLVIEW NEO, FiberTech Co., Chiba, Japan) is performed while coronary blood flow was interrupted by inflating the balloon, and blood is cleared away by the injection of 5–10 ml of lactated Ringer's or 3 % dextran solution. On the other hand, the non-balloon occlusion type (FiberTech Co.) is designed for pullback visualization without balloon occlusion, while flushing with 3 % dextran solution through a flushing catheter.

10.3 Angioscopic Findings

10.3.1 Characteristics of Plaque Morphology

From a pathological point of view, atherosclerotic plaques can be classified into two components. These include an atheromatous and a fibrous plaque, which are generally consistent with vulnerable and stable plaques, respectively [9]. Of course, ACS patients have more plaques with characteristics of vulnerability, leading to plaque disruption and thrombosis [3]. From an angioscopic findings, vulnerable plaques show plaque disruption which is defined as having high-yellow color intensity plaque and a mural thrombus formation. Plaque disruption is further classified into two types of plaque morphology such as plaque rupture and erosion [10, 11].

Angioscopically, plaque rupture is defined as the plaque showing dissection, fissuring, ulceration, or confirmed atheroma contents [11]. Plaque erosion is defined as eroded if it shows only reddening and erosion with no evidence of dissection, cleft, or depressed ulceration [11]. On the other hand, plaques in SAP patients usually have a smooth surface with white or light yellow color and no thrombi [12]. Representative image of plaque rupture, erosion, and stable plaque is shown in Fig. 10.1.

10.3.2 Grading of Plaque Color

Plaque color differs in patients with ACS and SAP. According to the relationship between the color of the plaque and its histopathological features, deep-yellow and yellow-red lesions represent either atheroma (53 %) or degenerated plaque (42 %), whereas pate-yellow or gray-yellow lesions were predominantly with degenerated plaque (64 %) and, to a lesser extent, with fibrous plaque (14 %) or atheroma (14 %) [13]. In SAP patients, both types of lesions, smooth gray-white and yellow lesions, were found to be equally distributed [13]. On the other hand, in ACS patients, the yellow color and plaque rupture were frequently found [13]. A previous

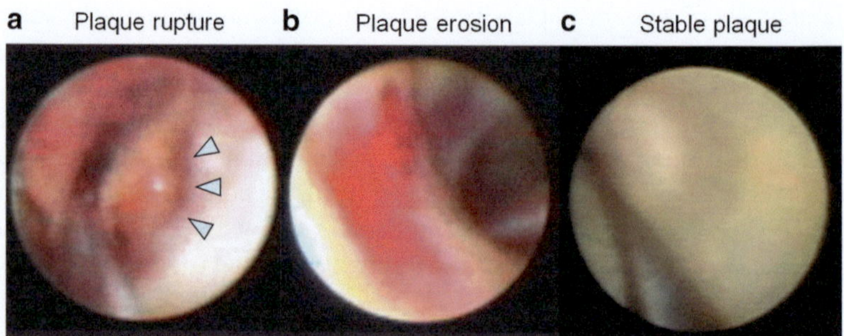

Fig. 10.1 Representative image of plaque morphology by angioscopy. (**a**) Angioscopic image showed a cleft with intensive yellow plaque and a mixed thrombus. (**b**) Angioscopic image showed erosion on a light-yellow plaque with no evidence of dissection. (**c**) Angioscopic image showed a smooth surface of light-yellow plaque without thrombus

angioscopic study reported that the number of yellow plaques in a coronary artery is an independent future risk of cardiovascular events and that patients with multiple yellow plaques per vessel have 2.2-fold higher risk of suffering ACS than patients with no or a single yellow plaque per vessel [14].

Recently, yellow plaques were further classified according to yellow color intensity: grade 0, white; grade1, light yellow; grade2, yellow; and grade3, intensive yellow (Fig. 10.2) [15]. Several studies reported that yellow color intensity was associated with plaque vulnerability. Uchida et al. reported that ACS events occurred in 3.3 % of white plaque, 7.6 % of non-glistening yellow plaque, and 68.4 % of glistening yellow plaque [16]. Ueda et al. demonstrated that yellow plaques with higher color grade have a higher incidence of thrombus on the plaque (Fig. 10.3) [15]. Furthermore, Kubo et al. revealed that there was a significant negative correlation between yellow color intensity and fibrous cap thickness evaluated by angioscopy and OCT (Fig. 10.4) [17]. Therefore, it is considered that plaque color grade assessed by angioscopy showed a good correlation with plaque stability or instability. Based on these findings, the relationship between plaque color changes and effect of statin therapy was evaluated using angioscopy. The TWINS (evaluaTion With simultaneous angIoscopy and iNtravascular ultraSound) study and TOGETHAR trial demonstrated that reduction of yellow grade detected by angioscopy occurred independently of volumetric plaque change by statin therapy [18, 19].

The major limitation of angioscopic evaluation is that color grading is often different from each observer. Therefore, in order to avoid this problem, Okada and Ishibashi, et al. have attempted a quantitative assessment color analysis using colorimetry apparatus [20, 21].

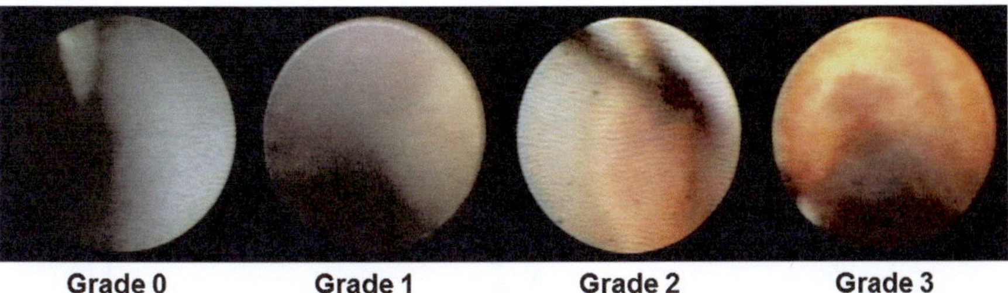

Fig. 10.2 Angioscopic color grading of plaque. Grade 0, *white*; grade 1, *light yellow*; grade 2, *yellow*; grade 3, *intensive yellow*

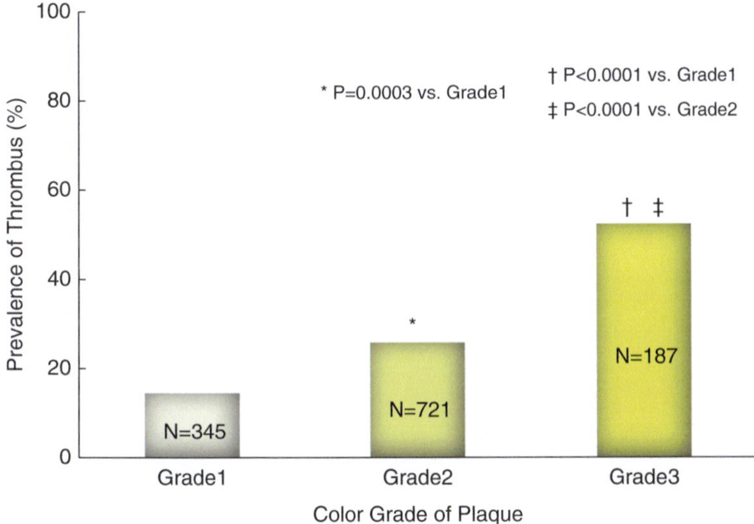

Fig. 10.3 Relation between color grade of plaque and prevalence of thrombus. *Yellow color intensity of plaque is associated with the prevalence of thrombus.* (Reproduced with permission from Ref. Ueda et al. [15])

10.3.3   Characteristics of Thrombus

Angioscopy is superior to other imaging modalities for detecting thrombus. In angioscopic image, thrombus is usually adhering to the intima or protruding into the lumen, which persists even after flushing with lactated Ringer's or dextran solution. Thrombi were further classified by color such as solid red, mixed red, and white mass, although the relationship between thrombus color and clinical outcome is uncertain [22–24]. A white thrombus was defined as a shaggy, irregular, and cotton-wool-like mass in which white area occupies more than two thirds. The majority of red thrombus was solid and globular, and red area occupies more than two thirds.

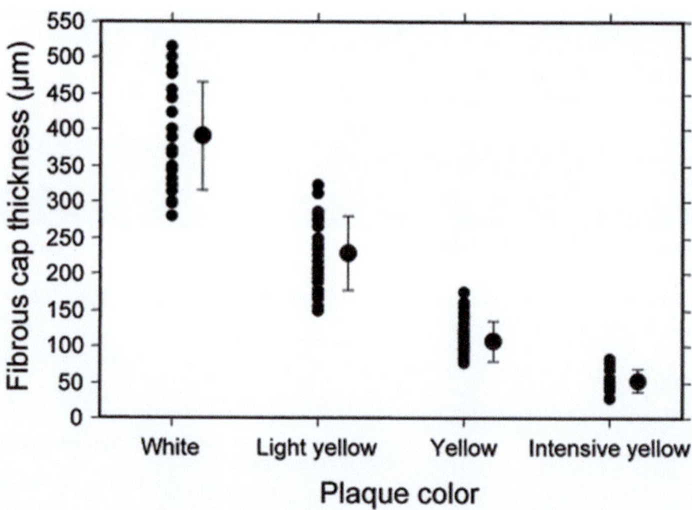

Fig. 10.4 Relation between color grade of plaque and fibrous cap thickness by optical coherence of tomography. There was a significant negative correlation between yellow color intensity and fibrous cap thickness ($P < 0.0001$). (Reproduced with permission from Ref. Kubo et al. [17])

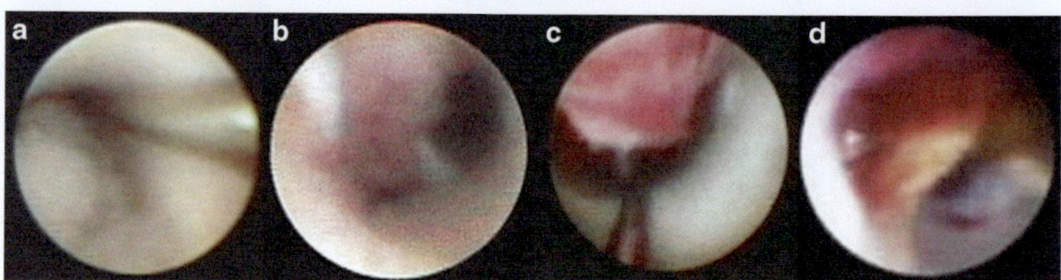

Fig. 10.5 Representative image of thrombus by angioscopy. (**a**) White thrombus, (**b**) mixed thrombus (white > red thrombus), (**c**) mixed thrombus (red > white thrombus), (**d**) red thrombus

Mixed thrombus was defined as white and red in a mosaic pattern (one third to two thirds are red) [25]. Representative images of thrombus are shown in Fig. 10.5.

A previous study reported that plaque rupture and thrombus were present in 17 % of SAP and 68 % of ACS evaluated by angioscopy, respectively [26]. However, the presence of thrombus detected by angioscopy do not necessary lead to the clinical manifestation of an ACS, although the prevalence of thrombus is higher in patients with ACS.

10.4 Summary

The prevalence of cardiovascular disease is growing rapidly, leading to an increasing incidence of ACS. Therefore, it is important to predict individuals at risk of plaque rupture and developing an ACS using novel modalities. Currently, several invasive and noninvasive modalities are under investigation. Coronary angioscopy gives us both plaque characteristics and the presence of thrombus as direct visualized information, which are helpful to assess the effect of preventive treatment and to make a treatment strategy of PCI such as distal protection. However, there are several limitations to perform coronary angioscopy such as the need for an invasive procedure, limited visual field, and induction of myocardial ischemia during the procedure.

Based on clinical findings using invasive imaging modalities such as angioscopy and IVUS, noninvasive screening tests for preventing ACS are developing including MRI detection of plaque inflammation, contrast-enhanced CT for assessment of noncalcified plaques, and positron emission tomography-CT for combined assessment of plaque burden and activity of the inflamed plaques. In the near future, further investigation will develop novel diagnostic procedure for plaque morphology both invasively and noninvasively.

References

1. Juul-Möller S, Edvardsson N, Jahnmatz B, Rosén A, Sørensen S, Omblus R. Double-blind trial of aspirin in primary prevention of myocardial infarction in patients with stable chronic angina pectoris. The Swedish Angina Pectoris Aspirin Trial (SAPAT) Group. Lancet. 1992;340:1421–5.
2. Yeghiazarians Y, Braunstein JB, Askari A, Stone PH. Unstable angina pectoris. N Engl J Med. 2000;342:101–14.
3. Fuster V, Badimon L, Badimon JJ, Chesebro JH. The pathogenesis of coronary artery disease and the acute coronary syndromes. N Engl J Med. 1992;326(242–50):310–18.
4. Hamdan A, Assali A, Fuchs S, Battler A, Kornowski R. Imaging of vulnerable coronary artery plaques. Catheter Cardiovasc Interv. 2007;70:65–74.
5. MacNeill BD, Lowe HC, Takano M, Fuster V, Jang IK. Intravascular modalities for detection of vulnerable plaque: current status. Arterioscler Thromb Vasc Biol. 2003;23:1333–42.
6. Nakamura M, Nishikawa H, Mukai S, Setsuda M, Nakajima K, Tamada H, Suzuki H, Ohnishi T, Kakuta Y, Nakano T, Yeung AC. Impact of coronary artery remodeling on clinical presentation of coronary artery disease: an intravascular ultrasound study. J Am Coll Cardiol. 2001;37:63–9.
7. Lee SY, Mintz GS, Kim SY, Hong YJ, Kim SW, Okabe T, Pichard AD, Satler LF, Kent KM, Suddath WO, Waksman R, Weissman NJ. Attenuated plaque detected by intravascular ultrasound: clinical, angiographic, and morphologic features and post-percutaneous coronary intervention complications in patients with acute coronary syndromes. JACC Cardiovasc Interv. 2009;2:65–72.
8. Jang IK, Tearney GJ, MacNeill B, Takano M, Moselewski F, Iftima N, Shishkov M, Houser S, Aretz HT, Halpern EF, Bouma BE. In vivo characterization of coronary atherosclerotic plaque by use of optical coherence tomography. Circulation. 2005;111:1551–5.

9. Falk E, Shah PK, Fuster V. Coronary plaque disruption. Circulation. 1995;92:657–71.
10. Naghavi M, Libby P, Falk E, Casscells SW, Litovsky S, Rumberger J, Badimon JJ, Stefanadis C, Moreno P, Pasterkamp G, Fayad Z, Stone PH, Waxman S, Raggi P, Madjid M, Zarrabi A, Burke A, Yuan C, Fitzgerald PJ, Siscovick DS, de Korte CL, Aikawa M, Juhani Airaksinen KE, Assmann G, Becker CR, Chesebro JH, Farb A, Galis ZS, Jackson C, Jang IK, Koenig W, Lodder RA, March K, Demirovic J, Navab M, Priori SG, Rekhter MD, Bahr R, Grundy SM, Mehran R, Colombo A, Boerwinkle E, Ballantyne C, Insull Jr W, Schwartz RS, Vogel R, Serruys PW, Hansson GK, Faxon DP, Kaul S, Drexler H, Greenland P, Muller JE, Virmani R, Ridker PM, Zipes DP, Shah PK, Willerson JT. From vulnerable plaque to vulnerable patient: a call for new definitions and risk assessment strategies: Part I. Circulation. 2003;108:1664–72.
11. Hayashi T, Kiyoshima T, Matsuura M, Ueno M, Kobayashi N, Yabushita H, Kurooka A, Taniguchi M, Miyataka M, Kimura A, Ishikawa K. Plaque erosion in the culprit lesion is prone to develop a smaller myocardial infarction size compared with plaque rupture. Am Heart J. 2005;149:284–90.
12. Takano M, Mizuno K, Okamatsu K, Yokoyama S, Ohba T, Sakai S. Mechanical and structural characteristics of vulnerable plaques: analysis by coronary angioscopy and intravascular ultrasound. J Am Coll Cardiol. 2001;38:99–104.
13. Thieme T, Wernecke KD, Meyer R, Brandenstein E, Habedank D, Hinz A, Felix SB, Baumann G, Kleber FX. Angioscopic evaluation of atherosclerotic plaques: validation by histomorphologic analysis and association with stable and unstable coronary syndromes. J Am Coll Cardiol. 1996;28:1–6.
14. Ohtani T, Ueda Y, Mizote I, Oyabu J, Okada K, Hirayama A, Kodama K. Number of yellow plaques detected in a coronary artery is associated with future risk of acute coronary syndrome: detection of vulnerable patients by angioscopy. J Am Coll Cardiol. 2006;47:2194–200.
15. Ueda Y, Ohtani T, Shimizu M, Hirayama A, Kodama K. Assessment of plaque vulnerability by angioscopic classification of plaque color. Am Heart J. 2004;148:333–5.
16. Uchida Y, Nakamura F, Tomaru T, Morita T, Oshima T, Sasaki T, Morizuki S, Hirose J. Prediction of acute coronary syndromes by percutaneous coronary angioscopy in patients with stable angina. Am Heart J. 1995;130:195–203.
17. Kubo T, Imanishi T, Takarada S, Kuroi A, Ueno S, Yamano T, Tanimoto T, Matsuo Y, Masho T, Kitabata H, Tanaka A, Nakamura N, Mizukoshi M, Tomobuchi Y, Akasaka T. Implication of plaque color classification for assessing plaque vulnerability: a coronary angioscopy and optical coherence tomography investigation. JACC Cardiovasc Interv. 2008;1:74–80.
18. Okada K, Ueda Y, Takayama T, Honye J, Komatsu S, Yamaguchi O, Li Y, Yajima J, Takazawa K, Nanto S, Saito S, Hirayama A, Kodama K. Influence of achieved low-density lipoprotein cholesterol level with atorvastatin therapy on stabilization of coronary plaques: sub-analysis of the TWINS study. Circ J. 2012;76:1197–202.
19. Kodama K, Komatsu S, Ueda Y, Takayama T, Yajima J, Nanto S, Matsuoka H, Saito S, Hirayama A. A Stabilization and regression of coronary plaques treated with pitavastatin proven by angioscopy and intravascular ultrasound–the TOGETHAR trial. Circ J. 2010;74:1922–8.
20. Okada K, Ueda Y, Oyabu J, Ogasawara N, Hirayama A, Kodama K. Plaque color analysis by the conventional yellow-color grading system and quantitative measurement using LCH color space. J Interv Cardiol. 2007;20:324–34.
21. Ishibashi F, Mizuno K, Kawamura A, Singh PP, Nesto RW, Waxman S. High yellow color intensity by angioscopy with quantitative colorimetry to identify high-risk features in culprit lesions of patients with acute coronary syndromes. Am J Cardiol. 2007;100:1207–11.
22. Mizuno K, Satomura K, Miyamoto A, Arakawa K, Shibuya T, Arai T, Kurita A, Nakamura H, Ambrose JA. Angioscopic evaluation of coronary-artery thrombi in acute coronary syndromes. N Engl J Med. 1992;326:287–91.
23. Lehmann KG, van Suylen RJ, Stibbe J, Slager CJ, Oomen JA, Maas A, di Mario C, deFeyter P, Serruys PW. Composition of human thrombus assessed by quantitative colorimetric angioscopic analysis. Circulation. 1997;96:3030–41.

24. Abela GS, Eisenberg JD, Mittleman MA, Nesto RW, Leeman D, Zarich S, Waxman S, Prieto AR, Manzo KS. Detecting and differentiating white from red coronary thrombus by angiography in angina pectoris and in acute myocardial infarction. Am J Cardiol. 1999;83:94–7.
25. Uchida Y, Uchida Y, Sakurai T, Kanai M, Shirai S, Morita T. Characterization of coronary fibrin thrombus in patients with acute coronary syndrome using dye-staining angioscopy. Arterioscler Thromb Vasc Biol. 2011;31:1452–60.
26. Hong MK, Mintz GS, Lee CW, Kim YH, Lee SW, Song JM, Han KH, Kang DH, Song JK, Kim JJ, Park SW, Park SJ. Comparison of coronary plaque rupture between stable angina and acute myocardial infarction: a three-vessel intravascular ultrasound study in 235 patients. Circulation. 2004;110:928–33.

Chapter 11
Angioscopy of Saphenous Vein Graft

Nobuyuki Komiyama

Abstract Histology of saphenous vein graft (SVG) serially changes after coronary artery bypass grafting (CABG). In the early stage (within 1 year) after CABG, fibrointimal thickening of SVG is initialized and angioscopy shows whitish and smooth surface at angiographically normal site and whitish and smooth but tapered lumen at narrowed site corresponding to fibrointimal hyperplasia. In the middle stage (1–2 years) after CABG, angioscopy still reveals whitish and smooth luminal narrowing in angiographically stenosed site, also meaning excess proliferation of fibrointima. In the late stage (several years) after CABG, angioscopy demonstrates whitish and smooth surface at angiographically normal site where diffuse, concentric, and circumferential fibrointimal proliferation is revealed in ex vivo study. However, angioscopy shows yellow atheromatous plaque with friability, ulceration, or red thrombus at angiographically narrowed site corresponding to lipid-rich or necrosed atheroma and thrombus in histology. Thus, angioscopy is useful to identify the morphologic changes of SVG at different points after CABG. Such changes of SVG can be also demonstrated by other invasive imaging modalities of intravascular ultrasound and optical coherent tomography as well as angioscopy.

Keywords Fibrointimal proliferation • Yellow plaque • Friability • Ulceration • Red thrombus

11.1   Introduction

Clinical application of angioscopy with flexible fiberoptic endoscope was begun as an adjunctive invasive imaging of peripheral arteries and veins at laser recanalization or in situ saphenous vein grafting for peripheral arterial occlusive disease [1, 2]. In a couple of decades, efficacy of angioscopy assistance in preparation of saphenous veins for in situ saphenous vein grafting had been demonstrated to improve outcome

N. Komiyama, M.D., Ph.D. (✉)
Cardiovascular Center, Matsudo City Hospital / Saitama Medical University,
4005 Kami-Hongo, Matsudo, Chiba 271-8511, Japan
e-mail: nobu.komiyama@dream.com

© Springer Japan 2015
K. Mizuno, M. Takano (eds.), *Coronary Angioscopy*,
DOI 10.1007/978-4-431-55546-9_11

in terms of graft patency [3]. Intraoperative angioscopy in coronary artery bypass grafting (CABG) was also reported to evaluate saphenous vein grafts as well as coronary arteries at almost the same time [4].

On the other hand, CABG has been one of the most important developments in the treatment of coronary artery disease and saphenous vein graft (SVG) has been the graft most commonly used especially for complete revascularization in CABG. However, SVG may become occluded or stenosed at several years after CABG and the morphologic changes in the SVG which have been delineated with in vitro techniques are likely associated with the connection of the venous conduit to the high-pressure arterial system. Recently, various techniques in percutaneous coronary intervention (PCI) for the SVG disease have been developed with interpretation of pathological changes revealed by invasive imaging modalities such as angioscopy as well as in vitro techniques in the pathology. Relation between angioscopic findings and pathohistology of SVG disease will be reviewed and the efficacy of angioscopy in the treatment of SVG disease will be discussed in this chapter.

11.2 Pathology of SVG Disease

11.2.1 The Normal Saphenous Vein

The normal histologic findings of newly harvested saphenous vein contain tunica intima, tunica media, and tunica adventitia. The intima is thin and consists of relatively acellular fibrous tissue covered by a single layer of endothelial cells separated from the media by a rudimentary internal elastic membrane. The media consists of multiple layers of smooth muscle cells separated by bundles of collagen, ground substances, and occasional short elastic fibers. Most medial smooth muscle layers have a circular orientation. The adventitia is composed of bundles of collagen with scattered fascicles of longitudinally oriented smooth muscle cells. Broad, loose bands of elastic fibers are present in abundance. Vasa vasorum are present and may extend into the outermost portion of the media [5, 6] (Fig. 11.1).

11.2.2 Early Changes in Saphenous Vein Graft

Depending upon the harvesting technique, denudation of endothelial cells is frequent in freshly harvested veins before their insertion. The endothelium often appears disrupted and the intimal surface is usually covered, partially or completely, by fibrin. Endothelial injury exposes the thrombogenic subendothelium and media to circulating blood. Platelets become activated at the site of injury and play a central role in the initiation and progression of mural platelet thrombosis. Also, platelet activation leads to release enough platelet-derived growth factors to stimulate the

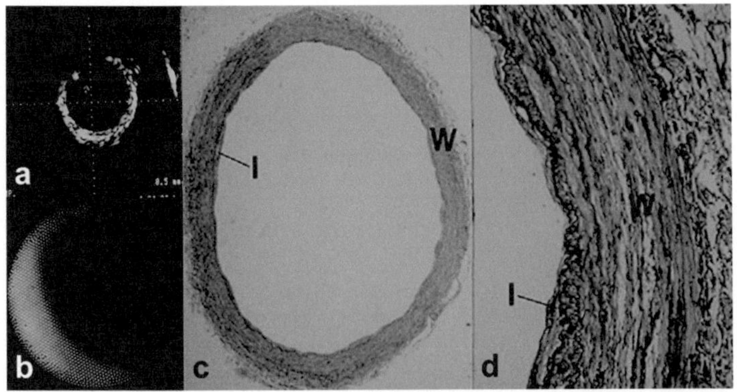

Fig. 11.1 Intravascular images (**a, b**) and histologic sections (**c, d**) of a newly harvested saphenous vein in ex vivo study [5]. Intravascular ultrasound (**a**) shows single-layered appearance. Angioscopy (**b**) shows whitish and smooth surface. Corresponding histologic sections (**c, d**) demonstrate thin intima (*I*) and vessel wall (*W*) mainly consisting of smooth muscle cells and collagen fibers (elastic van Gieson stain)

slow and gradual process of primary intimal smooth muscle cell proliferation and secondary smooth muscle cell proliferation, the cell migrated from the media to the intima [7, 8]

Minimal medial edema and disruption of adventitia occur just after harvesting SVG. Mural edema becomes more pronounced, some medial smooth muscle cells become necrotic, and inflammatory infiltrates are present in the next 2 weeks. The smooth muscle fibers of the media gradually diminish in number and are replaced, in part or in whole, by fibrous tissue.

Fibrous tissue also increases in the adventitia, and its elastic fibers become severely disrupted or disappear completely. Organizing fibrin on the external surface of the SVG probably contributes to the adventitial fibrosis. Thus, the SVG becomes a fibrous-tissue conduit [6].

11.2.3 Late Changes in Saphenous Vein Graft

The principal changes of SVG body at more than 2 years after CABG are concentric circumferential *fibrointimal proliferation* and fibrotic-atrophied medial layer at angiographically normal sites (Fig. 11.2) [5].

Further, atherosclerotic changes can be seen in SVG bodies with irregular luminal border, luminal narrowing, or occlusion in angiography. *Lipid* is present as intracellular lipid (foam cells, i.e., lipid-laden macrophages) located near the luminal surfaces of the intimal fibrous tissue, which does not narrow the lumen appreciably, and extracellular lipid deposits located deeper in the plaque, separated from the lumen by a layer of fibrous tissue, which significantly contribute to luminal narrowing. *Hemorrhage into plaque* is found into the lipid portion only and luminal

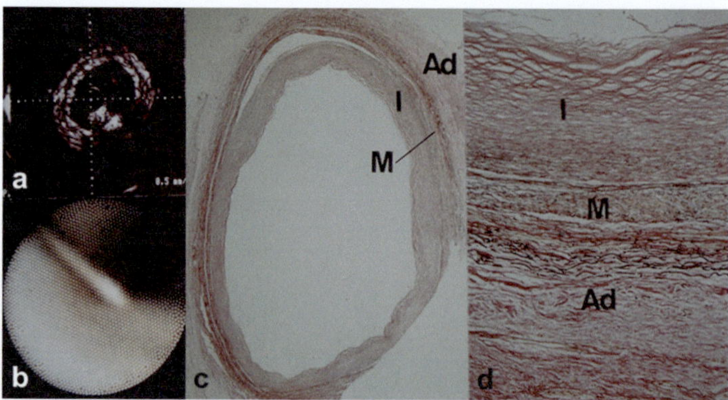

Fig. 11.2 Intravascular images (**a, b**) and histologic sections (**c, d**) of the late stage saphenous vein graft in ex vivo study [5]. Intravascular ultrasound (**a**) shows triple-layered appearance. Angioscopy (**b**) shows whitish and smooth surface. Corresponding histologic sections (**c, d**) demonstrate concentric circumferential fibrointimal proliferation (*I*), fibrotic-atrophied media (*M*), and adventitia (*Ad*) (elastic van Gieson stain)

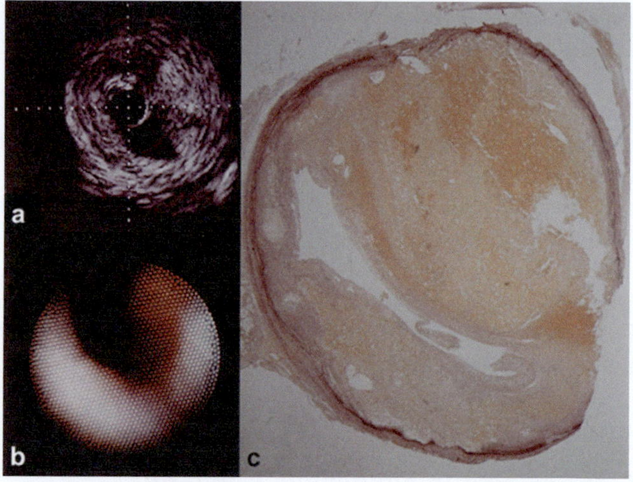

Fig. 11.3 Intravascular images (**a, b**) and histologic sections (**c**) of the late stage saphenous vein graft in ex vivo study. Intravascular ultrasound (**a**) shows eccentric plaque. Angioscopy (**b**) shows localized yellow plaque. Corresponding histologic section (**c**) demonstrates large atheromatous plaque (elastic van Gieson stain)

narrowing is more common in SVGs with plaque hemorrhage than in those without. *Luminal thrombus* is sometimes present and small *calcium deposit* can be seen but it is not so often [6] (Fig. 11.3).

11.3 Angioscopic Findings of Saphenous Vein Graft

11.3.1 Early Stage

Angioscopy demonstrates whitish and smooth surface of lumen in a newly harvested SVG without fibrointimal proliferation (Fig. 11.1) and angiographically normal SVG within 1 year after CABG (Fig. 11.4). SVG has sometimes discrete or diffuse narrowing even in the early stage after CABG, where angioscopy shows whitish and smooth luminal narrowing indicating excessive fibrointimal proliferation in the SVG (Fig. 11.5) [5].

11.3.2 Middle Stage

Angioscopy also reveals whitish and smooth surface of the lumen in angiographically normal SVG at 1–2 years after CABG and whitish and smooth tapered lumen at stenosis of the SVG, where histology of tissue resected by directional coronary atherectomy demonstrates fibrointimal proliferation containing elastic fibers (Fig. 11.6) [5].

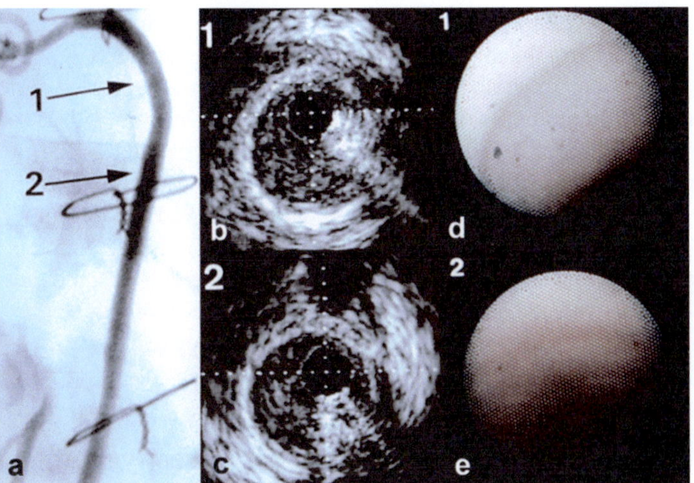

Fig. 11.4 An angiogram (**a**) and intravascular images (**b**–**e**) of the early stage saphenous vein graft [5]. Intravascular ultrasound (**b**, **c**) shows single-layered appearance at the sites in the angiogram (*1*, *2*). Angioscopy (**d**, **e**) shows whitish and smooth wall

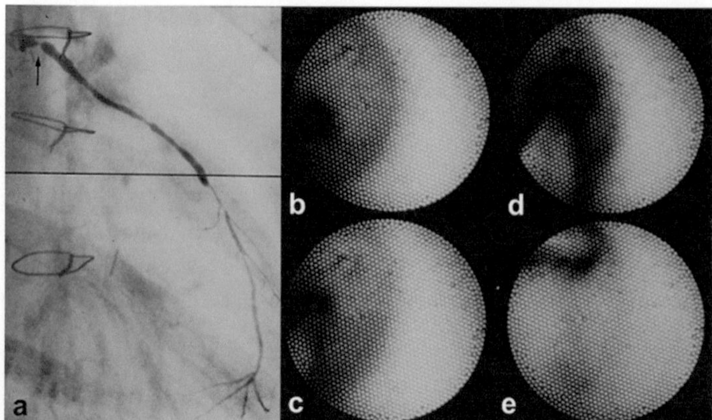

Fig. 11.5 An angiogram (**a**) and angioscopic images (**b–e**) of narrowed saphenous vein graft at the early stage. An angiogram shows stenosis (*arrow*) at proximal portion of the SVG. Angioscopy (**b–e**) demonstrates whitish and smooth luminal narrowing at the same site

11.3.3 Late Stage

Angioscopy shows whitish and smooth luminal surface in angiographically normal SVG even at several years after CABG, where diffuse and circumferential intimal proliferation is revealed by ex vivo evaluation of the histology (Figs. 11.2 and 11.7) [5]. In angiographically irregular or narrowed sites in the SVGs, angioscopy reveals yellow atheromatous plaques with smooth surface or sometimes friable appearance corresponding to lipid-rich atheroma with necrosed tissue shown by histology (Figs. 11.2, 11.8 and 11.9) [5]. Friability is defined as the presence of fragmented and loosely adherent plaque lining the vessel wall corresponding to mass of foam cells or lipid debris with very thin or partially lacked fibrous cap (Figs. 11.10 and 11.11) [9]. This is a specific finding in the vein graft disease which is absent in the culprit lesion of native coronary artery in patients with unstable angina [10]. Also, ulceration with or without red thrombus and white thrombus or mass of fibrin floating in blood-flushing fluid can be seen by angioscopy (Fig. 11.12).

11.4 Comparison of the Findings in Angioscopy with Other Invasive Imaging Modalities

11.4.1 Intravascular Ultrasound

Intravascular ultrasound (IVUS) is a catheter-based, real-time imaging technology with high-frequency ultrasound (20–45 MHz) and the maximal spatial resolution of around 100 μm. It can provide us with morphological information in the vessel wall as well as the luminal surface using both qualitative and quantitative manners.

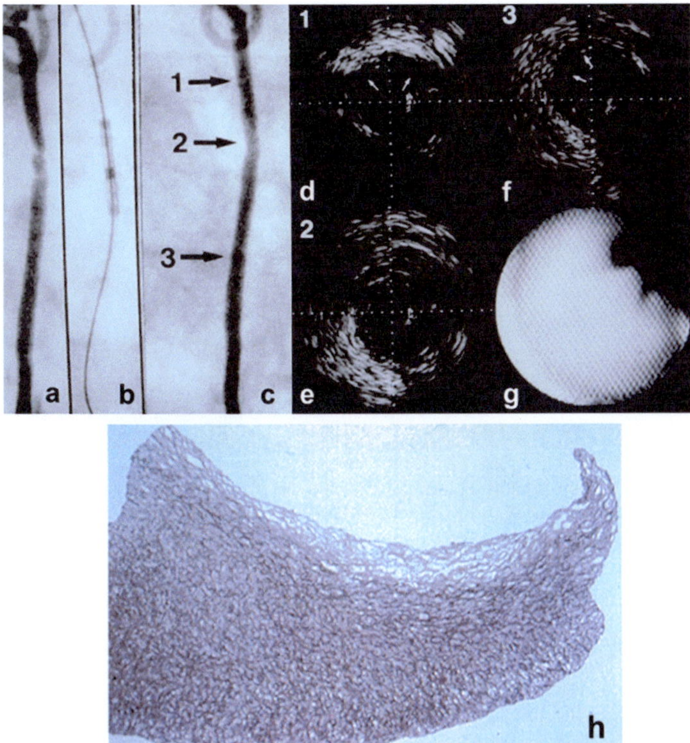

Fig. 11.6 An angiogram (**a–c**), intravascular images (**d–g**) and corresponding histologic section (**h**) resected by directional coronary atherectomy in the middle-stage saphenous vein graft [5]. An angiogram (**a**) shows a discrete stenotic lesion (*thick arrow*). Angioscopy (**g**) shows whitish luminal narrowing. Intravascular ultrasound reveals triple-layered appearance (**d, f**) (*small arrows*) at site *1, 2* and residual plaque (**e**) with homogeneous dense echo at site *2* after directional coronary atherectomy (**b, c**). Histology of resected specimen (**h**) demonstrates thickened intima with elastic fibers (elastic van Gieson stain)

In a newly harvested SVG or an angiographically normal SVG at the early stage after CABG, IVUS demonstrates an echogenic and single-layered vessel wall (Figs. 11.1 and 11.4). In a SVG at the middle stage after CABG, IVUS sometimes shows triple-layered appearance at the site without narrowing where single-layered appearance is demonstrated more often, and it reveals a thick internal layer with a homogeneous and relatively dense echo pattern at stenosed site corresponding to fibrointimal proliferation (Fig. 11.6). In an angiographically normal SVG at the late stage after CABG, IVUS shows the triple-layered appearance without a plaque structure which consists of inner and outer echogenic layers and a medial echolucent layer, mimicking the IVUS images of native coronary arteries with normal or mildly thickened intima (Fig. 11.7). In comparison with histology in ex vivo study, the triple-layered appearance in the IVUS image of SVG at the late stage should be derived from diffuse and circumferential fibrointimal proliferation (Fig. 11.2). At

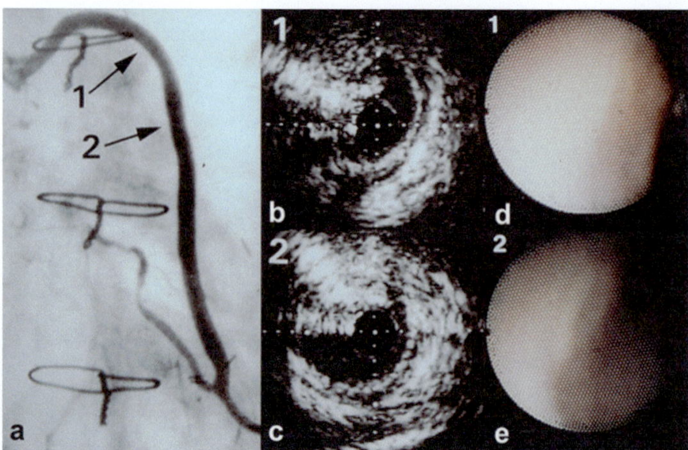

Fig. 11.7 An angiogram (**a**) and intravascular images (**b–e**) of the late stage saphenous vein graft [5]. Intravascular ultrasound (**b, c**) shows triple-layered appearance at the sites in the angiogram (*1, 2*). Angioscopy (**d, e**) shows whitish and smooth surface structure

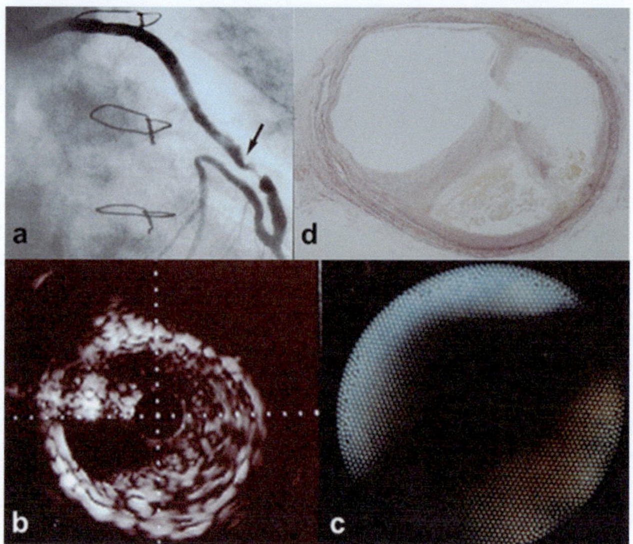

Fig. 11.8 An angiogram (**a**), intravascular images (**b, c**) and corresponding histologic section (**d**) of the late stage saphenous vein graft in ex vivo study [5]. At a site (*arrow*) of eccentric stenosis on angiogram (**a**), intravascular ultrasound reveals eccentric plaque with heterogeneous echo pattern (**b**) and angioscopy demonstrates yellowish atheromatous plaque (**c**). Histology (**d**) shows lipid-rich eccentric atheroma with necrosed tissue (elastic van Gieson stain)

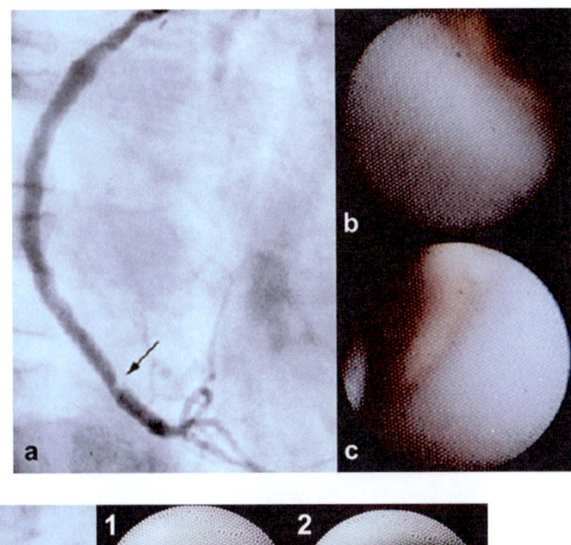

Fig. 11.9 An angiogram (**a**) and angioscopic images (**b**, **c**) of the late stage saphenous vein graft. At a site (*arrow*) of mild stenosis on angiogram (**a**), angioscopy shows yellow atheromatous plaques (**b**, **c**)

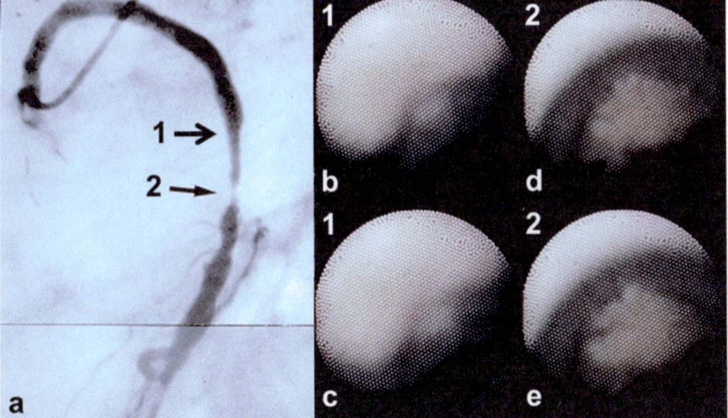

Fig. 11.10 An angiogram (**a**) and angioscopic images (**b–e**) of the late stage saphenous vein graft [5]. At sites of broad-based stenosis on angiogram (**a**), angioscopy demonstrates relatively whitish smooth plaque at site *1* (**b**, **c**) and yellowish atheromatous plaque with friable surface at site *2* (**d**, **e**)

angiographically irregular or narrowed sites in the SVG of the late stage, IVUS reveals eccentric plaques with heterogeneous and relatively echolucent and without the triple-layered appearance, corresponding to eccentric lipid-rich atheroma with necrosed tissue in an ex vivo histologic study (Fig. 11.8) [5].

11.4.2 Optical Coherent Tomography

Optical coherent tomography (OCT) is also a catheter-based, real-time imaging technology with broadband infrared light and the maximal spatial resolution is approximate 10 μm. OCT can provide us with more accurate morphologic

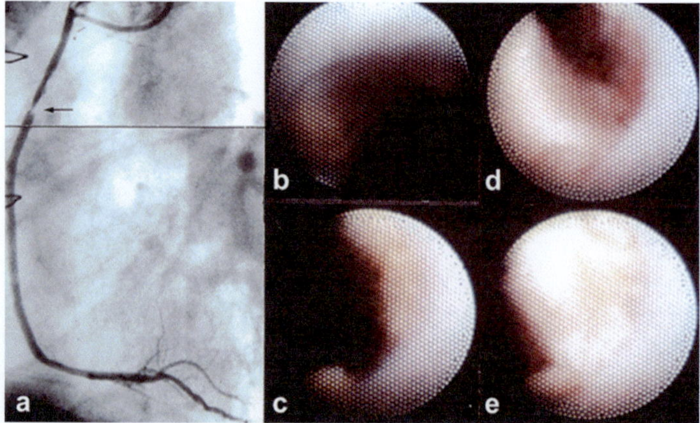

Fig. 11.11 An angiogram (**a**) and angioscopic images (**b–e**) of the late stage saphenous vein graft. At a site (*arrow*) of eccentric discrete stenosis on angiogram (**a**), angioscopy shows yellow atheromatous plaques with friable surface (**b–e**)

Fig. 11.12 An angiogram (**a**) and angioscopic images (**b, c**) of the late stage saphenous vein graft [5]. At a site (*arrow head*) of ulcer-like lesion on angiogram (**a**), angioscopy (**b, c**) reveals ulceration with red thrombus

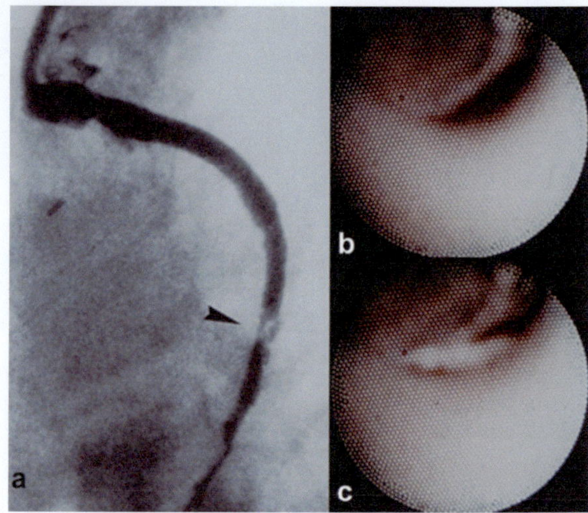

information about vessel surface and wall structures than IVUS, but its penetration depth in radial direction is quite less than IVUS.

OCT demonstrates thin-cap fibroatheroma, ulceration or rupture of intima, red or white thrombus, friable plaque (loose fibroatheromatous debris), calcium deposit, and neovascularization (small cavity in the plaque) at the culprit site of late-stage SVG in patients with acute coronary syndrome [11].

Comparison of image findings of SVG among various imaging modalities are shown in Table 11.1.

Table 11.1 Comparison of findings in SVG among invasive imaging modalities and histology

Stage after CABG	Angiography	Angioscopy	Intravascular ultrasound	Optical coherent tomography	Histology
Early (<1 year)	Normal	Whitish	Single-layer appearance		Initial intimal thickening
	Diffuse narrowing	Whitish	Intimal thickening (homogeneous dense echo)		Excess fibrointimal thickening
	Discrete stenosis (anastomosed site)	Sometimes, red thrombus	Thrombus		Thrombus at anastomosed site
Middle (1–2, 3 years)	Normal	Whitish	Sometimes, triple-layer		Homogeneous intimal thickening
	Diffuse narrowing	Whitish, smooth surface, tapered lumen	Intimal thickening (homogeneous dense echo)		Excess fibrointimal thickening
	Discrete stenosis				
Late (several years)	Normal	Whitish	Triple-layer	Fibrous	Excess and homogeneous fibrointimal thickening
				Fatty	
				TCFA	
				Thrombus	
	Irregular	Yellow plaque	Plaque (heterogeneous loose echo)	Plaque rupture	Atheroma (lipid-rich, necrosed)
				Friability	
				Calcification	Ulcer formation
				Neovascularization	Thrombus
	Narrowing, eccentric or ulcer-like	Yellow plaque, friability, ulceration, red or white thrombus	Plaque (heterogeneous loose echo, eccentric), calcification, thrombus, impaired vessel remodeling	(At culprit lesion of ACS)	Excess fibrosis in adventitia

Abbreviation: *SVG* saphenous vein graft, *CABG* coronary artery bypass grafting, *ACS* acute coronary syndrome, *TCFA* thin-cap fibroatheroma

11.5 Clinical Impact of Angioscopy for Percutaneous SVG Intervention

Percutaneous coronary intervention (PCI) is one of effective therapeutic strategies for vein graft disease although PCI for chronic SVG occlusion is not recommended because of low success rates, high complication rates and poor long-term patency rates according to the guidelines [12]. PCI can be performed to discrete or not so diffuse narrowings in SVG at both early and late stages after CABG. In addition, the guidelines recommend using embolic protection device (EPD) during PCI procedure for the lesions in the late stage SVG where angioscopy often demonstrates friable atheromatous plaque or thrombus, which should be causes of distal embolization. On the other hand, EPD should not be necessary during PCI for the lesions in the early stage SVG where angioscopy reveals white and smooth tapered lumen indicating the stenosis caused by fibrointimal proliferation. Thus, angioscopy can be used to evaluate the target lesion characteristics and it should become an effective guide to decide whether additional devices should be used to prevent complications in PCI for vein graft disease.

References

1. Litvack F, Grundfest WS, Lee ME, Carroll RM, Foran R, Chaux A, Berci G, Rose HB, Matloff JM, Forrester JS. Angioscopic visualization of blood vessel interior in animals and humans. Clin Cardiol. 1985;8:65–70.
2. Seegar JM, Abela GS. Angioscopy as an adjunct to arterial reconstructive surgery: a preliminary report. J Vasc Surg. 1986;4:315–20.
3. Thorne J, Danielsson G, Danielsson P, Jonung T, Norgren L, Ribbe E, Zdanowski Z. Intraoperative angioscopy may improve the outcome of in situ saphenous vein bypass grafting: a prospective study. J Vasc Surg. 2002;35:759–65.
4. Sanborn TA, Rygaard JA, Westbrook BM, Lazar HL, McCormick JR, Roberts AJ. Intraoperative angioscopy of saphenous vein and coronary arteries. J Thorac Cardiovasc Surg. 1986;91:339–43.
5. Komiyama N, Nakanishi S, Nishiyama S, Seki A. Intravascular imaging of serial changes of disease in saphenous vein grafts after coronary artery bypass grafting. Am Heart J. 1996;132:30–40.
6. Roberts WC. Changes in venous autografts used as aortocoronary conduits. In: Bates ER, Holmes DR, editors. Saphenous vein bypass graft disease. New York: Marcel Dekker; 1998. p. 77–89.
7. Solymoss BC, Leung TK, Pelletier LC, Campeau L. Pathologic changes in coronary artery saphenous vein grafts and related etiologic factors. In: Water DD, Bourassa MG, editors. Care of the patient with previous coronary bypass surgery. Philadelphia: F. A. Davis Company; 1991. p. 45–65.
8. Lam JYT, Solymoss BC, Campeuu L. Platelets and thrombosis in vein graft occlusion: role and prevention. In: Water DD, Bourassa MG, editors. Care of the patient with previous coronary bypass surgery. Philadelphia: F. A. Davis Company; 1991. p. 67–81.
9. White CJ, Ramee SR, Collins TJ, Mesa J, Jain A. Percutaneous angioscopy of saphenous vein coronary bypass grafts. J Am Coll Cardiol. 1993;21:1181–5.

10. Silva JA, White CJ, Collins TJ, Ramee SR. Morphologic comparison of atherosclerotic lesions in native coronary arteries and saphenous vein grafts with intracoronary angioscopy in patients with unstable angina. Am Heart J. 1998;136:156–63.
11. Davlouros P, Damelou A, Kalantalis V, Xanthopoulou I, Mavronasiou E, Tsigkas G, Hahalis G, Alexopoulos D. Evaluation of culprit saphenous vein graft lesions with optical coherence tomography in patients with acute coronary syndromes. J Am Coll Cardiol Intv. 2011;4:683–93.
12. Levine GN, Bates ER, Blankenship JC. 2011 ACCF/AHA/SCAI guideline for percutaneous coronary intervention. J Am Coll Cardiol. 2011;58:e44–e122.

Chapter 12
Other Vessels

Takanobu Tomaru, Kazuhiro Shimizu, Takeshi Sakurai, Kei-ichi Tokuhiro, Fumitaka Nakamura, Toshihiro Morita, and Yasumi Uchida

Abstract Angioscopy system for the visualization of peripheral artery disease (PAD), veins, and/or pulmonary arteries has been developed, using a special balloon guiding catheter that provides direct color images of thrombus. Our previous studies demonstrated that this is very useful for accurate diagnosis and treatment in patients with venous thromboembolism. Since angioscopy is the most accurate imaging modality for the evaluation of inner surface or internal surface of plaque in patients with PAD, this has been shown to be useful for improving diagnosis and treatment of PAD.

Keywords Pulmonary embolism • Deep venous thrombosis • Peripheral artery disease

12.1   Introduction

Visualization of the internal surface of vessels using fiber-optic angioscopy started in the mid-1980s [1, 2]. Using a fiber-optic angioscope, thrombus and the pathomorphology of vessel walls could be clearly evaluated, and angioscopy was shown

T. Tomaru, M.D., Ph.D. (✉) • K. Shimizu, M.D. • T. Sakurai, M.D.
Cardiovascular Center, Toho University Medical Center Sakura Hospital, Shimoshizu 564-1, Sakura, Chiba 285-8741, Japan
e-mail: tomaru-t@sakura.med.toho-u.ac.jp

K.-i. Tokuhiro, M.D.
Cardiovascular Surgery, Misato Memorial Hospital, Misato, Japan

F. Nakamura, M.D.
The Third Department of Internal Medicine, Teikyo University Chiba Medical Center, Anesaki 3426-3, Ichihara, Chiba 299-0111, Japan

T. Morita, M.D.
Cardiology, Tokyo University Medical School, Tokyo, Japan

Y. Uchida, M.D.
Public Trust Cardiovascular Fund, Shiba 3-33-1, Minato-Ku, Tokyo 105-8574, Japan

© Springer Japan 2015

131

K. Mizuno, M. Takano (eds.), *Coronary Angioscopy*,
DOI 10.1007/978-4-431-55546-9_12

to be more sensitive for the detection of thrombus than angiography [3, 4]. In this chapter, we describe the application of angioscopy to veins and peripheral arteries.

12.2 Veins and Pulmonary Arteries

The major diseases of the peripheral venous system are varicose veins caused by valve insufficiency with or without thrombosis, thrombophlebitis, and cancer. Another important venous disease is thrombosis, which may cause pulmonary emboli [5].

For the diagnosis of deep venous thrombosis (DVT), various medical techniques have been used. At first, the patient can be suspected on the basis of symptoms and physical examination. Venous ultrasonography is then used for direct imaging of thrombus, compression, and loss of flow by Doppler color imaging. Contrast-enhanced computed tomography (CT) scanning or magnetic resonance (MR) venography is used for imaging thrombus. Venography or laboratory tests, including the D-dimer test, are also important. However, these methods cannot provide accurate imaging of thrombus. Small-size or fragile thrombi cannot be detected.

On the other hand, angioscopy can provide direct color imaging of thrombus. Angioscopy system for the visualization of veins and/or pulmonary arteries has been developed using a special balloon guiding catheter [6, 7]. Using such a guiding catheter, angioscopy was safely performed for the visualization of venous thrombus. Furthermore, angioscopy was also performed for the evaluation of pulmonary thrombus.

Intravascular imaging methods such as angioscopy and intravascular ultrasound (IVUS) have been used for the evaluation of venous diseases, and the usefulness of angioscopy has been reported [8]. Fifty-three patients (50 patients with chronic venous insufficiency and 3 patients with deep vein thrombosis) were diagnosed and visualized using angioscopy (Olympus OES) and IVUS. Only 21 valves (24 %) were visualized by IVUS among the 88 valves observed at angioscopy. Thus, the intravascular imaging method of angioscopy has been shown to be more suitable for observing valves and obtaining intraluminal views compared with IVUS, whereas IVUS is more suitable for observing the cross-sectional venous walls.

Angioscopy has also been used for the visualization of thrombus in patients with chronic pulmonary embolic obstruction of the pulmonary arteries [7, 9].

Angioscopy preceded by ventilation/perfusion lung scans, right heart catheterization, and pulmonary angiography resulted in diagnostic changes in 4 of 8 patients: from pulmonary artery agenesis to chronic emboli, from chronic emboli to normal pulmonary arterial intima (primary pulmonary hypertension), from chronic pulmonary emboli to extrinsic compression of a major pulmonary artery (fibrosing mediastinitis), and from suspected agenesis or chronic emboli to a tumor (fibrosarcoma) of the pulmonary artery. Angioscopy also provided the accurate extent and surgical accessibility of chronic embolic obstruction in 5 patients. Thus, the direct visualization capability of angioscopy has been shown to contribute significantly to the diagnostic evaluation of chronic pulmonary arterial obstruction.

Chronic thromboembolic pulmonary hypertension (CTEPH) is a debilitating disease caused by chronic obstruction of pulmonary artery branches following pulmonary embolism [10]. Chest radiography and echocardiography have been used for diagnosis, but their diagnostic accuracy is limited. CTEPH may be diagnosed by the presence of a mismatched wedge-shaped perfusion deficit during ventilation/perfusion scintigraphy or characteristic findings during computed tomography (CT) angiography, including a mosaic perfusion pattern, dilated pulmonary arteries and right heart, and vascular obstruction.

Pulmonary angiography and right heart catheterization can be a definitive diagnostic technique to indicate the site and accessibility of the obstruction. Pulmonary angioscopy is not routinely used in the diagnosis of CTEPH, but can help to resolve the differential diagnosis between primary PH and distal/small-vessel pulmonary thromboembolic disease [11].

As previous studies have shown, venous thrombi are classified as mural, often overlooked by phlebography, and globular. Further, they are classified as fresh or organized. When examined using angioscopy, superficial various veins often contain fresh or organized thrombi [9].

Our angioscopy system comprises a light source, 1.7–4.5 F fiberscope, 6–9 F guiding balloon catheter, intensified chilled coupled device (ICCD) camera, camera controller, image divider, DVD recorder, and television monitor [12]. Usually, a 4.5 F fiberscope and 9 F balloon guide catheter are used for the observation of large-diameter vessels. Figure 12.1 shows the whole angioscopy system. The 4.5 F fiberscope (AF 14, Olympus Corporation, Tokyo) contains 3,000 glass fibers for image guidance and 300 glass fibers for light guidance. The fiberscope is passed through a 9 F balloon guide catheter (Clinical Supply Company, Gifu, Japan) (Fig. 12.2). The balloon is inflated with CO_2. The catheter has a Y-connector at the proximal end: one channel for fiberscope insertion and another for saline flushing. The white balance of the AS is adjusted using white gauze immersed in saline solution.

We evaluated the usefulness of angioscopy for the diagnosis of deep venous thrombosis (DVT) in the selected patients. Seven patients (age 37–76 years old, mean 62.1 years, 2 males, 5 females) were studied. Lesions: I.V.C. [2] Rt.C.I.V. [1] Lt.C.I.V. [4] Thrombus: acute [3] acute on chronic [1], chronic [3]. Compressibility was evaluated by B-mode ultrasonography. Color Doppler flow image is obtained by milking of the leg. Table 12.1 shows the profile of all 7 patients. Angioscopy was performed at 1 week to 2 years after the onset of DVT. In 3 patients who underwent angioscopy at 1 or 2 weeks after the onset, angioscopy demonstrated red thrombus in two of them (Fig. 12.3) and white one in 1 (Fig. 12.4). In these patients, thrombolysis therapy using urokinase was performed, and thrombus disappeared in the patients with red thrombus.

Diagnosis of acute pulmonary embolism (PE) is commonly done by contrast CT, angiography, or MRI, but these methods can only provide indirect imaging

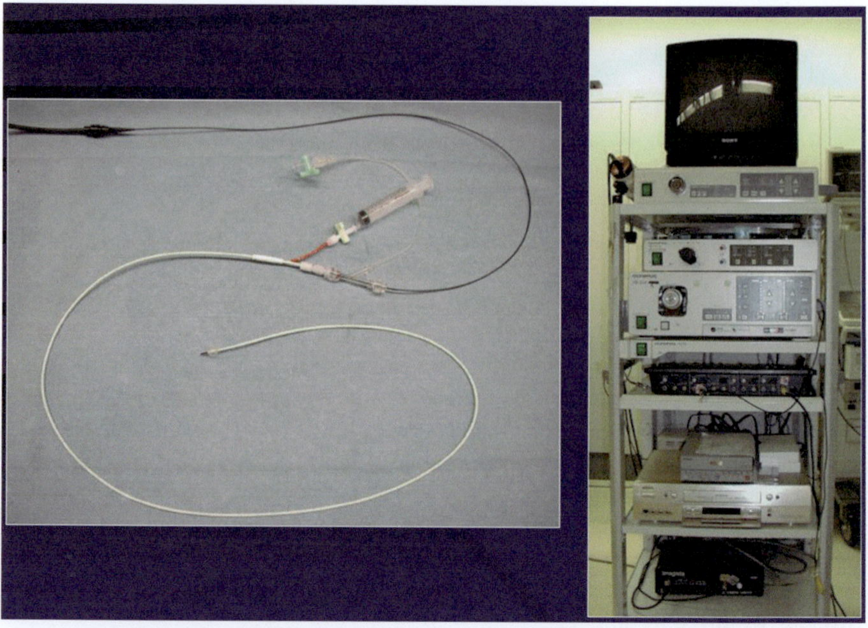

Fig. 12.1 Photo of whole angioscopy system

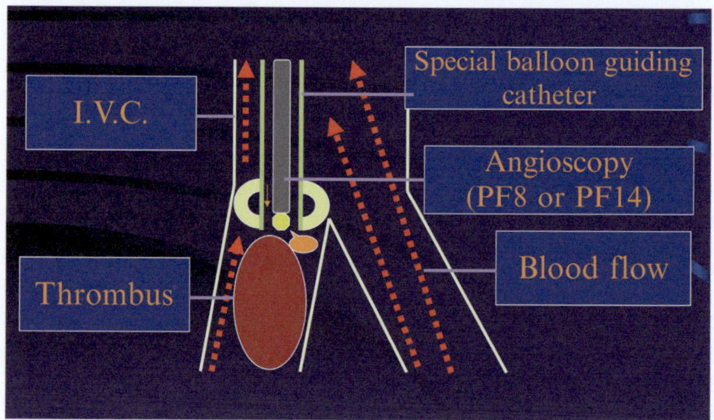

Fig. 12.2 Visualization of deep venous thrombus by using angioscope. A guiding balloon catheter is inserted through brachial or cervical vein, and heparinized saline was infused to replace blood for angioscopic visualization of thrombus

of thrombus. On the other hand, angioscopy can provide direct visualization of pulmonary thrombus. We performed angioscopy in 32 patients [13]. There were 6 patients of less than 1 week after onset, 7 of 1–4 weeks, 8 of 1–3 months, 6 of more than 3 months, and 4 with recurrent PTE. A 1.4 mm angioscope with 9 F guiding

Table 12.1 Follow-up of patients with DVT

Case	Angioscopy	Region	Color	D-dimer	TAT	Urokinase	Follow-up
66 F	1 W	Rt.CIV	Red	19	9.3	○	No thromb
58 M	2 W	IVC	Red	16.6	11.3	○	No thromb
73 F	1 W	Lt.CIV	White	21.6	9.0	○	No change
61 F	3 W	Lt.CIV	White	6.8	5.5	×	Size down
74 F	2Y	Lt.CIV	White	0.5	0.6	×	Size down
37 M	2 M	IVC	White	1.4	1.6	×	No change
66 F	6 M	Lt.CIV	Red	0.5	3.6	○	Size down

D-dimer (μg/ml), *TAT* thrombin antithrombin complex (ng/ml)

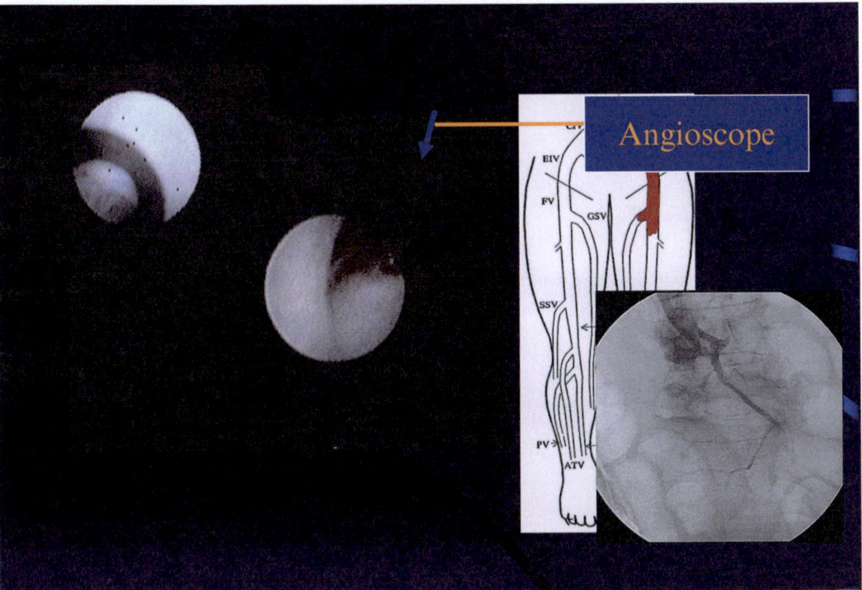

Fig. 12.3 Angioscopic image of red thrombus. Pathohistology shows red cell-rich fresh thrombus

catheter was used. In the patients within 1week from onset, there were 1 patient with red thrombus and 3 with white thrombus. In those from 1 week to 1 month after onset, there were 1 red and 2 white. In those of more than 1 month after onset, all patients had yellow or red yellow thrombus. Angiography could diagnose pulmonary thromboembolism in 11 of 16 patients with globular thrombus and 1 of 5 with mural thrombus. In a few cases, we performed thrombolysis with urokinase (Fig. 12.5). Therefore, mural small thrombus visualized by angioscopy cannot be detected by angiography. Angioscopy may provide a final diagnosis of PE in patients suspected for PE.

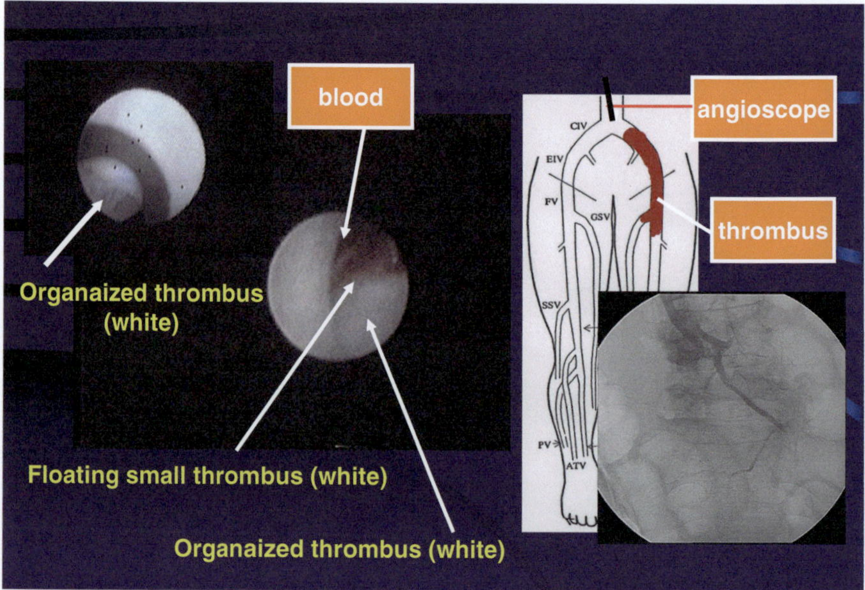

Fig. 12.4 Angioscopic image of white thrombus

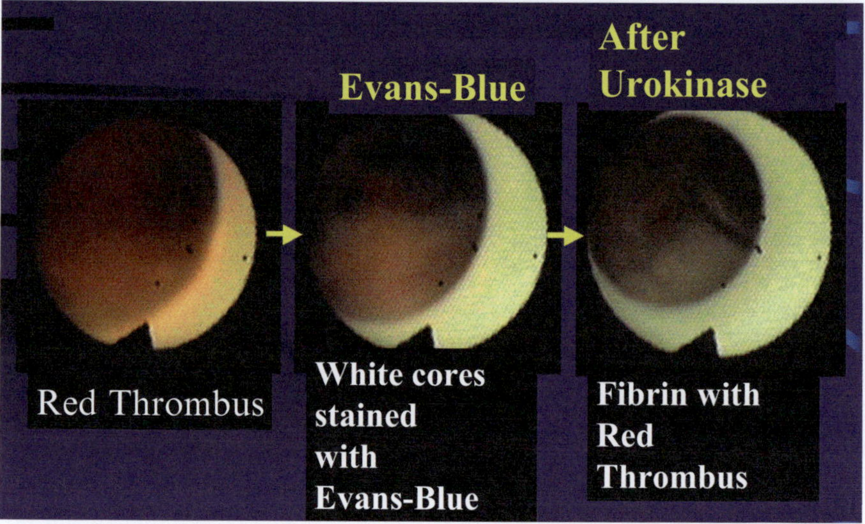

Fig. 12.5 Pulmonary angioscopic observation of thrombolysis. Infusion of urokinase could result in thrombolysis of fresh red pulmonary thrombus. Evans blue-stained fibrin nets

12.3 Peripheral Artery Disease

Peripheral artery disease (PAD) is a disease with obstruction of the blood supply to the lower or upper extremities and is caused not only by arteriosclerosis but also has other etiologies, including chronic inflammation [14, 15]. It is commonly caused by atherosclerosis and may also result from vasculitis, thromboembolism, fibromuscular dysplasia, or entrapment. In general practice, PAD is usually underdiagnosed due to the difficulty of diagnosing it.

The simplest test for the diagnosis of PAD is a segmental pressure measurement; however, an ankle-brachial pressure index (ABI) is considered to be more accurate and useful. A Doppler ultrasound probe is placed over the dorsalis pedis and posterior tibial arteries to measure ankle blood pressure. Brachial artery systolic pressure can be measured in a routine manner. The normal ABI should be 1.0 or greater. An ABI of less than 0.9 is considered abnormal. However, this method cannot be reliably applied to calcified vessels.

Duplex ultrasonography (DUS) enables a direct noninvasive assessment of the anatomic characteristics of peripheral arteries and the functional significance of arterial stenoses. Color-assisted duplex ultrasound imaging is a useful method of localizing peripheral arteries. DUS imaging has approximately 80–98 % sensitivity and 89–99 % specificity for the identification of significant stenosis [16, 17]. Angiography has been used for the diagnosis of peripheral artery diseases, and this is a golden standard for the evaluation of arterial stenosis. However, computed tomography angiography (CTA) is now used as the new alternative imaging modality and is considered to be as reliable as angiography. CTA is also a useful follow-up modality after percutaneous transluminal angioplasty (PTA).

Compared with angiography, angioscopy is superior for the evaluation of internal surfaces of peripheral arteries [18]. Angioscopy revealed that the luminal surface of a non-stenotic peripheral artery by angiography is smooth and milky white or light yellow in color due to fat. According to surface morphology of angioscopy, atherosclerotic plaques in diseased vessels are classified into regular (non-ruptured) and complex (ruptured) and according to color into white and yellow, as for coronary plaques. Spiral folds in luminal surface are often observed in apparently normal arteries on angiography [19].

Thrombus is observed in 20–40 % of cases in the superficial femoral or iliac arterial plaque. Thrombus appeared to be thin at the narrowed outlet of the residual lumen or minuscule and globular at the stenotic inlet. These thrombi cannot be detected by using angiography.

In patients with peripheral artery disease, percutaneous transluminal angioplasty (PTA) has been performed for the treatment of occluded arteries. However, the restenosis rate was very high in the patients with calcified complex lesions. To minimize restenosis, laser angioplasty was applied, but its preventive effect has been limited [20, 21]. Recently, stenting has been used for the prevention of restenosis. The enhanced flexibility and superior fracture resistance of the latest stent generation could enable the endovascular treatment of more difficult and

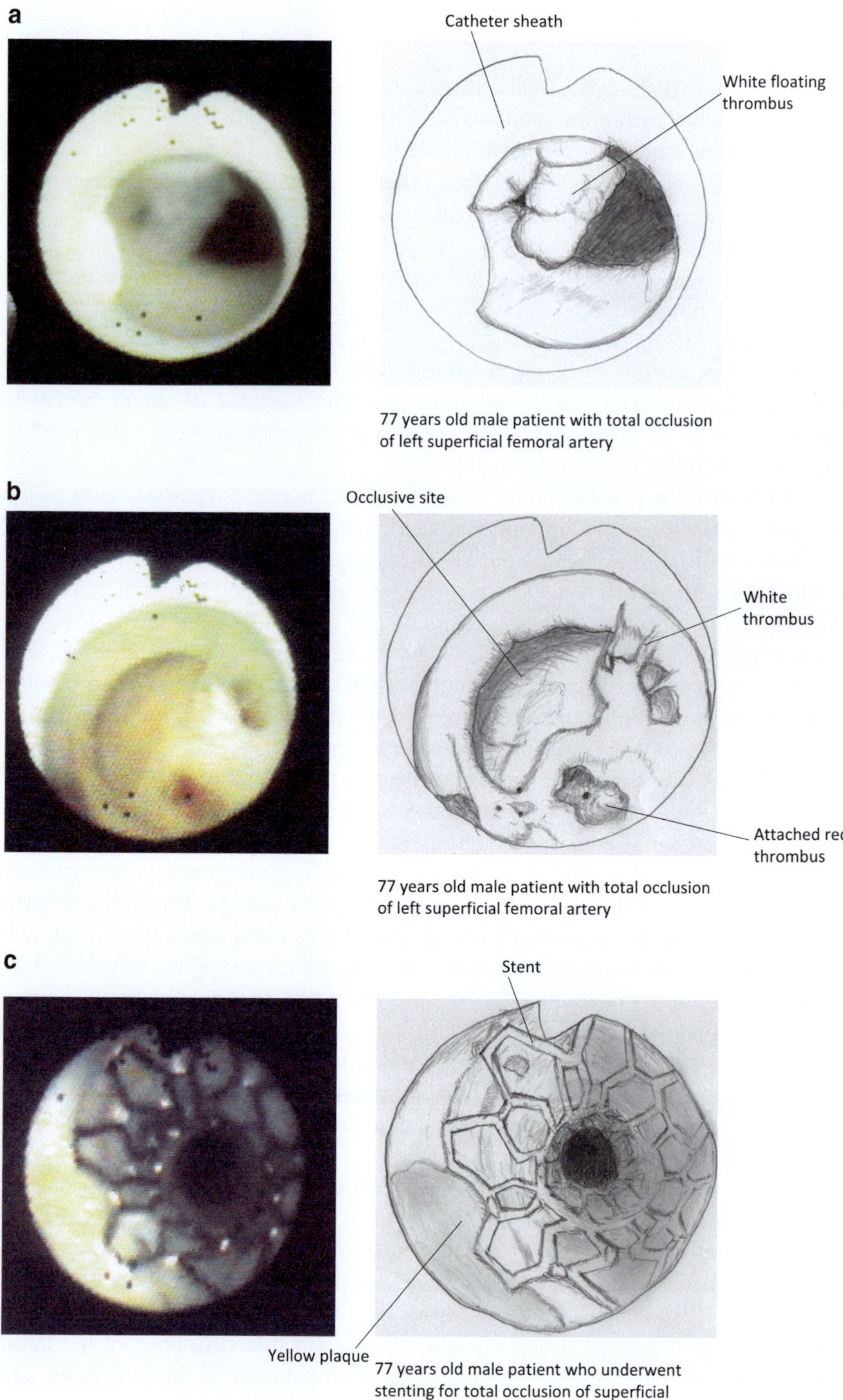

Fig. 12.6 Angioscopic observation of arterial lumen in patients with peripheral artery disease (Illustrations by K Tokuhuro)

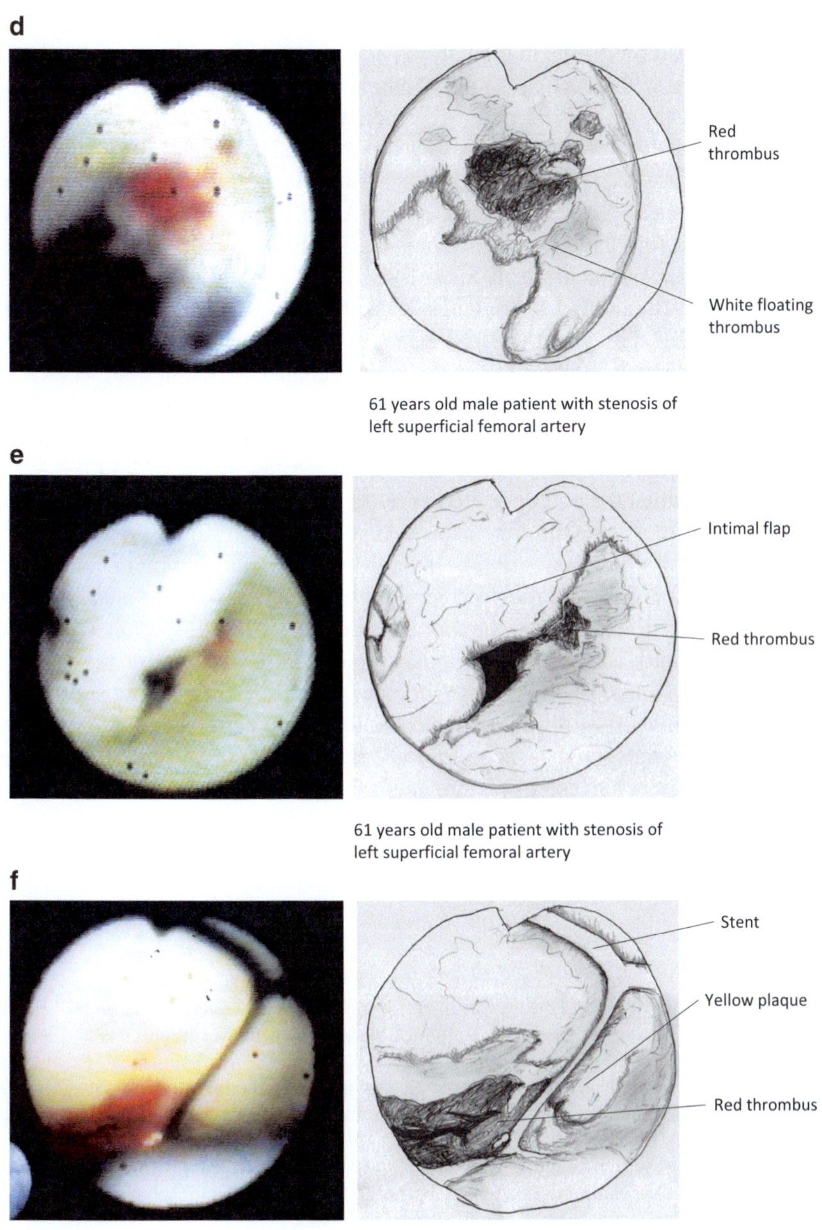

d

61 years old male patient with stenosis of left superficial femoral artery

e

61 years old male patient with stenosis of left superficial femoral artery

f

54 years old male patient who underwent stenting for right iliac artery

Fig. 12.6 (continued)

complex lesions. Recent registry studies suggest that the newer stent designs may have better long-term results in the femoral artery than before [22].

In our patients with total occlusion or complex calcified lesion, stenting following PTA decreased the restenosis rate. We studied paired scans (DUS and CTA) in 75 patients with PAD who were treated by PTA [23]. We had 43 patients with superficial femoral artery (SFA), 14 patients with iliac artery (IA), and 10 patients with both SFA and IA. In all patients with IA and/or SFA lesions, stenting was performed. In a few patients, angioscopy was performed during PTA. At 1-year follow-up, restenosis occurred in 5 (17.9 %) of 28 SFA cases and 1 (7.1 %) of 14 IA cases with calcified lesions. On the other hand, restenosis occurred in 3 (12 %) of 25 SFA cases and 0 of 10 IA cases without calcification. Angioscopy demonstrated plaque characteristics and luminal changes after stenting (Fig. 12.6) and also revealed minor thrombus formation at the injured sites or stent edge (Fig. 12.6f), which could not be detected by angiography. If the stenosed lesion is successfully dilated with stenting, calcification in the lesion or number of risk factor may not affect the outcome. However, angioscopic evaluation after PTA may be helpful to predict acute thrombosis. In PAD patients, angioscopy is useful for the accurate evaluation of plaque morphology, thrombosis, and luminal changes after PTA and can be a useful modality to predict acute thrombosis or inadequate stenting.

Angioscopy is useful for the evaluation of luminal surface of peripheral arteries, veins, or pulmonary arteries. Since angioscopy is more sensitive for the detection of thrombus than angiography or other imaging modalities, it is very useful for the final diagnosis of venous thromboembolism and the prediction of acute thrombosis after PTA. Since angioscopy is the most accurate imaging modality for the detection of thrombus or inner surface of plaque, this can be useful for improving diagnosis and treatment of PAD or venous diseases.

References

1. Litvack F, Grundfest WS, Lee ME, Carrol RM, Fran R, Chaux A, Berci G, Rose HB, Matroff JM, Forrester JS. Angioscopic visualization of blood vessel interior in animals and humans. Clin Cardiol. 1985;8:65–70.
2. Uchida Y, Tomaru T, Nakamura F, Sonoki H, Sugimoto T. Fiberoptic angioscopy of cardiac chambers, valves and great vessels using a guiding balloon catheter in dogs. Am Heart J. 1988;118:1297–302.
3. Sherman CT, Litvak F, Brundfest W, Lee M, Hickey A, Chaux A, Kass R, Blanche C, Matroff JM, Morgenstein L, Ganz W, Swan HJC, Forrester JS. Coronary angioscopy in patients with unstable angina pectoris. N Engl J Med. 1986;315:909–19.
4. Tomaru T, Nakamura F, Fujimori Y, Omata M, Kawai S, Okada R, Murata Y, Uchida Y. Local treatment with antithrombotic drugs can prevent thrombus formation: an angioscopic and angiographic study. J Am Coll Cardiol. 1995;26:1325–32.
5. Hirsh J, Hoak J. Management of deep vein thrombosis and pulmonary embolism. A statement for healthcare professionals from the Council on Thrombosis (in Consultation with the Council on Cardiovascular Radiology) American Heart Association. Circulation. 1996;93:2212–45.

6. Uchida Y, Tomaru T, Kato S. Percutaneous pulmonary angioscopy using a guiding balloon catheter. Clin Cardiol. 1988;11:143–8.

7. Shure D, Gregoratos G, Moser KM. Fiberoptic angioscopy: role in the diagnosis of chronic pulmonary arterial obstruction. Ann Intern Med. 1985;103:844–50.

8. Satokawa H, Hoshino S, Iwaya F, Igari T, Midorikawa H, Ogawa T. Intravascular imaging methods for venous disorders. Int J Angiol. 2000;9:117–21.

9. Uchida Y. Venous disease. In: Uchida Y, editor. Atlas of cardioangioscopy. Tokyo: Medical View; 1995. p. 206–16.

10. Moser KM, Auger WR, Fedullo PF. Chronic major-vessel thromboembolic pulmonary hypertension. Circulation. 1990;81:1735–43.

11. Riedel M, Stanek V, Widimsky J, et al. Longterm follow-up of patients with pulmonary thromboembolism – late prognosis and evolution of hemodynamic and respiratory data. Chest. 1982;81:151–8.

12. Uchida Y. Angioscopy systems and their manipulation. In: Uchida Y, editor. Coronary angioscopy. Armonk: Futura Publishing; 2001. p. 7–24.

13. Tomaru T. Application of angioscopy for diagnosis and treatment of venous thromboembolism. J Heart Dis. 2007;5(Suppl):4.

14. Criqui MH, Langer RD, Fronek A, Feigelson HS, Klauber MR, McCann TJ, Browner D. Mortality over a period of 10 years in patients with peripheral arterial disease. N Engl J Med. 1992;326:381–6.

15. Brevetti G, Giugliano G, Brevetti L, Hiatt WR. Inflammation in peripheral artery disease. Circulation. 2010;122:1862–75.

16. Shareghi S, Gopal A, Gul K, Matchinson JC, Wong CB, Weinberg N, Lensky M, Budoff MJ, Shavelle DM. Diagnostic accuracy of 64 multidetector computed tomographic angiography in peripheral vascular disease. Catheter Cardiovasc Interv. 2010;75(1):23–31.

17. Olin JW, Sealove BA. Peripheral artery disease: current insight into the disease and its diagnosis and management. Mayo Clin Proc. 2010;85:678–92.

18. Uchida Y, Uchida Y. Advances in angioscopic imaging of vascular disease. World J Cardiovasc Surg. 2012;2:114–31.

19. Uchida Y, Nakamura F, Tomaru T. Rheological significance of tandem lesions of the coronary artery. Heart Vessel. 1995;10:106–10.

20. Uchida Y, Fujimori Y, Tomaru T, Oshima O, Hi-Rose J. Percutaneous angioplasty of chronic obstruction of peripheral arteries by a temperature-controlled Nd-YAG laser system. J Interv Cardiol. 1992;5:301–8.

21. Geschwind HJ, Aptecar E, Boussignac G, Dubois-Randé JL, Zelinsky R, Poirot G, Tomaru T. Results and follow-up after percutaneous pulsed laser-assisted balloon angioplasty guided by spectroscopy. Circulation. 1991;83:787–96.

22. Scheinert D, Grummt L, Piorkowski M, Sax J, Scheinert S, Ulrich M, Werner M, Bausback Y, Braunlich S, Schmidt A. A novel self-expanding interwoven nitinol stent for complex femoropopliteal lesions: 24-month results of the SUPERA SFA registry. J Endovasc Ther. 2011;18:745–52.

23. Tomaru T. Polyvascular disease. J Heart Dis. 2014;11(Suppl):49.

Chapter 13
Quantification of Angioscopy

Kentaro Okamatsu

Abstract The greatest weakness of angioscopy is its limited ability of quantitative assessment for length, area, and volume, while the most unique aspect of angioscopy is the capability of assessing the true color of the intravascular structures. To intensify this aspect, a more objective and quantitative method of color evaluation has been studied. Particularly, a quantitative colorimetric system based on the $L^*a^*b^*$ color space enables us to detect a vulnerable plaque with angioscopy, and it has been applied to clinical use.

Keywords Quantitative colorimetry • Yellow plaque • Vulnerable plaque

13.1 Character of Angioscopy

Angioscopy can provide high-resolution, three-dimensional, and full-color images of the endoluminal surface of the blood vessels, and direct visualization of the lumen is applicable for macroscopic diagnosis of the intravascular structures including atherosclerotic plaque and thrombus based on color and morphology. Especially, the capability of assessing the true color of the intravascular structures is not found in any other cardiovascular imaging technique. In practice, coronary angioscopy is a sensitive method for detecting coronary thrombus, and it can also assess the composition of the thrombus from its color. Moreover, coronary angioscopy can evaluate the vulnerability of plaque based on its color. A major drawback of angioscopy, however, has been its limited ability to quantify the observed images.

Although preliminary efforts to accurately quantitate linear and volumetric measurements within angioscopic images were published in 1994 [1], this method was not put to practical use, because other devices such as intravascular ultrasounds (IVUS) were able to quantitate those more easily and exactly. While angioscopic

K. Okamatsu, M.D., Ph.D. (✉)
Division of Cardiology, Chiba Hokusoh Hospital, Nippon Medical School,
1715 Kamakari, Inzai, Chiba 270-1694, Japan

Division of Cardiology, Komagome Aoba Clinic, 1-38-2 Komagome,
Toshima, Tokyo 170-0003, Japan
e-mail: okamatsu@nms.ac.jp

© Springer Japan 2015
K. Mizuno, M. Takano (eds.), *Coronary Angioscopy*,
DOI 10.1007/978-4-431-55546-9_13

interpretation of color, the most unique aspect of angioscopy, was usually subjective or semiquantitative, angioscopic findings were tempered by substantial observer disagreement in the visual assessment of angioscopic color. Therefore, to make the angioscopic assessing the true color more sensitive and more reliable, a more objective and quantitative method of color evaluation has been required.

13.2   Quantification of Color and Composition of Thrombus

Mizuno et al. documented that reddish (erythrocyte-rich) thrombi were observed at the culprit lesions in almost all patients with acute myocardial infarction, as opposed to white (platelet-rich) thrombi observed in more than 70 % of individuals with unstable angina, using angioscopy [2]. Then, the angioscopic color of thrombus is considered to be an important factor that influences therapeutic decisions, as white platelet-rich thrombi appear to be much more resistant to pharmacologic thrombolysis than red erythrocyte-rich thrombi [3]. Therefore, Lehmann et al. studied quantitative colorimetry during angioscopy to differentiate thrombus based on color [4]. Their quantitative colorimetric system succeeded in providing quantitative information of thrombus composition (the concentration of erythrocytes), using the C1 (an intensity-independent red index)/C2 (an intensity-independent green index) chromaticity diagram which was developed in their laboratory specifically for angioscopic color of thrombus.

13.3   Quantification of Yellow Plaque

Postmortem pathological analysis has revealed that the main cause of acute coronary syndromes (ACS) is plaque rupture following thrombus formation; a plaque that is prone to rupture is characterized by having an abundant necrotic core beneath a thin fibrous cap [5]. In the human coronary artery, the plaques in ACS culprit lesions have been angioscopically identified as yellow [6, 7]. Histopathologic analysis of atherectomy specimens of coronary lesions from patients has supported the association of yellow plaque color with the presence of atheroma [8]. Moreover, prospective studies using angioscopy have shown that patients with yellow plaques more frequently suffer from ACS than patients with white plaques [9, 10]. However, all yellow plaques are not a vulnerable plaque, because ACS occurred in few of patients with yellow plaques in many angioscopic studies [11, 12]. To detect a vulnerable plaque, we need to differentiate yellow plaques more accurately and more reliably.

Yellow plaque color is due to the visualization of reflected light from the lipid core stained in yellow with beta-carotene through a thin fibrous cap. Miyamoto et al. have validated the nature of yellow color, using the experimental model that was constructed by injecting a yellow beta-carotene-lipid emulsion subendothelially into normal bovine aorta, and shown an inverse relationship between yellow color saturation and the cap thickness of fibroatheromas [13]. In their system, yellow saturation, derived from HIS color space, was used to represent yellow color intensity of plaques. However, yellow saturation may not ideally represent the gradations of yellow color intensity because of its nonlinear nature. In addition, the detailed process of optimization against the effect of variables unique to angioscopy was not examined in their system. Ishibashi et al. have developed a quantitative colorimetric system based on the $L*a*b*$ color space [14]. $L*a*b*$ color space is widely used to describe color differences because of its linear nature, that is, uniform color space, which is intended so that a color difference perceived as an equal dimension may correspond to an equal distance (Fig. 13.1). In their system, a yellow color intensity and brightness can be represented as simply the $b*$ value (yellow color intensity 0–100) and $L*$ value (brightness of the color −100 to 100). Their system can consistently measure yellow plaque color independent of such conditions as light intensity, the distance from lens of angioscope to the objective, and the angle of the angioscope to the region of interest, after proper adjustments for brightness ($L*$ value is within 40–80) (Figs. 13.2 and 13.3). Furthermore, they revealed that a plaque of $b*$ value >23 contains atheroma that has a fibrous cap thickness <100 μm, using ex vivo human tissue samples (Fig. 13.4). Thus, the intensive yellow color ($b*$ value >23) reflects a vulnerable plaque. This system based on $L*a*b*$ color space has been applied to clinical use. Ishibashi et al. have reported that plaques of $b*$ value >23 are more frequently observed in the culprit lesions of ACS than in the culprit lesions of SAP [15]. Yamamoto et al. have revealed that plaques of $b*$ value >23 are strongly correlated with the thin cap fibroatheroma determined by virtual histology IVUS [16]. Tajika et al. have shown that plaques of $b*$ value >23 are associated with elevated malondialdehyde-modified low-density lipoprotein levels, which has been reported to be detected in the plasma of patients with ACS [17].

Fig. 13.1 $L*a*b*$ color space

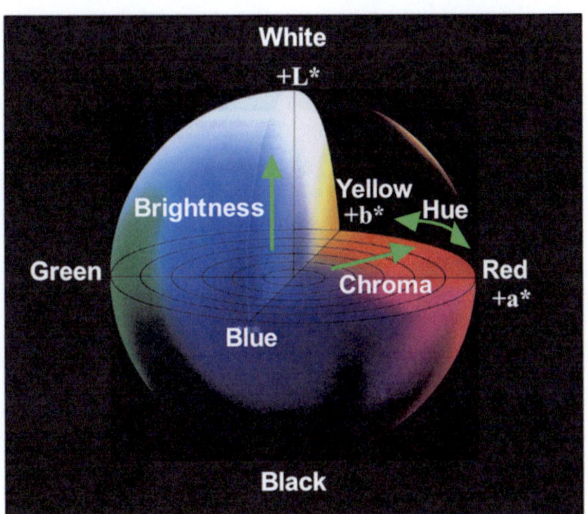

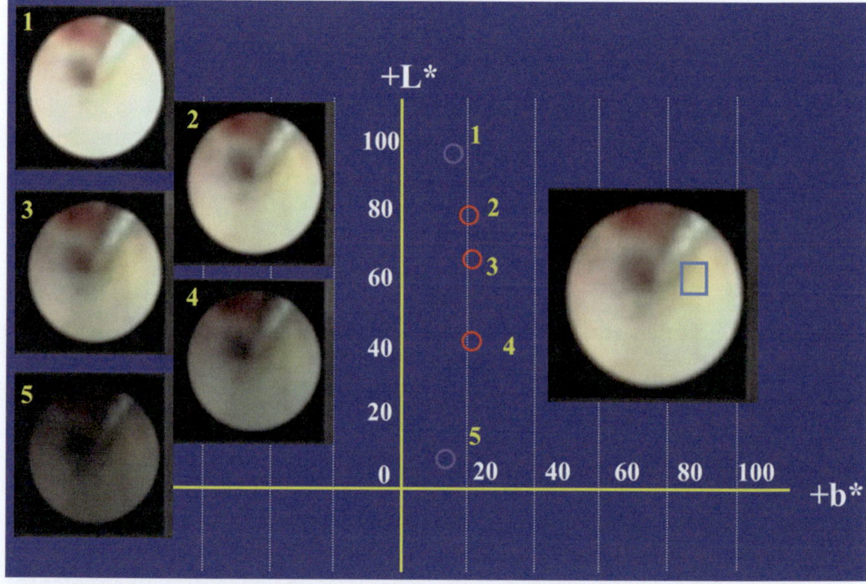

Fig. 13.2 $b*$ value with different light intensity levels. The $b*$ values of No. 2, No. 3, and No. 4 are the same after proper adjustments for brightness ($L*$ value is within 40–80)

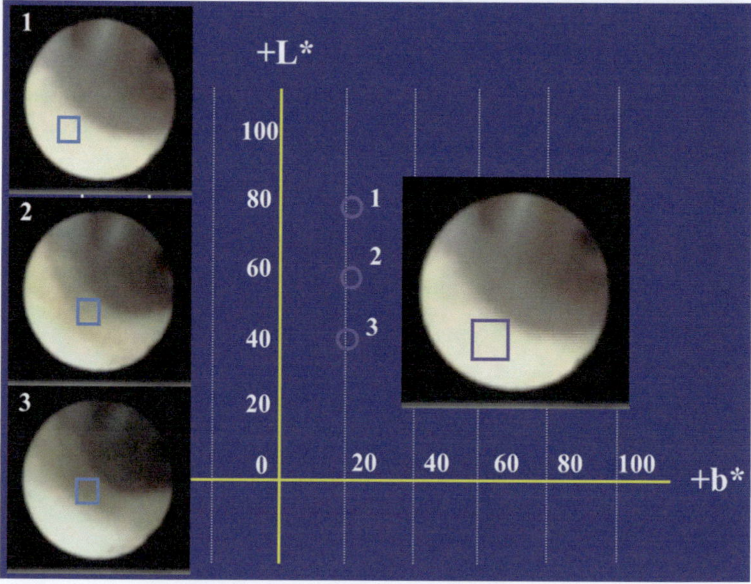

Fig. 13.3 $b*$ value with different distances from lens of angioscope to the region of interest. The $b*$ values of No. 1 (short distance), No. 2 (middle distance), and No. 3 (long distance) are the same after proper adjustments for brightness ($L*$ value is within 40–80)

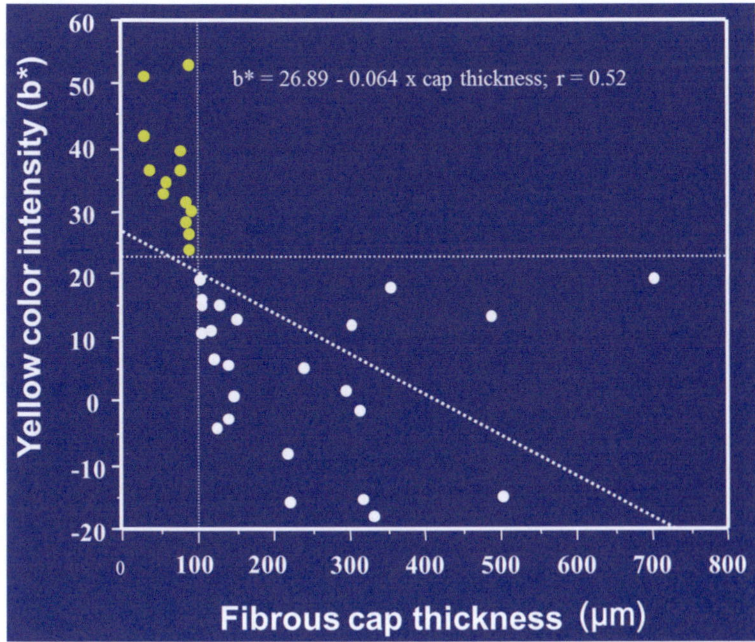

Fig. 13.4 The inverse linear correlation between b^* value and the fibrous cap thickness covering the lipid core. *Yellow* color intensity was high (b^* >23: represented by *yellow circles*) in all locations with the fibrous cap thickness <100 μm [14]

References

1. Spears JR, Ali M, Raza SJ, Iyer GS, Ravi S, Crilly RJ, Fromm B, Cheong WF. Quantitative angioscopy: a novel method of measurement of luminal dimensions during angioscopy with the use of a "lightwire". Cardiovasc Intervent Radiol. 1994;17:197–203.
2. Mizuno K, Satomura K, Miyamoto A, Arakawa K, Shibuya T, Arai T, Kurita A, Nakamura H, Ambrose JA. Angioscopic evaluation of coronary-artery thrombi in acute coronary syndromes. N Engl J Med. 1992;326:287–91.
3. Jang IK, Gold HK, Ziskind AA, Fallon JT, Holt RE, Leinbach RC, May JW, Collen D. Differential sensitivity of erythrocyte-rich and platelet-rich arterial thrombi to lysis with recombinant tissue-type plasminogen activator: a possible explanation for resistance to coronary thrombolysis. Circulation. 1989;79:920–8.
4. Lehmann KG, Oomen JA, Slager CJ, deFeyter PJ, Serruys PW. Chromatic distortion during angioscopy: assessment and correction by quantitative colorimetric angioscopic analysis. Catheter Cardiovasc Diagn. 1998;45:191–201.
5. Virmani R, Burke AP, Farb A, Kolodgie FD. Pathology of the vulnerable plaque. J Am Coll Cardiol. 2006;47:C13–18.
6. Mizuno K, Miyamoto A, Satomura K, Kurita A, Arai T, Sakurada M, Yanagida S, Nakamura H. Angioscopic coronary macromorphology in patients with acute coronary disorders. Lancet. 1991;337:809–12.
7. Okamatsu K, Takano M, Sakai S, Ishibashi F, Uemura R, Takano T, Mizuno K. Elevated troponin T levels and lesion characteristics in non-ST-elevation acute coronary syndromes. Circulation. 2004;109:465–70.

8. Thieme T, Wernecke KD, Meyer R, Brandenstein E, Habedank D, Hinz A, Felix SB, Baumann G, Kleber FX. Angioscopic evaluation of atherosclerotic plaques: validation by histomorphologic analysis and association with stable and unstable coronary syndromes. J Am Coll Cardiol. 1996;28:1–6.

9. Uchida Y, Nakamura F, Tomaru T, Morita T, Oshima T, Sasaki T, Morizuki S, Hirose J. Prediction of acute coronary syndromes by percutaneous coronary angioscopy in patients with stable angina. Am Heart J. 1995;130:195–203.

10. Ohtani T, Ueda Y, Mizote I, Oyabu J, Okada K, Hirayama A, Kodama K. Number of yellow plaques detected in a coronary artery is associated with future risk of acute coronary syndrome: detection of vulnerable patients by angioscopy. J Am Coll Cardiol. 2006;47:2194–200.

11. Takano M, Mizuno K, Yokoyama S, Seimiya K, Ishibashi F, Okamatsu K, Uemura R. Changes in coronary plaque color and morphology by lipid-lowering therapy with atorvastatin: serial evaluation by coronary angioscopy. J Am Coll Cardiol. 2003;42:680–6.

12. Asakura M, Ueda Y, Yamaguchi O, Adachi T, Hirayama A, Hori M, Kodama K. Extensive development of vulnerable plaques as a pan-coronary process in patients with myocardial infarction: an angioscopic study. J Am Coll Cardiol. 2001;37:1284–8.

13. Miyamoto A, Prieto AR, Friedl SE, Lin FC, Muller JE, Nesto RW, Abela 2nd GS. Atheromatous plaque cap thickness can be determined by quantitative color analysis during angioscopy: implications for identifying the vulnerable plaque. Clin Cardiol. 2004;27:9–15.

14. Ishibashi F, Yokoyama S, Miyahara K, Dabreo A, Weiss ER, Iafrati M, Takano M, Okamatsu K, Mizuno K, Waxman S. Quantitative colorimetry of atherosclerotic plaque using the L*a*b color space during angioscopy for the detection of lipid cores underneath thin fibrous cap. Int J Cardiovasc Imaging. 2007;23:679–91.

15. Ishibashi F, Mizuno K, Kawamura A, Singh PP, Nesto RW, Waxman S. High yellow color intensity by angioscopy with quantitative colorimetry to identify high-risk features in culprit lesions of patients with acute coronary syndromes. Am J Cardiol. 2007;100:1207–11.

16. Yamamoto M, Takano M, Okamatsu K, Murakami D, Inami S, Xie Y, Seimiya K, Ohba T, Seino Y, Mizuno K. Relationship between thin cap fibroatheroma identified by virtual histology and angioscopic yellow plaque in quantitative analysis with colorimetry. Circ J. 2009;73:497–502.

17. Tajika K, Okamatsu K, Takano M, Inami S, Yamamoto M, Murakami D, Kobayashi N, Ohba T, Hata N, Seino Y, Mizuno K. Malondialdehyde-modified low-density lipoprotein is a useful marker to identify patients with vulnerable plaque. Circ J. 2012;76:2211–17.

Part III
Angioscopic Findings After Stent- and Drug-Based Therapies

Chapter 14
Bare-Metal Stent

Toshiro Shinke

Abstract Bare-metal stent (BMS) has been widely used for the treatment of coronary artery disease. Tissue growth in response to implanted BMS forms relatively thick neointima and eventually seals and stabilizes vulnerable plaques containing thrombus. Recent pathological reports suggest that early neointimal growth peaked at 6 months and then the neointimas become thinner at 2–3 years and some of those eventually transform into atherosclerotic tissue (neoatherosclerosis) which mimics atherosclerosis in native coronary arteries. Full-color and 3-dimensional angioscopic images of the coronary lumen provide detailed information on the vessel walls, including the stent segment and atherosclerotic process beyond angiography. Angioscopy enables macroscopic pathological assessment of intra-stent tissue including early thick white neointima with embedded stent struts, thinner late phase neointima with transparent struts, and yellow neoatherosclerosis with newly formed intra-stent thrombus. Angioscopic assessment of serial changes after BMS implantation may have potential benefits on patient's management after coronary stenting.

Keywords Bare-metal stent • Histology • Neointima • Thrombus

14.1 Introduction

Recent postmortem histopathologic studies of patients dying after coronary stenting have shown that in-stent neointimal tissue growth results from smooth muscle cell proliferation and extracellular matrix formation. Angioscopy allows direct visualization of the arterial luminal surface and thereby supplies image information that cannot be provided by intravascular ultrasound or optical coherence tomography. Thus, angioscopy enables macroscopic pathological assessment of intra-stent tissue. Angioscopic assessment of serial changes after stent implantation may have potential benefits on patient's management after coronary stenting. In this chapter,

T. Shinke, M.D., Ph.D. (✉)
Division of Cardiovascular Medicine, Department of Internal Medicine, Kobe University
Graduate School of Medicine, 7-5-1, Kusunoki-cho, Chuo-ku, Kobe 650-0017, Japan
e-mail: shinke@med.kobe-u.ac.jp

© Springer Japan 2015
K. Mizuno, M. Takano (eds.), *Coronary Angioscopy*,
DOI 10.1007/978-4-431-55546-9_14

bare-metal stent (BMS), which has been widely used for the treatment of coronary artery disease, was focused to provide a comprehensive review of angioscopic assessment for intracoronary stent placement.

14.2 Vascular Response to BMS Implantation in Porcine Coronary Models

Stent implantation causes arterial injury, which can initiate neointimal growth. This process includes platelet deposition, thrombus, inflammation, migration of smooth muscle cells, smooth muscle cell proliferation, and extracellular matrix formation. Initially, platelet deposition and activation occur at the injury site, leading to the release of cell-signaling molecules. The cell-signaling molecules induce expression of cell surface receptors that bind to circulating inflammatory cells. The activated inflammatory cells secrete molecules that bind to specific receptors on smooth muscle cells. Bound smooth muscle cell receptors activate various intracellular smooth muscle cell proteins, causing the smooth muscle cells to undergo mitosis (i.e., cell proliferation). Proliferation of smooth muscle cells increases the cellular mass in the neointima, eventually leading to restenosis in some cases (Fig. 14.1) [1].

Comparative preclinical histologic studies remain the most effective method for assessing the healing characteristics of vascular stents. Porcine coronary models have been widely used for the evaluation of newly developed stent devices including drug-eluting stent (DES) [2]. Figure 14.2 demonstrated the hematoxylin-eosin staining histopathological cross sections in porcine coronary model at different time

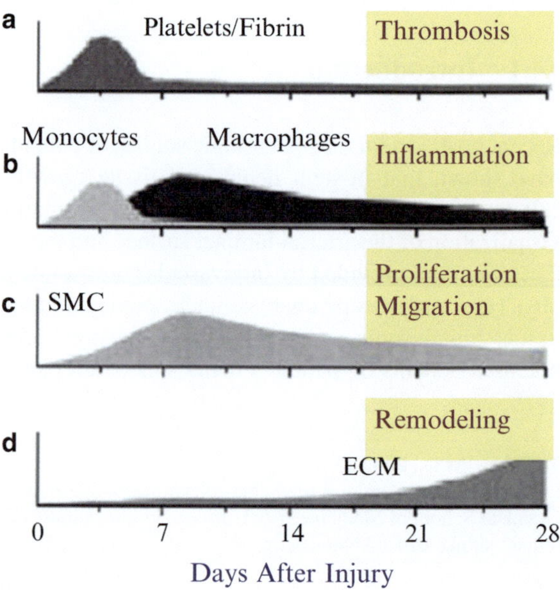

Fig. 14.1 Schematic presentation of time sequence after BMS implantation to coronary artery. Initially, platelet deposition and activation occur at the injury site, leading to activate inflammatory cells that secrete molecules that bind to specific receptors on smooth muscle cells. Migration and proliferation of smooth muscle cells increase the cellular mass in the neointima (Ref. [1])

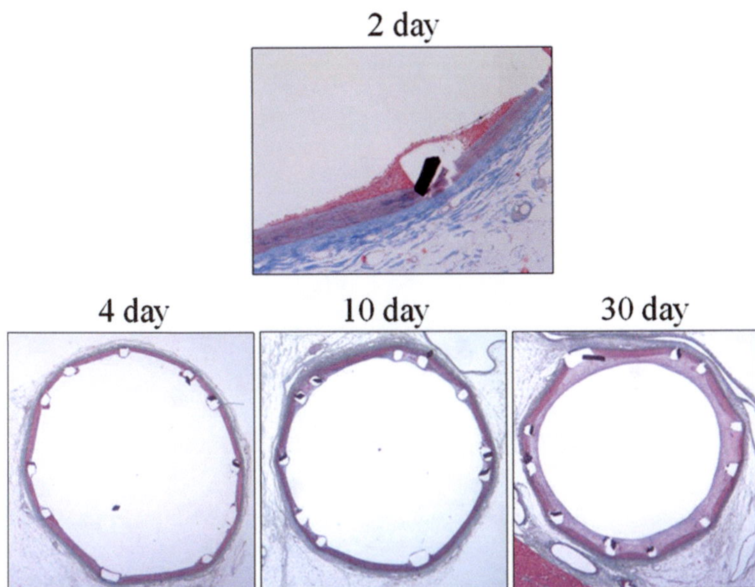

Fig. 14.2 Histopathological cross sections in porcine coronary model at different time points following BMS implantation. Initial thrombus formation at 2 days was followed by inflammatory cell infiltration and smooth muscle cell proliferation at 4–10 days. Finally, matured thick fibrocellular neointima was observed at 30 days

points following BMS implantation. As was shown in Fig. 14.1, initial thrombus formation at 2 days was followed by inflammatory cell infiltration and smooth muscle cell proliferation at 4–10 days. Finally, matured thick fibrocellular neointima was observed at 30 days.

We have evaluated angioscopic appearance of coronary arteries with BMS in parallel with assessment of arterial wall histological characteristics in nine porcine models at 30 days. It has been generally recognized that vascular response to stent implantation at 1 month in porcine is equivalent to 3–6 months in humans. So, this observation mimicked the midterm (6 months) follow-up angioscopy in human. Macroscopic images of vascular luminal surfaces of coronary segments showed BMS developed opaque white neointima, with virtual strut invisibility. Angioscopic finding was consistent with macroscopic images, and most of the stent strut embedded in the neointima was not visible at 30 days in porcine (Fig. 14.3) [3]. When angioscopic grading for neointimal coverage was classified into 4 semiquantitative grading categories, grade 0 = fully visible struts (similar to immediate post-implant); grade 1 = struts covered, but protruding into lumen, and transparently visible; grade 2 = struts embedded by neointima, but still translucent; and grade 3 = struts fully embedded and invisible, 93 % of BMS neointimal coverage was angioscopic grade 3, with invisible struts and overlying coverage of white, opaque neointima. 7 % and 0 % of BMS met criteria for grades 2 and 1, respectively (Fig. 14.4) [4]. Microscopic images of BMS segment exhibited well-

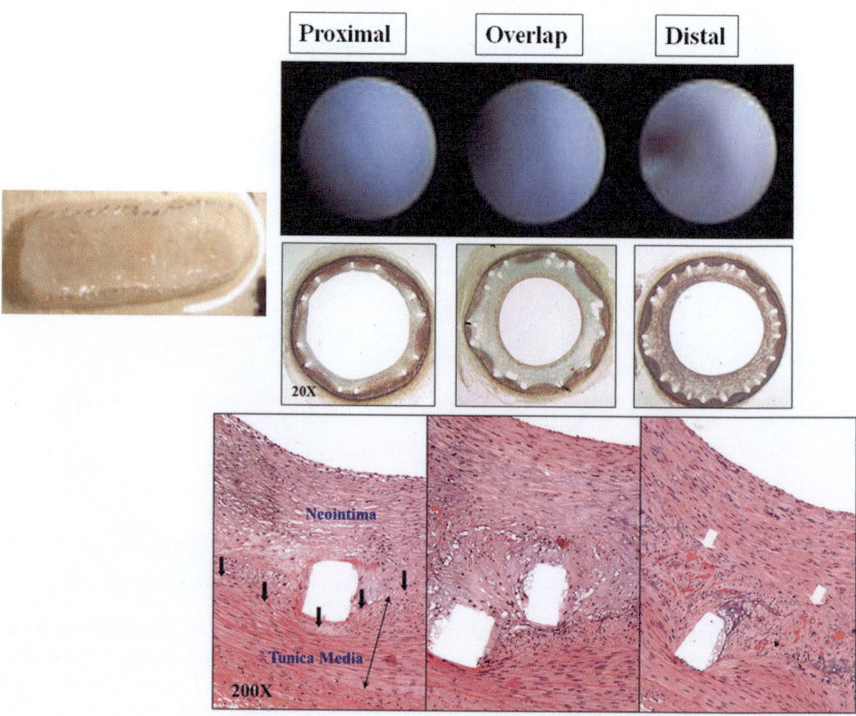

Fig. 14.3 Macroscopic images of vascular luminal surfaces of coronary segments implanted with BMS. BMS developed opaque white neointima, with virtual strut invisibility. Most of the stent struts embedded in the neointima were not visible by angioscopy. Movat pentachrome staining (20×) and hematoxylin-eosin staining (200×) showed BMS segment exhibited well-healed, thick fibrocellular neointima, completely covered with endothelial cells. Only minute deposits of inspissated thrombus and fibrin deposits were observed (Ref. [3])

healed, thick fibrocellular neointima, completely covered with endothelial cells. Only minute deposits of inspissated thrombus and fibrin deposits were observed (Fig. 14.3).

14.3 Time Course of Neointimal Growth After BMS Implantation in Human

The timing of healing response to stent placement may be difficult to translate from animal models to human; however, it has been suggested that the stages of healing are remarkably similar. Histological investigations using human autopsy samples have reported that migration of smooth muscle cells is identified around 2 weeks after BMS implantation and complete neointimal growth and endothelial coverage is achieved at 12 weeks [5, 6]. Angioscopy has been used to evaluate the time course of neointimal coverage of stents in human. According to the serial angioscopic

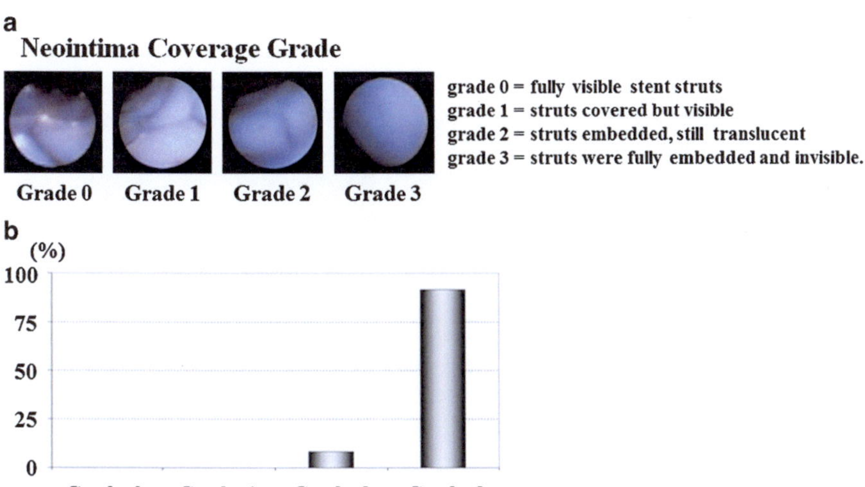

Fig. 14.4 (**a**) Strut coverage grade by angioscopy. Grade 0 was defined as stent struts that were fully visible, similar to immediately after implantation. Grade 1 was defined as stent struts that bulged into the lumen and, although covered, were still transparently visible. Grade 2 was defined as stent struts that were visible, but not clearly seen. Grade 3 was defined as stent struts that were not visible by angioscopy. (**b**) Proportion of neointimal coverage grade at BMS-implanted segment at 1 month in porcine coronary model. Most of the segments developed grade 3 coverage

study, no neointimal coverage was found angioscopically at 8–18 days post-implant [7]. Approximately 3 months were required for the completion of neointimal stent coverage after BMS implantation [7, 8]. Angioscopic study has shown complete neointimal coverage was observed in all of the BMS segments at 6 months [4]. Figure 14.5 demonstrates the angioscopic image of BMS-implanted segment at 6-month follow-up.

BMS have a plaque-healing/stabilizing effect. With BMS treatment, the unstable yellow plaque containing protruding mixed thrombus in infarction-related lesion changes to stable white plaque during 6-month follow-up [9]. Figure 14.6 shows the serial changes of angioscopic images at pre- and post-balloon inflation, post-stent placement, and 6-month follow-up after BMS implantation in patients with acute myocardial infarction (AMI). It is noteworthy that neointimal proliferation provides surface passivation of unstable plaques as well as the disappearance of early intra-stent thrombus [8]. Interestingly, plaque morphology on angioscopy may affect the artery healing process after BMS implantation. A serial angioscopic study of patients with AMI has demonstrated that the grade of neointimal stent coverage at 1-month follow-up is lower in the ruptured segment of infarct-related lesions than in the adjacent non-ruptured segment. Also the yellow grade of plaque color in ruptured segment was higher than that of non-ruptured segment immediately after stenting and at 1-month follow-up. Neointimal stent coverage and plaque color eventually became equivalent at 6 months [10]. These observations may in part support the rationale of recent guidelines regarding the duration of dual antiplatelet therapy after the onset of acute coronary syndrome [11].

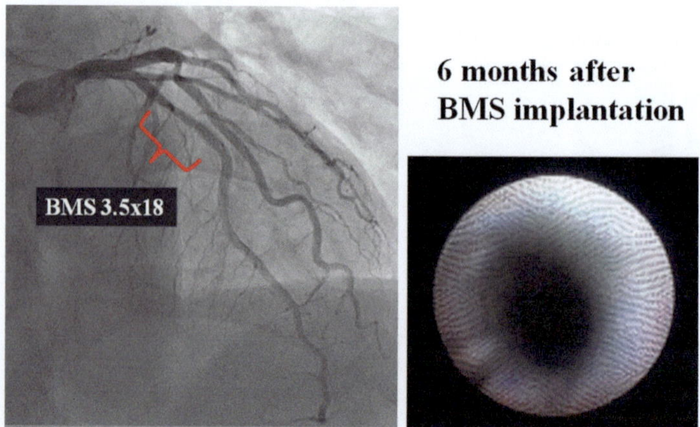

Fig. 14.5 Representative angiography and angioscopy images at 6 months after BMS implantation to stable coronary disease in human. Complete neointimal coverage was observed by angioscopy

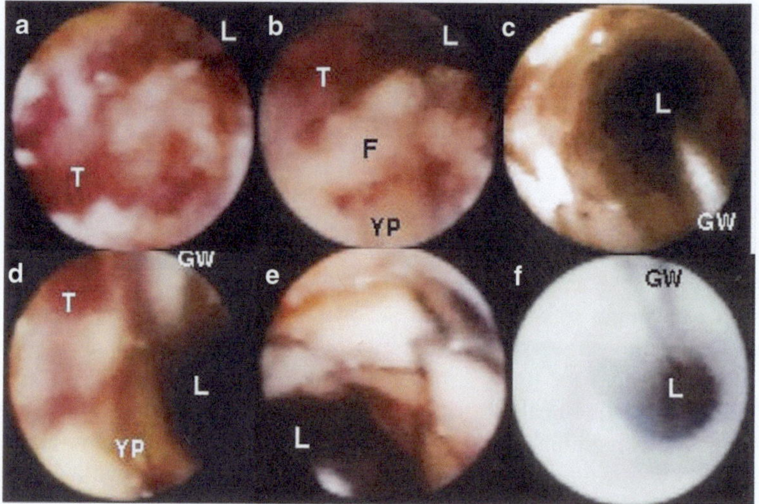

Fig. 14.6 Serial angioscopic images. (**a**) At baseline, a protruding mixed thrombus was seen. (**b**) Immediately after balloon angioplasty, a protruding thrombus and intimal flap were seen. (**c**) Immediately after stenting. (**d**) At 1-month follow-up, a lining thrombus was seen. (**e**) At 1-month follow-up, there was partial neointimal coverage. (**f**) At 6-month follow-up, there was smooth and white plaque without thrombus. *F* intimal flap, *GW* guide wire, *L* lumen, *Y* yellow plaque, *T* thrombus. (Ref. [9])

14.4 Transparency of Stent Struts According to Neointimal Thickness After BMS

Given the fact that the thickness of neointima was associated with transparency of stent struts underneath neointima assessed by angioscopy, there is a limited methodology to measure the thickness of neointima in vivo. Optical coherence

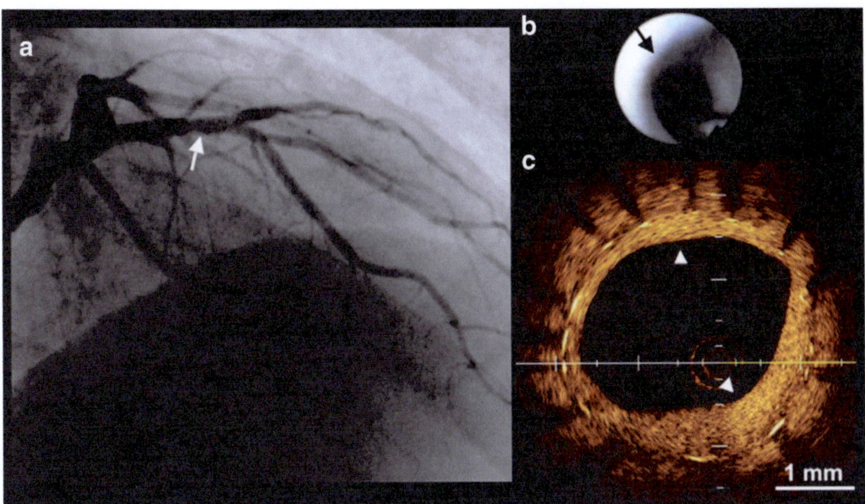

Fig. 14.7 Typical findings of angioscopy and optical coherence tomography after BMS implantation. (**a**) A 43-year-old man with stable angina pectoris received implantation of a BMS (3.5 mm × 13 mm) in the left anterior descending artery. Six-month follow-up angiogram shows no in-stent restenosis (*white arrow*). (**b**) Angioscopy shows white neointima covers completely over the BMS (*black arrow*) and the struts are invisible. (**c**) Circumferential stent struts with strong signals are identified by cross-sectional image of optical coherence tomography. Neointima inside the struts has uniform signals without their attenuation (*arrowheads*) (Ref. [12])

tomography (OCT) is a novel intracoronary imaging device that provides cross-sectional images with ultrahigh resolution. Murakami et al. presented the typical angioscopy and OCT images after BMS implantation (Fig. 14.7) [12]. Inoue et al. reported simultaneous angioscopy and OCT analysis for vascular response to stent placement [13]. Figure 14.8 shows neointimal thickness measured by OCT in each angioscopic grade of neointimal coverage. Neointimal thickness by OCT stepwisely increased as angioscopic neointimal grade increased (grade 0, 6 ± 4 μm; 1, 54 ± 25 μm; 2, 114 ± 68 μm; 3, 210 ± 136 μm). This suggests neointimal coverage grade assessed by angioscope is well correlated with OCT-derived thickness of neointima in vivo.

14.5 Long-Term Changes of Neointima Following BMS

The transparency of neointima under angioscopy, which was associated with the thickness of the neointima, gradually decreased from 3 to 6 months after BMS stenting. However, long-term follow-up with angioscopy revealed that thick nontransparent neointima shifts into thin and transparent appearance 3 years after stenting [14]. Similarly, Kimura et al. reported from serial angiographic follow-up that minimal lumen area decreased from post-stent placement to early restenosis phase until 6 months and then increased at intermediate-term regression phase from

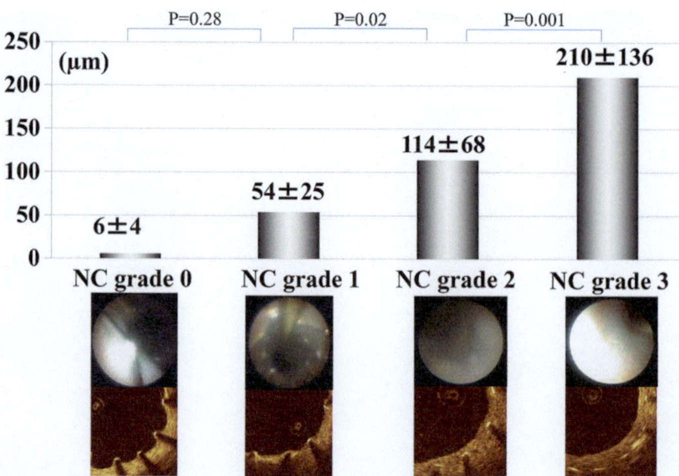

Fig. 14.8 Neointimal thickness measured by OCT in each angioscopic neointimal grade. Neointimal thickness measured by OCT stepwisely increased as angioscopic neointimal grade increased

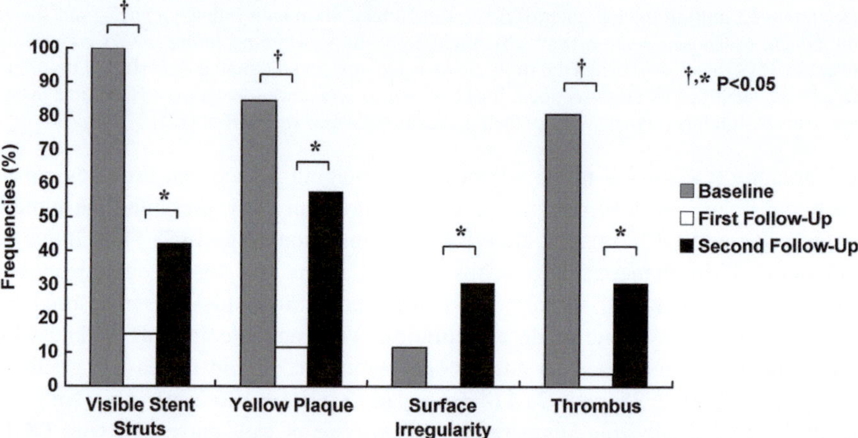

Fig. 14.9 Serial changes in visible stent struts, yellow plaque, lumen irregularity, and thrombus on angioscopy. The frequency of each angioscopic finding shows a biphasic response characterized by decreasing from baseline to the first follow-up and increasing from the first to second follow-ups (Ref. [17])

6 months to 3 years [15]. This regression process may be associated with decrease of cellular components and apoptosis as well as extracellular matrix [16].

Yokoyama et al. reported serial changes in angioscopic findings for BMS implanted in native coronary arteries [17]. The visible struts decreased from baseline to first follow-up at 6–12 months, but increased in the second follow-up at more than 4 years. Simultaneously, yellow plaques and thrombus had decreased from baseline to first follow-up, but those were increased from first to second follow-up (Fig. 14.9). The transparency And all of the yellow plaques in the second follow-up

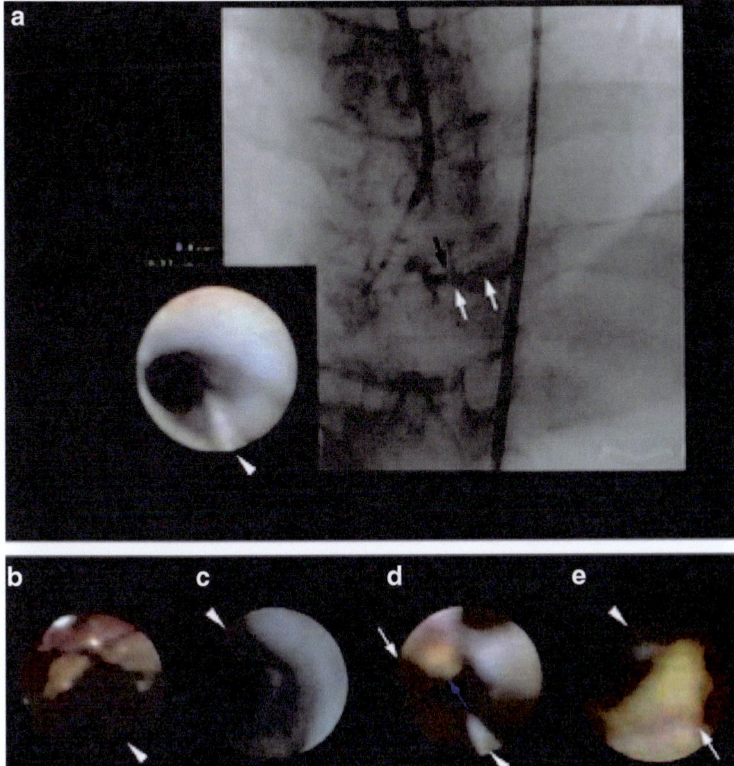

Fig. 14.10 Typical angioscopic findings after BMS implantation. (**a**) Image mixture system of fluoroscopy and angioscopy shows the precise positions of angioscopic images (*black arrow*) and implanted BMS (*white arrows*). (**b**) Immediately after BMS implantation, yellow plaque and red thrombus crushed out by the stent struts are seen. They are located outside the stent struts. (**c**) At the first follow-up, nontransparent white neointima completely covers over the stent struts. The stent struts are invisible, and the lumen surface is smooth. (**d**) At the second follow-up, irregular yellow plaque (*blue arrow*) is obviously protruding from the surrounding white intima into the lumen, and the plaque is accompanied with red thrombus (*white arrow*). The stent struts are invisible. (**e**) A yellow plaque is seen around the visible struts (*white arrow*) at the second follow-up. The plaque is clearly protruding from the struts. In this case, yellow plaque and visible struts simultaneously exist in the BMS segment. A white arrowhead indicates a guide wire (Ref. [17])

were protruding from the vessel wall into the lumen (Fig. 14.10). The important findings provided from this angioscopic follow-up study was that white neointima of BMS often changes into yellow plaque over an extended period of time, which may contribute to luminal narrowing and late stent failure. Long-term angiographic follow-up study also suggested triphasic luminal responses characterized by an early restenosis phase until 6 months, intermediate regression phase from 6 months to 3 years, and a late renarrowing phase beyond 4 years [15]. Pathological analysis using human autopsy samples reported newly formed atherosclerotic changes within neointima (neoatherosclerosis) both in BMS and drug-eluting stent. Most of neoatherosclerosis within BMS occurred at more than 3 years after implantation and located more frequently at proximal lesions than distal [18]. That is akin to the development of atherosclerosis in native coronary arteries. Recent studies have reported that one-third of patients with in-stent restenosis of BMS presented with acute coronary syndrome that is not regarded as clinically benign [19]. Angioscopy helps to detect atherosclerotic transformation from the healing response to BMS in vivo and may contribute to the better clinical management to improve long-term patients' outcome.

References

1. Fuster V, Falk E, Fallon JT, Badimon L, Chesebro JH, Badimon JJ. The three processes leading to post PTCA restenosis: dependence on the lesion substrate. Thromb Haemost. 1995;74:552–9.
2. Schwartz RS. Drug-eluting stents in preclinical studies: recommended evaluation from a Consensus Group. Circulation. 2002;106:1867–73.
3. Shinke T, Li J, Chen JP, et al. High incidence of intramural thrombus after overlapping paclitaxel-eluting stent implantation: angioscopic and histopathologic analysis in porcine coronary arteries. Circ Cardiovasc Interv. 2008;1:28–35.
4. Kotani J, Awata M, Nanto S, et al. Incomplete neointimal coverage of sirolimus-eluting stents: angioscopic findings. J Am Coll Cardiol. 2006;47:2108–11.
5. Grewe PH, Deneke T, Machraoui A, Barmeyer J, Muller KM. Acute and chronic tissue response to coronary stent implantation: pathologic findings in human specimen. J Am Coll Cardiol. 2000;35:157–63.
6. Komatsu R, Ueda M, Naruko T, Kojima A, Becker AE. Neointimal tissue response at sites of coronary stenting in humans: macroscopic, histological, and immunohistochemical analyses. Circulation. 1998;98:224–33.
7. Ueda Y, Nanto S, Komamura K, Kodama K. Neointimal coverage of stents in human coronary arteries observed by angioscopy. J Am Coll Cardiol. 1994;23:341–6.
8. Takano M, Ohba T, Inami S, Seimiya K, Sakai S, Mizuno K. Angioscopic differences in neointimal coverage and in persistence of thrombus between sirolimus-eluting stents and bare metal stents after a 6-month implantation. Eur Heart J. 2006;27:2189–95.
9. Sakai S, Mizumo K, Yokoyama S, et al. Morphologic changes in infarct-related plaque after coronary stent placement. A serial angioscopy study. J Am Coll Cardiol. 2003;42:1558–65.
10. Yokoyama S, Takano M, Sakai S, et al. Difference in neointimal proliferation between ruptured and non-ruptured segments after bare metal stent implantation. Int Heart J. 2010;51:7–12.
11. Hamm CW, Bassand JP, Agewall S, et al. ESC Guidelines for the management of acute coronary syndromes in patients presenting without persistent ST-segment elevation: the task force for the management of acute coronary syndromes (ACS) in patients presenting without persistent ST-segment elevation of the European Society of Cardiology (ESC). Eur Heart J. 2011;32:2999–3054.
12. Murakami D, Takano M, Yamamoto M, et al. Novel neointimal formation over sirolimus-eluting stents identified by coronary angioscopy and optical coherence tomography. J Cardiol. 2009;53:311–13.
13. Inoue T, Shinke T, Otake H, et al. Neoatherosclerosis and mural thrombus detection after sirolimus-eluting stent implantation. Circ J Off J Jpn Circ Soc. 2013;78:92–100.
14. Asakura M, Ueda Y, Nanto S, et al. Remodeling of in-stent neointima, which became thinner and transparent over 3 years: serial angiographic and angioscopic follow-up. Circulation. 1998;97:2003–6.

15. Kimura T. Long-term clinical and angiographic follow-up after coronary stent placement in native coronary arteries. Circulation. 2002;105:2986–91.
16. Robinson KA, Roubin G, King S, Siegel R, Rodgers G, Apkarian RP. Correlated microscopic observations of arterial responses to intravascular stenting. Scanning Microsc. 1989;3:665–78; discussion 678–9.
17. Yokoyama S, Takano M, Yamamoto M, et al. Extended follow-up by serial angioscopic observation for bare-metal stents in native coronary arteries: from healing response to atherosclerotic transformation of neointima. Circ Cardiovasc Interv. 2009;2:205–12.
18. Nakazawa G, Otsuka F, Nakano M, et al. The pathology of neoatherosclerosis in human coronary implants bare-metal and drug-eluting stents. J Am Coll Cardiol. 2011;57:1314–22.
19. Chen MS, John JM, Chew DP, Lee DS, Ellis SG, Bhatt DL. Bare metal stent restenosis is not a benign clinical entity. Am Heart J. 2006;151:1260–4.

Chapter 15
Coronary Angioscopic Insights into Several Drug-Eluting Stents of Different Platforms

Masaki Awata and Masaaki Uematsu

Abstract Several drug-eluting stents (DESs) of different platforms have been approved in the world, and comparisons of clinical outcomes with these <u>DESs</u> have raised much interest among coronary interventionists. Next-generation DESs have dramatically reduced the incidences of clinical events, especially late and very late stent thrombosis, which made it difficult to assess the safety thereof in a clinical study. On the other hand, coronary angioscopy allows the qualitative or semiquantitative assessment of arterial healing after *DES* implantation in patients with coronary artery disease.

In Japan, many investigators have already accumulated much coronary angioscopic evidence. Furthermore, those angioscopic studies have provided a great deal of information useful for the safe and effective use of DESs.

In this chapter, we present differences in angioscopic findings among several DESs of different platforms. Based on these findings, in addition, we also refer to technological innovations that are required for the future development of next-generation DESs.

Keywords Drug-eluting stent • Neointimal coverage • Late and very late stent thrombosis

15.1 Introduction

The advent of drug-eluting stents (DESs) substantially reduced the incidence of in-stent restenosis (ISR)—considered as the "Achilles tendon" of percutaneous coronary intervention (PCI). Instead of ISR, however, stent thrombosis subsequent to 1 month after implantation (late and very late stent thrombosis, LVLST) emerged

M. Awata, M.D., Ph.D. (✉)
Department of Advanced Cardiovascular Therapeutics, Osaka University Graduate School of Medicine, 2-2 Yamadaoka, Suita, Osaka 565-0871, Japan
e-mail: masaki@awata.jp

M. Uematsu, M.D., Ph.D., F.A.C.C.
Kansai Rosai Hospital Cardiovascular Center, 3-1-69 Inabaso, Amagasaki, Hyogo 660-8511, Japan

© Springer Japan 2015
K. Mizuno, M. Takano (eds.), *Coronary Angioscopy*,
DOI 10.1007/978-4-431-55546-9_15

as a new issue to be addressed. Several factors are considered to be involved in the pathogenesis of LVLST, among which incomplete neointimal coverage (NIC) and delayed reendothelialization are considered as its etiologies. Coronary angioscopy (CAS) is superior in qualitatively assessing the aspects of NIC at the site of DES implantation and also allows the detection of a microthrombus and a yellow plaque. Namely, CAS permits the qualitative assessment of a diversity of arterial healing processes after stent implantation that can never be captured by other intracoronary imaging modalities. We are willing to describe, based on findings obtained to date by CAS after DES implantation, the technological innovations that are required to develop next-generation DESs in the future.

15.2 Coronary Angioscopic Assessment of Arterial Healing After Stent Implantation

A variety of intravascular ultrasound (IVUS) studies have investigated arterial healing after bare-metal stent (BMS) implantation, especially neointimal proliferation at the site of stent implantation. However, the neointima became difficult to be identified by the IVUS observation of the implantation site of DESs that has potent neointimal proliferation-inhibitory activity. On the other hand, CAS of the relevant site allows the observation of various grades of NIC. We used the four-grade angioscopic scale to objectively assess the aspects of the neointima after stent implantation. NIC grades were defined as follows: grade 0, stent struts fully visible, similar to immediately after implantation; grade 1, stent struts bulged into the lumen and, although covered, were still transparently visible; grade 2, stent struts were embedded by the neointima but were seen translucently; and grade 3, stent struts fully embedded and invisible on coronary angioscopic images (Fig. 15.1) [1, 2]. In DESs except the paclitaxel-eluting stent (Taxus-PES), consequently, the

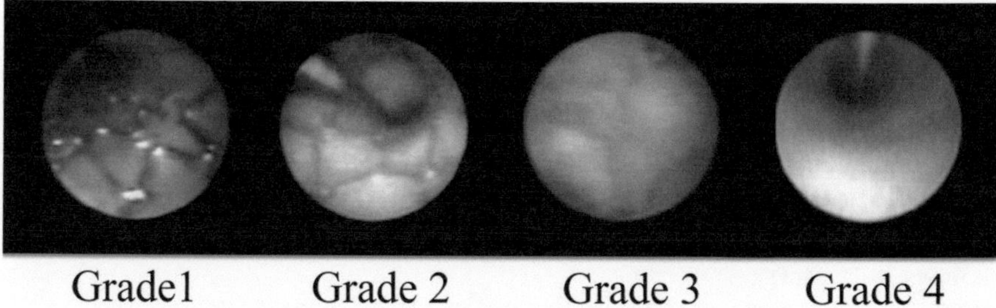

Fig. 15.1 Definitions of neointimal coverage grades. Neointimal coverage grades were defined as follows: grade 0, stent struts fully visible, similar to immediately after implantation; grade 1, stent struts bulged into the lumen and, although covered, were still transparently visible; grade 2, stent struts were embedded by the neointima but were seen translucently; grade 3, stent struts fully embedded and invisible on coronary (Reproduced with permission from the American College of Cardiology, partially modified [4])

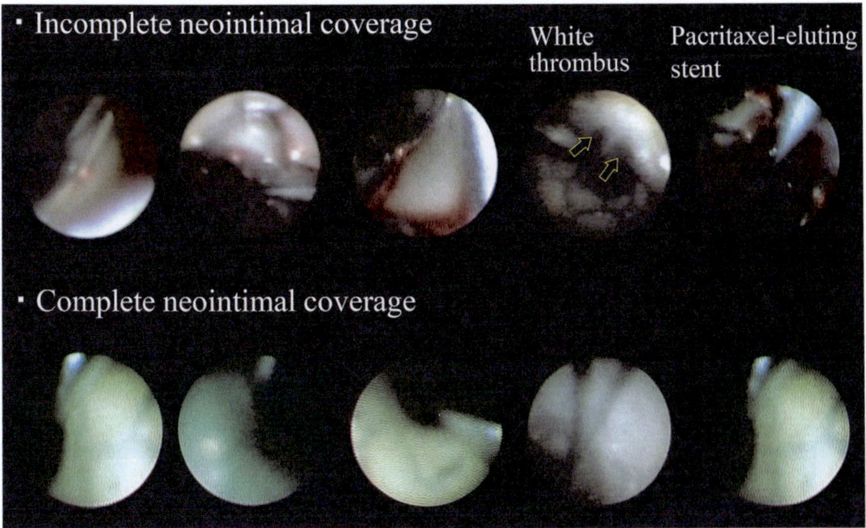

Fig. 15.2 Images of thrombi detected by coronary angioscopy. The *upper* images show thrombi adhering to the site of incomplete neointimal coverage (i.e., grade 0/1). The *lower* images show complete neointimal coverage (i.e., grade 2/3). Thrombus adhesion to the complete neointima is rare. White thrombi in Cypher-SES are indicated with open *yellow arrows*. Of note is the fact that thrombi observed with Taxus-PES in the *upper-right* panel show the extended areas of adhesion as compared with Cypher-SES. *SES* sirolimus-eluting stent, *PES* paclitaxel-eluting stent (Reproduced with permission from Medialpha (Coronary Intervention vol. 9, no. 1), partially modified)

incidence of thrombus adhesion was significantly higher at the site of NIC "grade 0/1 (incomplete NIC)" as compared with the site of NIC "grade 2/3 (complete NIC)" (Fig. 15.2) [3–8]. This fact leads us to expect that NIC grades as determined by CAS potentially enable the prediction of impaired reendothelialization. Mitsutake et al. conducted CAS and assessed vascular response by using acetylcholine at 9 months after first-generation DES implantation and reported the association between stents, whose incomplete NIC (i.e., grade 0/1) was dominant, and the presence of endothelial dysfunction [9].

The grades of not only NIC but also reendothelialization need to be determined to assess arterial healing because endothelial coverage rather than NIC is the goal after stent implantation. The presence or absence of endothelial cells is difficult to be assessed by CAS. As described above, nevertheless, CAS allows the indirect assessment of reendothelialization through the evaluation of NIC grade and thrombus adhesion. Finn et al. described that incomplete NIC, which is morphometrically quantified with the ratio of uncovered to total stent struts per section, is the most powerful morphologic surrogate indicator of endothelialization [10]. CAS is also a useful tool for evaluating the intravascular conditions at the site of abnormal vascular response after DES implantation, as typified by the peri-stent contrast staining [11].

15.3   Coronary Angioscopic Findings After Sirolimus-Eluding Stent (Cypher-SES) Implantation

A large number of studies are available that have reported on the first-generation DESs including Cypher-SES. We used the abovementioned grades of NIC to compare dominant NIC at 3–6 months after the implantation of Cypher-SES and BMS. Consequently, all 22 BMSs had complete NIC (grade 2/3) in contrast to Cypher-SES, in 87 % of which incomplete NIC (grade 0/1) was rated as dominant NIC (Fig. 15.3) [2]. Namely, the images of CAS were remarkably different between BMS and Cypher-SES. Furthermore, we observed time-course changes in NIC grades up to 2 years after Cypher-SES implantation. In consequence, we found no changes in NIC grades at 4 months to 1 year after implantation. Although a minority of Cypher-SES showed NIC grade progression at 1–2 years after implantation, 71 % of implanted Cypher-SES showed NIC grade 1 still at 2 years after implantation (Fig. 15.4) [3]. We found yellow plaques in 71 % of Cypher-SES at 4 months after implantation and observed the plaques also at 2 years after implantation. Takano

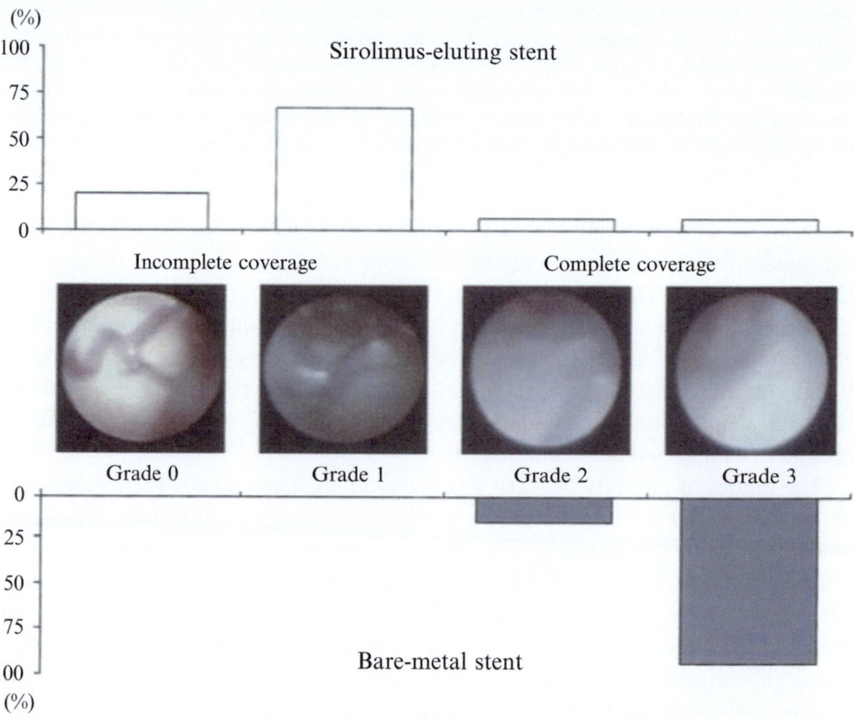

Fig. 15.3 Distributions of dominant neointimal coverage grades at 3–6 months after the implantation of BMS and SES. Neointimal coverage was more complete with bare-metal stent compared than with the sirolimus-eluting stent ($P < 0.000$). *BMS* bare-metal stent, *SES* sirolimus-eluting stent (Reproduced with permission from the American College of Cardiology [2])

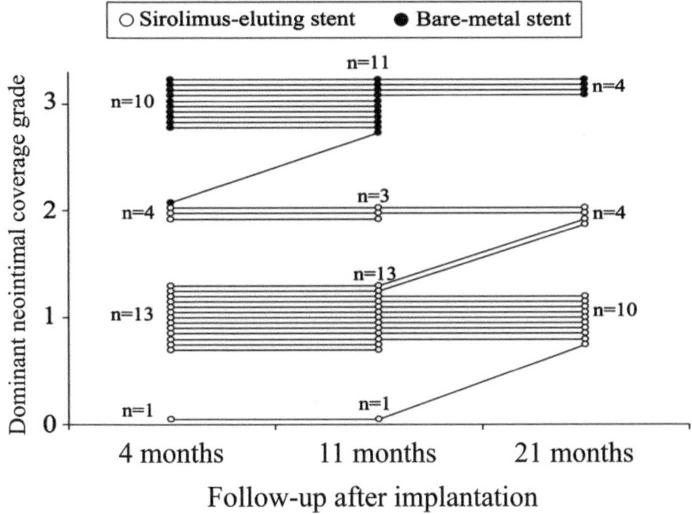

Fig. 15.4 Serial changes in neointimal coverage grades in 17 SESs and 11 BMSs. Seventy-six percent of SES showed NIC grade 1, while 91 % of BMS showed NIC grade 3 at the first follow-up. NIC grade 3 was noted with BMS at all follow-ups except for 1 stent that showed NIC grade 2. In contrast, the lower grades (0–2) of NIC were noted with SES. SES showed no increases in NIC grades at the second and third follow-ups. However, 3 SES showed one-grade increases in NIC grades at the third follow-up. *SES* sirolimus-eluting stent, *NIC* neointimal coverage, *BMS* bare-metal stent, *open circle*, SES ($n = 17$); *solid circle*, BMS ($n = 11$) (Reproduced with permission from American Heart Association, partially modified [3])

et al. also observed time-course changes in 20 Cypher-SES and found both 20 % of Cypher-SES uncovered and subclinical thrombus formation in 30 % of the Cypher-SES at 2 years after implantation [12]. It is very rare to find thrombus adhesion at the site of BMS implantation at this stage [13]. Furthermore, Oyabu et al. reported that thrombus adhesion after Cypher-SES implantation was found predominantly at the site where a substent yellow plaque was present [14]. Yellow plaques with thrombus seem to be more vulnerable than those without thrombus [15].

Pathological research has reported long-term incomplete reendothelialization by Cypher-SES [16] and inflammation induced by its polymer [17]. It is known that neoatherosclerosis progression is accelerated at the site of Cypher-SES implantation in association with these changes; this event is also considered as one of the contributing factors for LVLST [18]. The rapid progression of a yellow plaque underneath the stent struts and the presence of the yellow neointima on the stent were considered as the angioscopic manifestations of this event [19]. Attempts (e.g., employment of a highly biocompatible polymer) are being made to solve these issues in the development of next-generation DESs. The comparison of angioscopic findings between Cypher-SES and other DESs is useful for the assessment not only of arterial healing after DES implantation but also of these issues.

15.4 Can Cypher-SES Implantation Achieve the Plaque-Sealing Effect?

An intracoronary plaque with a more intense yellow tone is considered to involve a higher risk of developing acute coronary syndromes (ACS) because of the thinner fibrous cap covering lipid components [20]. The neointima formed after BMS implantation covers not only the stent but also the yellow plaque and thrombus that are present underneath the stent. The plaque present at the site of stent implantation is considered stabilized by this coverage as if being a plaque that is covered with a thick fibrous cap; this is called the plaque-sealing effect [21]. In fact, a study on the 5-year clinical outcomes of BMS-implanted patients with respect to the incidence of clinical events (death, myocardial infarction, revascularization, heart failure, or hospitalization for ACS), which were attributed to the implantation than non-implantation sites of BMS, described that the incidence was higher at the non-implantation site of BMS than at the implanted site of BMS at 1 or more years after implantation—the stage later than the phase of predilection for ISR [22]; we consider the involvement of the plaque-sealing effect after BMS implantation in this observation. Cypher-SES was successful in reducing the incidence of ISR by the suppression of neointimal proliferation but probably does not allow us to expect the plaque-sealing effect as suggested by coronary angioscopic findings. When Cypher-SES is implanted in a lipid-rich plaque and a ruptured plaque becomes bulged into the lumen, this highly thrombogenic plaque involves the risk of being uncovered by the neointima and consequently being exposed to the blood flow for a long time; this event is also considered as a contributing factor for LVLST. An observational study using Cypher-SES, which lasted as long as 5 years, described that the annual incidences of LVLST did not decrease with time, reaching 0.33 % [23]. Furthermore, an angioscopic study, which observed time-course changes in NIC at the stage later than 5 years after Cypher-SES implantation, indicated the persistence of incomplete NIC and subclinical thrombosis [24]. Delayed arterial healing as observed by CAS cannot be necessarily considered as a direct cause of LVLST [25]. However, we consider it essential to provide the long-term careful monitoring of Cypher-SES-implanted patients. In fact, we encountered a patient who developed very late stent thrombosis (VLST) at 5 years after Cypher-SES implantation, in whom we considered the uncovered stent struts as the main cause of VLST based on findings from CAS and optical coherence tomography [26].

15.5 Coronary Angioscopic Findings After Paclitaxel-Eluting Stent (Taxus-PES) Implantation

Taxus-PES, which became clinically applicable subsequently to Cypher-SES, showed a slightly greater in-stent late loss than that of Cypher-SES. We conducted CAS at 8 months after the implantation of 30 Taxus-PESs and compared them with

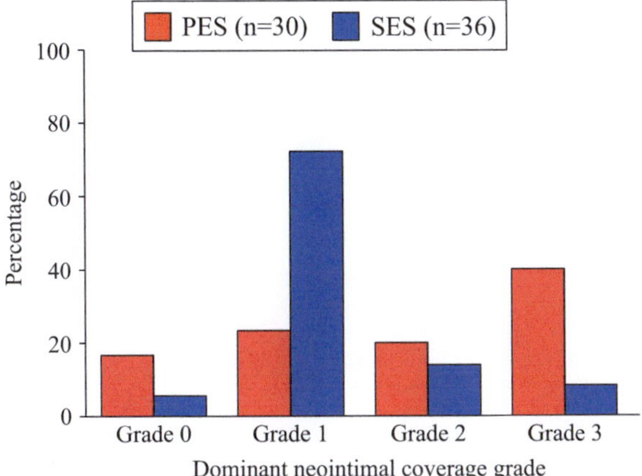

Fig. 15.5 Distributions of dominant neointimal coverage grades at 8 months after the implantation of PES and SES. Although 72 % of SES showed dominant NIC grade 1, PES showed the extended distributions of NIC grades. PES vs. SES, $P = 0.0006$ by chi-square test. *SES* sirolimus-eluting stent, *NIC* neointimal coverage, *PES* paclitaxel-eluting stent (Reproduced with permission from the American College of Cardiology [5])

36 Cypher-SESs. Consequently, the majority of Cypher-SES indicated NIC grade 1 in contrast to Taxus-PES, 40 % of which indicated NIC grade 3; NIC grades 0–2 were equally distributed in the remaining Taxus-PES (Fig. 15.5) [5]. As a characteristic finding, furthermore, Taxus-PES frequently exhibited heterogeneous NIC—the concomitant presence of different NIC grades—within the same stent. Takano et al. had previously pointed up the heterogeneous neointimal growth inside Cypher-SES [12]. We found the relevant heterogeneity in 47 % of Cypher-SES. In contrast, 74 % of Taxus-PES exhibited heterogeneous NIC; two-grade NIC differences were found in 26 % of this subgroup of Taxus-PES (Figs. 15.6 and 15.7) [5]. Thus, Taxus-PES indicated the high heterogeneity not only of dominant NIC among the stents but also of NIC within the same stents. Other investigators have also reported on this heterogeneous neointimal formation [6, 27]. The fact that paclitaxel has a narrow therapeutic window has been mentioned as a cause of heterogeneous neointimal formation. Namely, we consider that the profile of the drug—the potent suppression of neointimal proliferation by a high local concentration of paclitaxel and the insufficient suppression of the proliferation by a low local concentration of the drug—resulted to appear in a salient manner. We found the equivalent detection rates of yellow plaques (83 % and 78 % for Taxus-PES and Cypher-SES, respectively; $P = 0.76$) and the rather higher incidence of thrombus adhesion (43 % and 19 % for Taxus-PES and Cypher-SES, respectively; $P = 0.04$) [5]. Of particular note, furthermore, Cypher-SES showed thrombi that were mural, small, and localized. In contrast, Taxus-PES notably exhibited thrombi that extended more broadly as compared with Cypher-SES (Fig. 15.2). The follow-up assessments of serial CAS at 6 and 18 months after Taxus-PES implantation

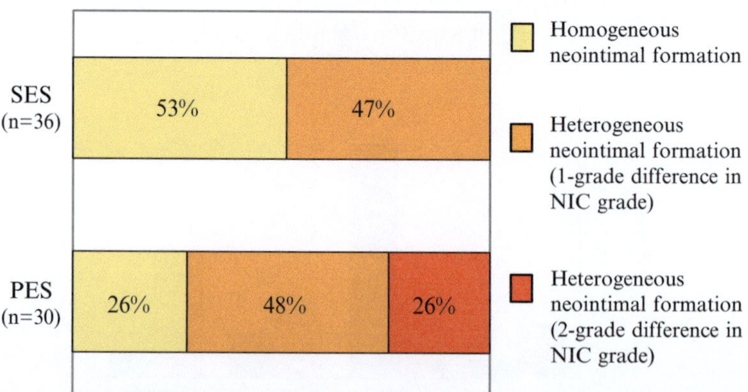

Fig. 15.6 Coronary angioscopically assessed homogeneous and heterogeneous neointimal formation of PES and SES. Forty-seven percent of SES showed the heterogeneous neointimal formation that was coronary angioscopically assessed as one-grade difference in NIC grade. Fifty-three percent demonstrated the homogeneity of NIC. In contrast, 74 % of PES showed heterogeneous NIC, 48 % showed one-grade difference in NIC grade, and 26 % showed two-grade difference in NIC grade. PES vs. SES, $P = 0.002$ by chi-square test. *SES* sirolimus-eluting stent, *NIC* neointimal coverage, *PES* paclitaxel-eluting stent (Reproduced with permission from the American College of Cardiology [5])

described the persistence of thrombus adhesion [28]. The significance of thrombus adhesion that is a characteristic of Taxus-PES is unknown. However, we deem it necessary to provide careful follow-up also for Taxus- or PES-implanted patients.

15.6 Coronary Angioscopic Findings After Zotarolimus-Eluting Stent (Endeavor-ZES) Implantation

Endeavor-ZES is a DES that has shown the greatest value of late loss among DESs ever examined. A foreign clinical study using Endeavor-ZES showed a late loss value of about 0.6 mm [29], and Endeavor-ZES has a greater incidence of target lesion revascularization (TLR) as compared with Cypher-SES [30]. Therefore, Endeavor-ZES turned to be a DES not for active use in the clinical settings. Nevertheless, we conjecture that Endeavor-ZES may indicate distinctive arterial healing because of its great late loss in comparison with other DESs. Hence, we conducted CAS in patients implanted with 14 Endeavor-ZES at 8 months after implantation. Consequently, 10 (71 %) and 4 (29 %) Endeavor-ZES exhibited NIC grade 3 and grade 2, respectively (Figs. 15.8 and 15.9). Furthermore, a yellow plaque and thrombus adhesion were observed only with 2 (14 %) and 1 (7 %), respectively [4]. Thus, Endeavor-ZES indicated findings similar to those of BMS. Furthermore, dominant NIC grade showed similar distributions at both 4 and 8 months after

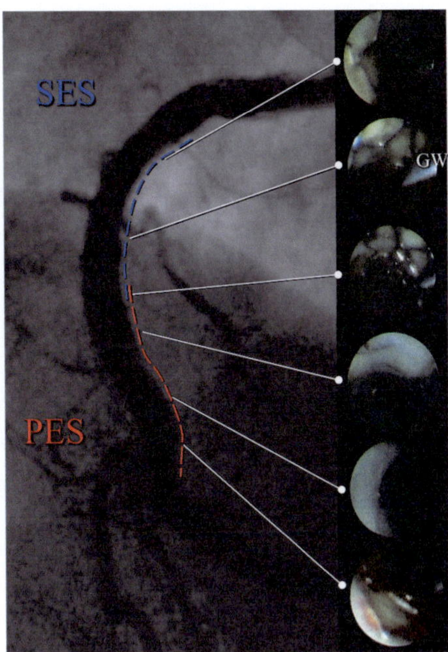

Fig. 15.7 Coronary angiograms and angioscopic images at 8 months after the tandem implantation of SES and PES. Coronary angiograms at follow-up revealed no restenosis at the segment of SES (3.5 mm × 23 mm) and PES (3.5 mm × 24 mm) implanted in tandem. The angioscopic images of SES showed the homogeneous neointimal formation angioscopically assessed as NIC grade 1. In contrast, PES showed the heterogeneous neointimal formation that was angioscopically assessed as two-grade difference in NIC grade; dominant NIC was grade 2 in PES; the distal segment showed NIC grade 0, with mural red thrombi adhered to yellow plaques and the naked stent struts. *SES* sirolimus-eluting stent, *PES* paclitaxel-eluting stent, *NIC* neointimal coverage. *Dashed blue line* = SES implantation site, *dashed red line* = PES implantation site. GW = guide wire (Reproduced with permission from the American College of Cardiology [5])

Endeavor-ZES implantation [8]. Studies have described that Endeavor-ZES, which allows the early achievement of complete NIC, also permits the attainment of early reendothelialization [31, 32]. Our previous study [8] supported the results from a study demonstrating that Endeavor-ZES enabled the shift from dual to single antiplatelet therapy at as early as 3 months after implantation and that the incidence of late stent thrombosis did not increase thereafter [33, 34]. We consider, based on coronary angioscopic findings, that Endeavor-ZES is a potential option to substitute BMS in high-risk patients for long-term dual antiplatelet therapy (DAPT).

We described above that arteriosclerosis progressed early at the site of Cypher-SES implantation and that the yellow tone of plaque intensified at the site of Cypher-SES implantation. Akazawa et al. reported that a yellow plaque underneath Endeavor-ZES was covered with the white thick neointima at the site of implantation [35]. This finding may hold promise for the plaque-sealing effect of Endeavor-ZES by means of NIC.

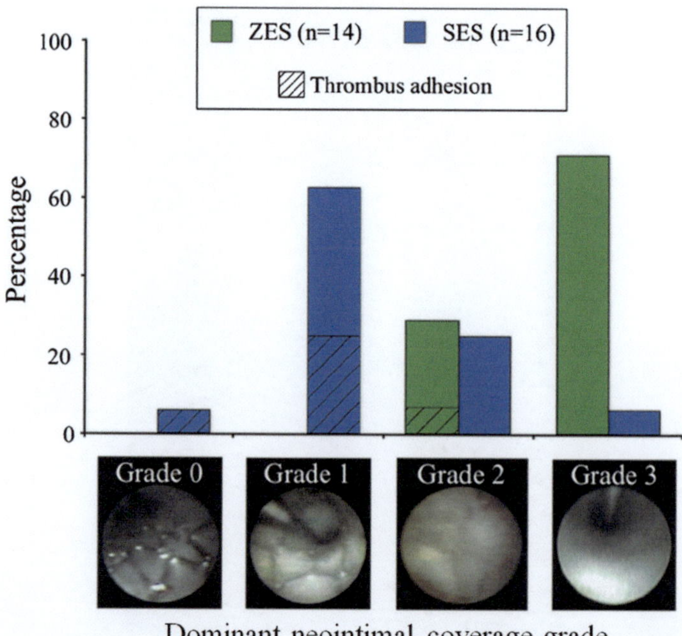

Fig. 15.8 Coronary angioscopic classification of neointimal coverage at 8 months after the implantation of ZES and SES. Seventy-one percent of ZES showed NIC grade 3, while 6 % of SES showed NIC grade 3. Neither grade 0 nor grade 1 was found with ZES. The *shadowed portion* indicates the incidence of thrombus adhesion. ZES vs. SES, $P = 0.0004$. *ZES* zotarolimus-eluting stent, *NIC* neointimal coverage, *SES* sirolimus-eluting stent (Reproduced with permission from the American College of Cardiology [4])

Endeavor-ZES has a higher TLR rate than that of first-generation DESs at 1 year after their implantation but is significantly lower than that of BMS [36]. Namely, we consider that Endeavor-ZES—which allows good arterial healing and a plaque-sealing effect at 4 months after implantation [8]—would have its particular existence value as, daringly to say, a "potent BMS" rather than as a DES with potent neointimal proliferation-inhibitory activity.

15.7 Coronary Angioscopic Findings After Biolimus-Eluting Stent (Nobori-BES) Implantation

Pathological research on Cypher-SES pointed out the potential induction of hypersensitivity reaction of the vessel walls to its polymer [17], which drove emphasis not only on drug class and stent design but also on polymer biocompatibility in the development of next-generation DESs. Therefore, Nobori-BES employed a

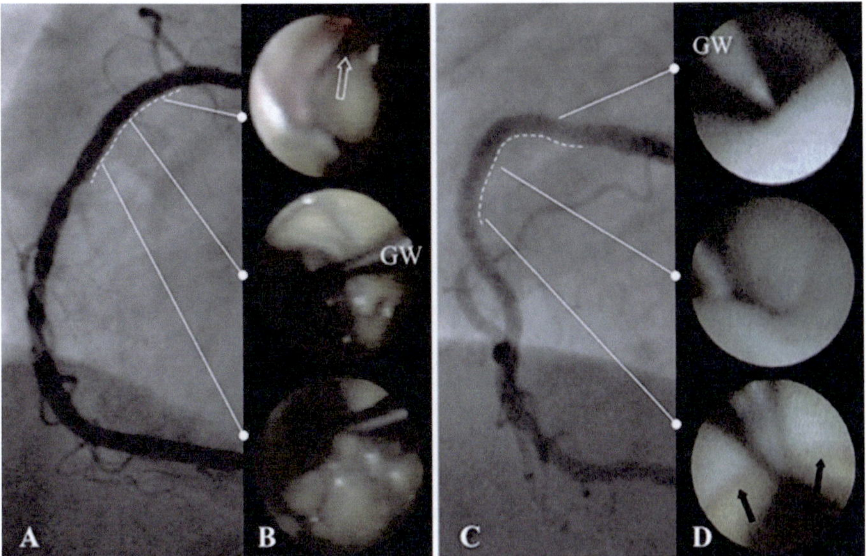

Fig. 15.9 Coronary angioscopic images at 8 months after the implantation of SES and ZES. The *left* panels (**a, b**) show a SES (3.5 mm × 23 mm), and the *right* panels (**c, d**) show a ZES (3.5 mm × 23 mm), both implanted at the proximal portion of the right coronary artery (**a, c**). Follow-up angiograms revealed no restenosis (**b**). The coronary angioscopic images of SES indicated NIC grade 1 along the entire segment of the stent, with mural red thrombus adhesion to the proximal end of the stent. Furthermore, yellow plaques were observed underneath the stent (the entire segment of the stent implanted in the vascular wall was yellow) (**d**). In contrast, ZES showed NIC grade 3 along its entire segment. Yellow plaques were present in the distal native coronary artery adjacent to the distal end of the stent. The vascular wall showed mild yellow saturation, while the stent was covered with the white-gray neointima showing no yellow plaques (**d**, *bottom image*). *SES* sirolimus-eluting stent; *ZES* zotarolimus-eluting stent; *NIC* neointimal coverage; *open arrow*, mural red thrombus; *solid arrow*, boundary line of NIC; *GW* guide wire (Reproduced with permission from the American College of Cardiology [4])

biodegradable polymer (polylactic acid). Furthermore, Nobori-BES is coated with its drug and polymer only on the surface in contact with the vessel walls (abluminal coating). The angioscopic observation of the stent interior at 8 months after Nobori-BES implantation revealed the more homogeneous NIC of the stent as compared with Cypher-SES (Fig. 15.10) [7]. Despite showing a small value of angiographic late loss as does Cypher-SES, Nobori-BES exhibited more homogeneous NIC. We speculate that the absence of drug coating on the surface in contact with the lumen may be mentioned as one of the reasons for this observation. Nevertheless, Nobori-BES also showed the distributions of most dominant NIC among the stents that did not largely differ from those of Cypher-SES, with great distribution biases (Fig. 15.11) [7].

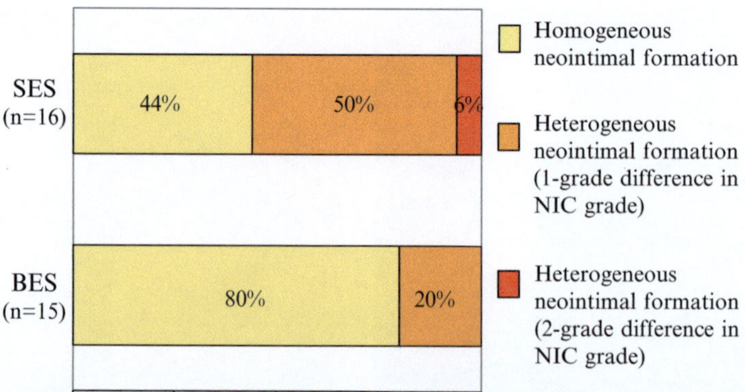

Fig. 15.10 Coronary angioscopically assessed homogeneous and heterogeneous neointimal formation of BES and SES. Eighty percent of BES showed homogeneous neointimal formation. The remaining 20 % of BES had heterogeneous neointimal formation that was coronary angioscopically assessed as a one-grade difference in NIC grade. In contrast, 56 % of SES demonstrated heterogeneous neointimal formation. *BES* biolimus-eluting stent, *SES* sirolimus-eluting stent (Reproduced with permission from the Japanese Circulation Society [7])

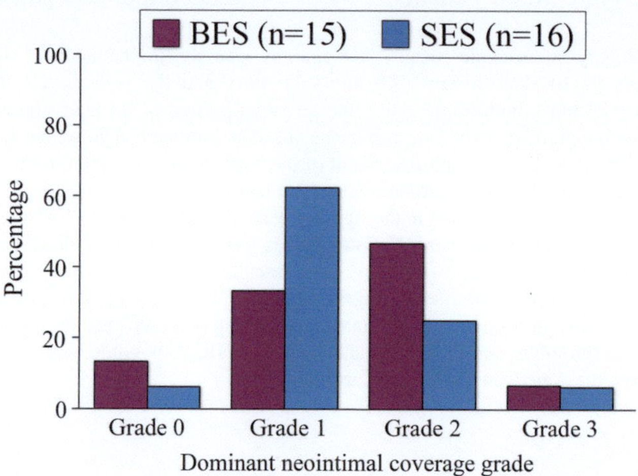

Fig. 15.11 Distributions of dominant neointimal coverage grades at 8 months after the implantation of BES and SES. Sixty-three percent of SES showed dominant NIC grade 1, while 47 % of BES showed dominant NIC grade 2. BES vs. SES, $P = 0.42$ by chi-square test. *SES* sirolimus-eluting stent, *NIC* neointimal coverage, *BES* biolimus-eluting stent (Reproduced with permission from the Japanese Circulation Society, partially modified [7])

15.8 Coronary Angioscopic Findings After Everolimus-Eluting Stent (Xience-EES) Implantation

Xience-EES has strut thickness as thin as 88 μm in comparison with other DESs mentioned above and also employs a biocompatible fluoropolymer. Therefore, Xience-EES holds promise for good arterial healing after implantation. There are

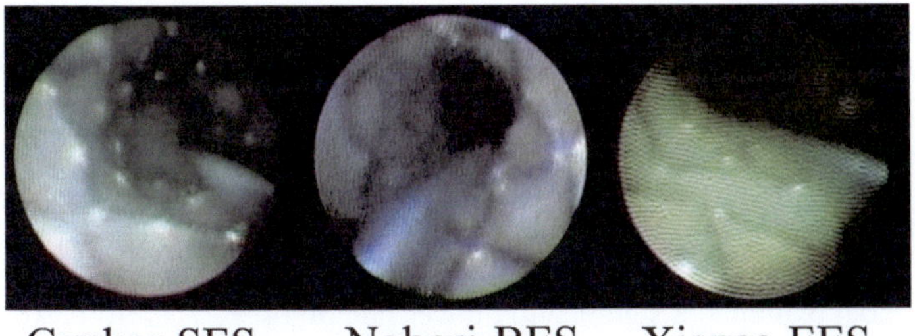

Fig. 15.12 Strut bulge into the lumen of SES, BES, and EES showing neointimal coverage grade 1. The strut bulge into the lumen is less pronounced for Xience-EES with the thin struts than for Cypher-SES and Nobori-BES with the thicker stent struts, although all these drug-eluting stents similarly indicate NIC grade 1. *EES* everolimus-eluting stent, *SES* sirolimus-eluting stent, *BES* biolimus-eluting stent, *NIC* neointimal coverage (Reproduced with permission from Medialpha (Coronary Intervention vol. 9, no. 1), partially modified)

two angioscopic studies using Xience-EES and Cypher-SES that have examined and compared NIC grades at 8 months after implantation [37, 38]. Regarding dominant NIC, these studies showed no significant difference in the distributions of NIC grades between Xience-EES and Cypher-SES. However, thrombus adhesion is considered to occur less frequently with Xience-EES than with Cypher-SES. Furthermore, Dai et al. described the low detection rate of a yellow plaque at the site of Xience-EES implantation as compared with Cypher-SES [37]. Akazawa et al. conducted CAS at 1 year after Xience-EES implantation and did not find any intensified yellow tone of plaque in comparison with the plaque observed at the time of stent implantation, as found with Cypher-SES [35]. The lower incidence of thrombus adhesion suggests the achievement of good reendothelialization, while the presence of a less yellow plaque holds promise for solving the issue of neoatherosclerosis. Figure 15.12 shows the angioscopic images of Cypher-SES, Nobori-BES, and Xience-EES that were assessed to be grade 1. Although being the same low-grade NIC, thinning of strut thickness makes the strut bulge into the lumen less pronounced with Xience-EES than with the other stents. This contributes to a reduction in turbulence around the struts [39] and to the achievement of reendothelialization. Thin strut thickness may be one of the reasons why thrombus adhesion after stent implantation occurs less frequently with Xience-EES than with Cypher-SES [39].

15.9   Optimal Implantation of DESs Based on Coronary Angioscopic Findings

Whether or not better arterial healing can be achieved by PCI maneuvers at the time of stent implantation constitutes a therapeutic issue to be addressed. For this purpose, we examined the association between IVUS findings after Cypher-SES implantation and coronary angioscopic findings obtained at the time of follow-up coronary angiography [40]. Regarding the relevant coronary angioscopic findings, we compared the stent expansion indexes at the time of stent implantation between the groups of NIC grades 0/1 and 2/3. Consequently, the latter group showed the significantly greater stent expansion indexes (minimum stent area-to-reference vessel area ratios) [40]. Cypher-SES with a stent expansion index of ≥ 0.4 showed the NIC grade 2/3 a rate of 57 % at the chronic stage, while Cypher-SES with an index of <0.4 exhibited a significantly lower rate of 14 %. Therefore, we consider that the IVUS-guided implantation of DESs, in consideration of "optimal stent expansion" and for the objective of attaining good NIC is one of the means to achieve good arterial healing.

15.10 Technological Innovations Required for the Future Development of Next-Generation DESs

Coronary angioscopic studies have demonstrated that the drug-induced, excessive suppression of neointimal formation and reendothelialization concurrently involves the risk of provoking incomplete NIC and neoatherosclerosis [19], apart from the suppression of stent restenosis. Concerning the next-generation DESs, this issue can be addressed by assessing the incidence of thrombus adhesion, the intensification of yellow tone of a plaque underneath the stent struts, and the presence or absence of the yellow neointima. Furthermore, the coronary angioscopic observations of Endeavor-ZES have revealed that DESs leading to the formation of the neointima of appropriate thickness hold promise for the plaque-sealing effect [4, 35]. We consider that the heterogeneous neointimal formation by Taxus-PES [5] and the homogeneous neointimal formation by Nobori-BES [7] hide the clues for the achievement of the homogenous neointimal formation by next-generation DESs to be developed. Angioscopic findings suggested that the thin strut platform, which Xience-EES employed, induced better arterial healing as compared with DESs of thick strut platform. As mentioned above, these findings will greatly contribute to the future development of next-generation DESs.

References

1. Awata M, Kotani J, Nanto S, Uematsu M, Morozumi T, Hori M, Nagata S. Sustained attenuation of neointimal coverage over the stent following brachytherapy for in-stent restenosis: angioscopic findings. Circ J. 2006;70(7):846–50.
2. Kotani J, Awata M, Nanto S, Uematsu M, Oshima F, Minamiguchi H, Mintz GS, Nagata S. Incomplete neointimal coverage of sirolimus-eluting stents: angioscopic findings. J Am Coll Cardiol. 2006;47(10):2108–11. doi:10.1016/j.jacc.2005.11.092.
3. Awata M, Kotani J, Uematsu M, Morozumi T, Watanabe T, Onishi T, Iida O, Sera F, Nanto S, Hori M, Nagata S. Serial angioscopic evidence of incomplete neointimal coverage after sirolimus-eluting stent implantation: comparison with bare-metal stents. Circulation. 2007;116(8):910–16. doi:10.1161/CIRCULATIONAHA.105.609057.

4. Awata M, Nanto S, Uematsu M, Morozumi T, Watanabe T, Onishi T, Iida O, Sera F, Kotani J, Hori M, Nagata S. Angioscopic comparison of neointimal coverage between zotarolimus- and sirolimus-eluting stents. J Am Coll Cardiol. 2008;52(9):789–90. doi:10.1016/j.jacc.2008. 07.007.

5. Awata M, Nanto S, Uematsu M, Morozumi T, Watanabe T, Onishi T, Iida O, Sera F, Minamiguchi H, Kotani J, Nagata S. Heterogeneous arterial healing in patients following paclitaxel-eluting stent implantation: comparison with sirolimus-eluting stents. J Am Coll Cardiol Intv. 2009;2(5):453–8. doi:10.1016/j.jcin.2009.03.005.

6. Takano M, Yamamoto M, Murakami D, Inami S, Okamatsu K, Seimiya K, Ohba T, Seino Y, Mizuno K. Lack of association between large angiographic late loss and low risk of in-stent thrombus: angioscopic comparison between paclitaxel- and sirolimus-eluting stents. Circ Cardiovasc Interv. 2008;1(1):20–7. doi:10.1161/CIRCINTERVENTIONS.108.769448.

7. Awata M, Uematsu M, Sera F, Ishihara T, Watanabe T, Fujita M, Onishi T, Iida O, Ishida Y, Nanto S, Nagata S. Angioscopic assessment of arterial repair following biodegradable polymer-coated biolimus A9-eluting stent implantation. Circ J. 2011;75(5):1113–19. doi:10. 1253/circj.CJ-10-0776.

8. Ishihara T, Awata M, Sera F, Fujita M, Watanabe T, Iida O, Ishida Y, Nanto S, Uematsu M. Arterial repair 4 months after zotarolimus-eluting stent implantation observed on angioscopy. Circ J. 2013;77(5):1186–92. doi:10.1253/circj.CJ-12-1369.

9. Mitsutake Y, Ueno T, Yokoyama S, Sasaki K, Sugi Y, Toyama Y, Koiwaya H, Ohtsuka M, Nakayoshi T, Itaya N, Chibana H, Kakuma T, Imaizumi T. Coronary endothelial dysfunction distal to stent of first-generation drug-eluting stents. J Am Coll Cardiol Intv. 2012;5(9):966–73. doi:10.1016/j.jcin.2012.06.010.

10. Finn AV, Joner M, Nakazawa G, Kolodgie F, Newell J, John MC, Gold HK, Virmani R. Pathological correlates of late drug-eluting stent thrombosis: strut coverage as a marker of endothelialization. Circulation. 2007;115(18):2435–41. doi:10.1161/CIRCULATIONAHA. 107.693739.

11. Ishihara T, Awata M, Fujita M, Watanabe T, Iida O, Ishida Y, Nanto S, Uematsu M. Angio-scopic assessment of peri-stent contrast staining following drug-eluting stent implantation. Circ J. 2014;78(1):122–7. doi:10.1253/circj.CJ-13-0464.

12. Takano M, Yamamoto M, Xie Y, Murakami D, Inami S, Okamatsu K, Seimiya K, Ohba T, Seino Y, Mizuno K. Serial long-term evaluation of neointimal stent coverage and thrombus after sirolimus-eluting stent implantation by use of coronary angioscopy. Heart. 2007;93(12):1533–6. doi:10.1136/hrt.2007.131714.

13. Asakura M, Ueda Y, Nanto S, Hirayama A, Adachi T, Kitakaze M, Hori M, Kodama K. Remodeling of in-stent neointima, which became thinner and transparent over 3 years: serial angiographic and angioscopic follow-up. Circulation. 1998;97(20):2003–6.

14. Oyabu J, Ueda Y, Ogasawara N, Okada K, Hirayama A, Kodama K. Angioscopic evaluation of neointima coverage: sirolimus drug-eluting stent versus bare metal stent. Am Heart J. 2006;152(6):1168–74. doi:10.1016/j.ahj.2006.07.025.

15. Ueda Y, Ohtani T, Shimizu M, Hirayama A, Kodama K. Assessment of plaque vulnerability by angioscopic classification of plaque color. Am Heart J. 2004;148(2):333–5. doi:10.1016/j.ahj. 2004.03.047.

16. Joner M, Finn AV, Farb A, Mont EK, Kolodgie FD, Ladich E, Kutys R, Skorija K, Gold HK, Virmani R. Pathology of drug-eluting stents in humans: delayed healing and late thrombotic risk. J Am Coll Cardiol. 2006;48(1):193–202. doi:10.1016/j.jacc.2006.03.042.

17. Virmani R, Guagliumi G, Farb A, Musumeci G, Grieco N, Motta T, Mihalcsik L, Tespili M, Valsecchi O, Kolodgie FD. Localized hypersensitivity and late coronary thrombosis secondary to a sirolimus-eluting stent: should we be cautious? Circulation. 2004;109(6):701–5. doi:10. 1161/01.CIR.0000116202.41966.D4.

18. Nakazawa G, Otsuka F, Nakano M, Vorpahl M, Yazdani SK, Ladich E, Kolodgie FD, Finn AV, Virmani R. The pathology of neoatherosclerosis in human coronary implants bare-metal and drug-eluting stents. J Am Coll Cardiol. 2011;57(11):1314–22. doi:10.1016/j.jacc.2011.01. 011.

19. Higo T, Ueda Y, Oyabu J, Okada K, Nishio M, Hirata A, Kashiwase K, Ogasawara N, Hirotani S, Kodama K. Atherosclerotic and thrombogenic neointima formed over sirolimus drug-eluting stent: an angioscopic study. J Am Coll Cardiol Img. 2009;2(5):616–24. doi:10.1016/j.jcmg. 2008.12.026.
20. Takano M, Jang IK, Inami S, Yamamoto M, Murakami D, Okamatsu K, Seimiya K, Ohba T, Mizuno K. In vivo comparison of optical coherence tomography and angioscopy for the evaluation of coronary plaque characteristics. Am J Cardiol. 2008;101(4):471–6. doi:10.1016/j.amjcard.2007.09.106.
21. Sakai S, Mizuno K, Yokoyama S, Tanabe J, Shinada T, Seimiya K, Takano M, Ohba T, Tomimura M, Uemura R, Imaizumi T. Morphologic changes in infarct-related plaque after coronary stent placement: a serial angioscopy study. J Am Coll Cardiol. 2003;42(9):1558–65.
22. Cutlip DE, Chhabra AG, Baim DS, Chauhan MS, Marulkar S, Massaro J, Bakhai A, Cohen DJ, Kuntz RE, Ho KK. Beyond restenosis: five-year clinical outcomes from second-generation coronary stent trials. Circulation. 2004;110(10):1226–30. doi:10.1161/01.CIR.0000140721. 27004.4B.
23. Kimura T, Morimoto T, Nakagawa Y, Kawai K, Miyazaki S, Muramatsu T, Shiode N, Namura M, Sone T, Oshima S, Nishikawa H, Hiasa Y, Hayashi Y, Nobuyoshi M, Mitudo K, j-Cypher Registry I. Very late stent thrombosis and late target lesion revascularization after sirolimus-eluting stent implantation: five-year outcome of the j-Cypher Registry. Circulation. 2012;125(4):584–91. doi:10.1161/CIRCULATIONAHA.111.046599.
24. Yamamoto M, Takano M, Murakami D, Inami T, Kobayashi N, Inami S, Okamatsu K, Ohba T, Ibuki C, Hata N, Seino Y, Jang IK, Mizuno K. The possibility of delayed arterial healing 5 years after implantation of sirolimus-eluting stents: serial observations by coronary angioscopy. Am Heart J. 2011;161(6):1200–6. doi:10.1016/j.ahj.2011.03.006.
25. Nishino M, Yoshimura T, Nakamura D, Lee Y, Taniike M, Makino N, Kato H, Egami Y, Shutta R, Tanouchi J, Yamada Y. Comparison of angioscopic findings and three-year cardiac events between sirolimus-eluting stent and bare-metal stent in acute myocardial infarction. Am J Cardiol. 2011;108(9):1238–43. doi:10.1016/j.amjcard.2011.06.038.
26. Ishihara T, Awata M, Fujita M, Watanabe T, Iida O, Ishida Y, Nanto S, Uematsu M. Very late stent thrombosis 5 years after implantation of a sirolimus-eluting stent observed by angioscopy and optical coherence tomography. J Am Coll Cardiol Intv. 2013;6(5):e28–30. doi:10.1016/j. jcin.2012.12.127.
27. Hara M, Nishino M, Taniike M, Makino N, Kato H, Egami Y, Shutta R, Yamaguchi H, Tanouchi J, Yamada Y. High incidence of thrombus formation at 18 months after paclitaxel-eluting stent implantation: angioscopic comparison with sirolimus-eluting stent. Am Heart J. 2010;159(5):905–10. doi:10.1016/j.ahj.2010.02.032.
28. Hara M, Nishino M, Taniike M, Makino N, Kato H, Egami Y, Shutta R, Tanouchi J, Yamada Y. Serial angioscopic evaluation of neointimal coverage and incidence of thrombus formation after Paclitaxel-eluting stent implantation: comparison between 6- and 18-month follow-up. Clin Cardiol. 2011;34(5):322–6. doi:10.1002/clc.20881.
29. Mauri L, Orav EJ, Candia SC, Cutlip DE, Kuntz RE. Robustness of late lumen loss in discriminating drug-eluting stents across variable observational and randomized trials. Circulation. 2005;112(18):2833–9. doi:10.1161/CIRCULATIONAHA105.570093.
30. Maeng M, Tilsted HH, Jensen LO, Kaltoft A, Kelbaek H, Abildgaard U, Villadsen AB, Krusell LR, Ravkilde J, Hansen KN, Christiansen EH, Aaroe J, Jensen JS, Kristensen SD, Botker HE, Madsen M, Thayssen P, Sorensen HT, Thuesen L, Lassen JF. 3-Year clinical outcomes in the randomized SORT OUT III superiority trial comparing zotarolimus- and sirolimus-eluting coronary stents. J Am Coll Cardiol Intv. 2012;5(8):812–18. doi:10.1016/j.jcin.2012.04.008.
31. Hamilos M, Sarma J, Ostojic M, Cuisset T, Sarno G, Melikian N, Ntalianis A, Muller O, Barbato E, Beleslin B, Sagic D, De Bruyne B, Bartunek J, Wijns W. Interference of drug-eluting stents with endothelium-dependent coronary vasomotion: evidence for device-specific responses. Circ Cardiovasc Interv. 2008;1(3):193–200. doi:10.1161/CIRCINTERVENTIONS. 108.797928.

32. Joner M, Nakazawa G, Finn AV, Quee SC, Coleman L, Acampado E, Wilson PS, Skorija K, Cheng Q, Xu X, Gold HK, Kolodgie FD, Virmani R. Endothelial cell recovery between comparator polymer-based drug-eluting stents. J Am Coll Cardiol. 2008;52(5):333–42. doi:10.1016/j.jacc.2008.04.030.
33. Kim BK, Hong MK, Shin DH, Nam CM, Kim JS, Ko YG, Choi D, Kang TS, Park BE, Kang WC, Lee SH, Yoon JH, Hong BK, Kwon HM, Jang Y, Investigators R. A new strategy for discontinuation of dual antiplatelet therapy: the RESET Trial (REal Safety and Efficacy of 3-month dual antiplatelet Therapy following Endeavor zotarolimus-eluting stent implantation). J Am Coll Cardiol. 2012;60(15):1340–8. doi:10.1016/j.jacc.2012.06.043.
34. Feres F, Costa RA, Abizaid A, Leon MB, Marin-Neto JA, Botelho RV, King 3rd SB, Negoita M, Liu M, de Paula JE, Mangione JA, Meireles GX, Castello Jr HJ, Nicolela Jr EL, Perin MA, Devito FS, Labrunie A, Salvadori Jr D, Gusmao M, Staico R, Costa Jr JR, de Castro JP, Abizaid AS, Bhatt DL, Investigators OT. Three vs twelve months of dual antiplatelet therapy after zotarolimus-eluting stents: the OPTIMIZE randomized trial. J Am Med Assoc. 2013;310(23):2510–22. doi:10.1001/jama.2013.282183.
35. Akazawa Y, Matsuo K, Ueda Y, Nishio M, Hirata A, Asai M, Nemoto T, Wada M, Murakami A, Kashiwase K, Kodama K. Atherosclerotic change at one year after implantation of endeavor zotarolimus-eluting stent vs. everolimus-eluting stent. Circ J. 2014;78(6):1428–36. doi:10.1253/circj.CJ-14-0085.
36. Kandzari DE, Leon MB, Meredith I, Fajadet J, Wijns W, Mauri L. Final 5-year outcomes from the Endeavor zotarolimus-eluting stent clinical trial program: comparison of safety and efficacy with first-generation drug-eluting and bare-metal stents. J Am Coll Cardiol Intv. 2013;6(5):504–12. doi:10.1016/j.jcin.2012.12.125.
37. Dai K, Ishihara M, Inoue I, Kawagoe T, Shimatani Y, Miura F, Nakama Y, Otani T, Ooi K, Ikenaga H, Nakamura M, Miki T, Kishimoto S, Sumimoto Y. Coronary angioscopic findings 9 months after everolimus-eluting stent implantation compared with sirolimus-eluting stents. J Cardiol. 2013;61(1):22–30. doi:10.1016/j.jjcc.2012.08.011.
38. Sawada T, Shinke T, Otake H, Mizoguchi T, Iwasaki M, Emoto T, Terashita D, Mizuguchi T, Okamoto H, Matsuo Y, Kim SK, Takarada A, Yokoyama M. Comparisons of detailed arterial healing response at seven months following implantation of an everolimus- or sirolimus-eluting stent in patients with ST-segment elevation myocardial infarction. Int J Cardiol. 2013;168(2):960–6. doi:10.1016/j.ijcard.2012.10.043.
39. Kolandaivelu K, Swaminathan R, Gibson WJ, Kolachalama VB, Nguyen-Ehrenreich KL, Giddings VL, Coleman L, Wong GK, Edelman ER. Stent thrombogenicity early in high-risk interventional settings is driven by stent design and deployment and protected by polymer-drug coatings. Circulation. 2011;123(13):1400–9. doi:10.1161/CIRCULATIONAHA.110.003210.
40. Sera F, Awata M, Uematsu M, Kotani J, Nanto S, Nagata S. Optimal stent-sizing with intravascular ultrasound contributes to complete neointimal coverage after sirolimus-eluting stent implantation assessed by angioscopy. J Am Coll Cardiol Intv. 2009;2(10):989–94. doi:10.1016/j.jcin.2009.07.006.

Chapter 16
Peri-stent Contrast Staining

Kazuoki Dai and Masaharu Ishihara

Abstract Lack of contact between stent struts and underlying vessel surface, described as stent malapposition, is observed more frequently after implantation of drug-eluting stent (DES) than that of bare-metal stent. Several studies have suggested the potential relationship between the stent malapposition and late stent thrombosis (LST). On the coronary angiography, stent malapposition is recognized as peri-stent staining (PSS) that is contrast staining outside of the stent contour. Intravascular imaging modalities, including intravascular ultrasound and optical coherence tomography, can detect less extensive stent malapposition by their high resolution and the ability to provide the cross-sectional images of the vessel. Coronary angioscopy, the intravascular imaging of a different dimension, permits the direct visualization of the intimal surface and provides an opportunity to understand pathogenesis and clinical implication of PSS. Pathological examination showed hypersensitivities mainly composed of inflammation at the site of stent malapposition. Coronary angioscopy shows yellow plaque and thrombus at PSS site, suggesting underlying inflammation and high thrombogenicity. These findings support the relation of PSS to LST. Careful medications, including dual antiplatelet therapy and intensive statin therapy, should be warranted for prevention of LST in patients with PSS.

Keywords Peri-stent contrast staining • Stent thrombosis • Inflammation

Drug-eluting stents (DES) have dramatically reduced the incidence of restenosis and target vessel revascularization as compared with bare-metal stents (BMS) [1, 2]. Although DES has been used prevalently in the world, concern about the increased risk of late stent thrombosis (LST) after DES implantation is raised [3, 4].

K. Dai, M.D.
Department of Cardiology, Hiroshima City Hospital, 7-33 Motomachi, Naka-ku Hiroshima-shi, Hiroshima 730-8518, Japan

M. Ishihara, M.D., Ph.D., FACC (✉)
Division of Coronary Heart Disease, Hyogo College of Medicine, 1-1, Mukogawa-cho, Nishinomiya, Hyogo 663-8501, Japan
e-mail: ishifami@fb3.so-net.ne.jp

© Springer Japan 2015
K. Mizuno, M. Takano (eds.), *Coronary Angioscopy*,
DOI 10.1007/978-4-431-55546-9_16

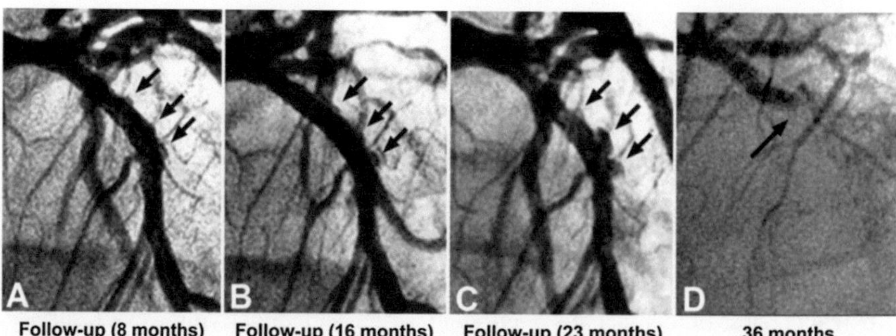

Fig. 16.1 Serial changes of contrast staining outside the sirolimus-eluting stent [7]. A 69-year-old man was treated with a SES (3.0 mm diameter × 33 mm long) implantation for chronic total occlusion lesion of LAD. (**a**) At 16 months after stenting, coronary angiography showed the areas of contrast staining outside the stent contour (PSS) (**b**) which increased in size at 23 months. (**c**) At 36 months after stenting, VLST of the SES occurred (**d**)

Lack of contact between stent struts and underlying vessel surface, so-called stent malapposition, is observed more frequently after implantation of DES than that of BMS. [5] Several studies have suggested the potential relation between stent malapposition and LST. [6] On the findings of coronary angiography, stent malapposition is recognized as peri-stent staining (PSS) that is contrast staining outside of the stent contour. Kon et al. reported that LST occurred several years after a sirolimus-eluting stent (SES) implantation in a patient with contrast staining outside a SES at follow-up coronary angiography (Fig. 16.1) [7]. Hypersensitivity reaction and chronic inflammation were found in the stent segment according to a pathological examination [7]. Previous study demonstrated that PSS was associated with late adverse events, such as restenosis or LST (Fig. 16.2) [8].

Intravascular imaging modalities, including intravascular ultrasound (IVUS) and optical coherence tomography (OCT), can detect less extensive stent malapposition due to their high resolution and the ability to provide the cross-sectional images of the vessel. On IVUS examination, PSS was recognized as stent malapposition, which was defined as separation of stent struts from the arterial wall with evidence of blood flow behind the strut except for a vessel bifurcation. Stent malapposition in late phase is formed by positive arterial remodeling, dissolution of residual thrombus or plaque debris, and chronic stent recoil [9, 10]. Previous IVUS studies showed that late acquired stent malapposition with positive remodeling was seen in 5–13 % of lesions treated with DES [11–13], and the stent malapposition was associated with the occurrence of LST. [6] On OCT examination, PSS was recognized as cavities between and outside the stent struts (Fig. 16.3). These cavities, uncovered struts, and red thrombus were frequently observed in the lesions with PSS compared with those without PSS. These findings suggested that PSS was associated with delayed healing and could be a risk factor for stent thrombosis.

Coronary angioscopy, the intravascular imaging of a different dimension, permits the direct visualization of the intimal surface and provides an opportunity to

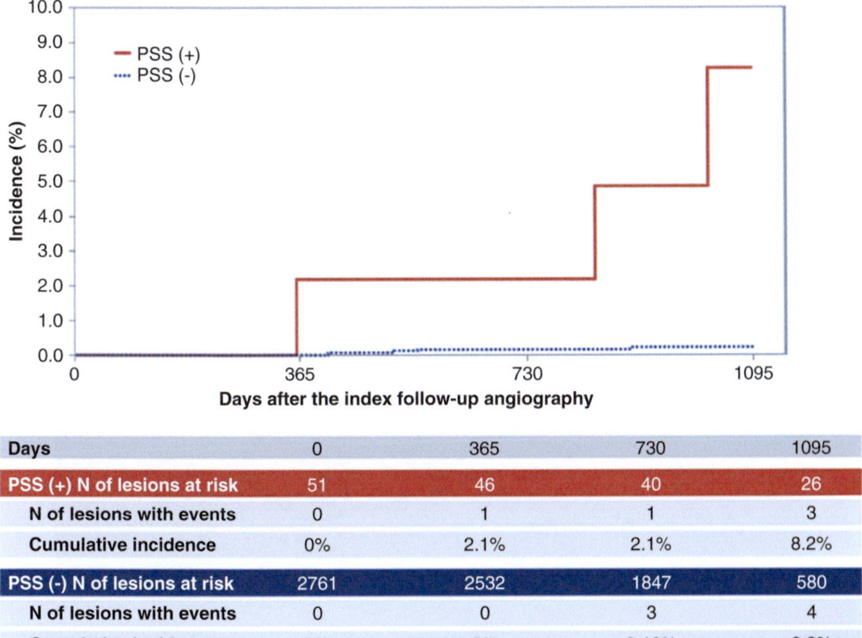

Days	0	365	730	1095
PSS (+) N of lesions at risk	51	46	40	26
N of lesions with events	0	1	1	3
Cumulative incidence	0%	2.1%	2.1%	8.2%
PSS (-) N of lesions at risk	2761	2532	1847	580
N of lesions with events	0	0	3	4
Cumulative incidence	0%	0%	0.13%	0.2%

Fig. 16.2 Cumulative incidence of stent thrombosis after the index follow-up angiography: PSS group versus non-PSS group [8]. A 3-year cumulative incidence of subsequent definite stent thrombosis in the PSS group also was numerically higher than that in the non-PSS group (8.2 % vs. 0.2 %)

understand pathogenesis and clinical implication of PSS. We presented angioscopic images in two cases of PSS observed by coronary angiography. The first case is 77-year-old female with unstable angina pectoris who was treated with a paclitaxel-eluting stent (PES, 2.5 mm diameter × 20 mm long) at midportion of the left anterior descending artery 6 years ago. Follow-up coronary angiography showed no restenosis, but contrast staining outside the proximal site of stent segment, which is named PSS (Fig. 16.4). On coronary angioscopic examination, the struts at the proximal site of stent segment were exposed similar to immediately after implantation of the stent. Blood flow was observed behind stent struts. These findings showed that the struts were not covered by neointima and malapposed. Additionally, red thrombus on yellow plaque behind the malapposed struts was found. In the second case, 78-year-old female with stable angina pectoris was treated with SES (3.5 mm diameter × 18 mm long) implantation at midportion of right coronary artery 6 years ago. VLST unfortunately occurred during clinical follow-up in this case, and emergency coronary angiography at the time of VLST showed the occlusion of proximal site of the stent segment. After performing thrombus aspiration, coronary angiography showed TIMI-3 flow and appearance of PSS at proximal site of the stent segment (Fig. 16.5). Similar to the first case, coronary

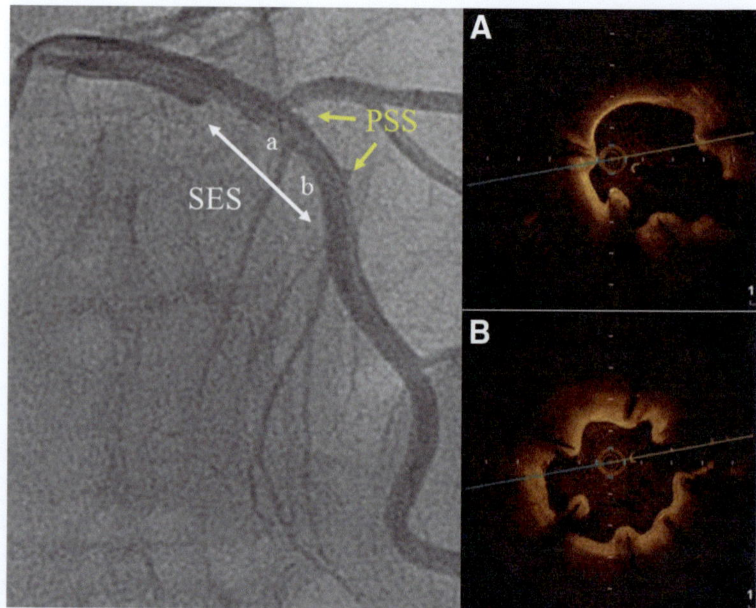

Fig. 16.3 Representative OCT findings at PSS sites. An 81-year-old male with acute myocardial infarction was treated with a SES (3.5 mm diameter × 18 mm long) at midportion of left anterior descending artery 10 years ago. Follow-up coronary angiography showed no restenosis, but contrast staining outside the proximal site of stent segment, which is named PSS. In OCT examination, many cavities between and outside the stent struts were observed

angioscopy showed that struts were uncovered and malapposed within the segment of PSS. There was red thrombus on yellow plaque behind the malapposed struts.

Ishihara et al. assessed angioscopic findings of 11 DES-implanted lesions of PSS on coronary angiography [14]. Neointimal coverage and existence of thrombus and/or yellow plaque were compared between PSS and non-PSS sites. Lower neointimal coverage and higher incidence of yellow plaque with thrombus were found at PSS sites compared with non-PSS sites. These findings suggested that delayed arterial healing and persisting inflammatory reaction resulted in thrombus formation at PSS sites. Also, they classified angiocsopic findings of PSS into 3 types. First, stent struts at PSS sites were not covered by neointima. Second, stent struts were covered by neointima, which could be seen only on the struts. Third, stent struts were covered by neointima, which was also observed between struts, but was partially absent. In the absence of neointimal coverage, blood flow between the stent and vessel wall was found and their space formed a cavity.

Pathological examination showed hypersensitivities mainly composed of inflammation at the site of late acquired stent malapposition [15, 16]. Coronary angioscopy shows yellow plaque and thrombus at PSS site, suggesting underlying inflammation and high thrombogenicity. These findings support the relationship between PSS and LST.

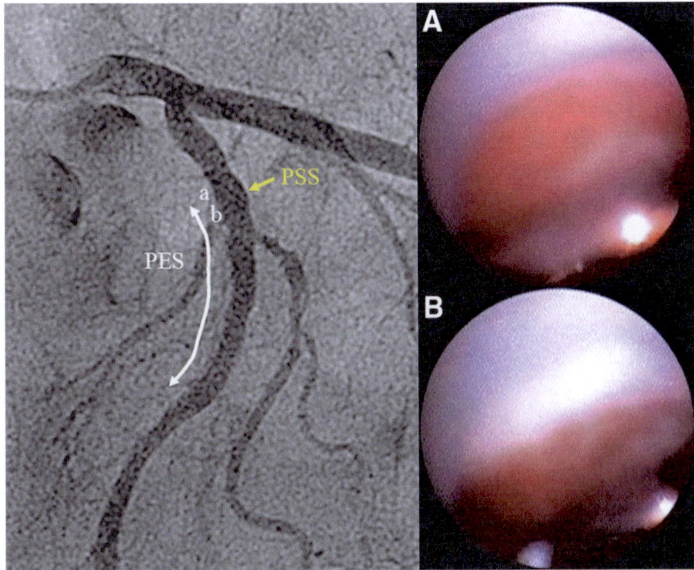

Fig. 16.4 Representative angioscopic findings at a PSS site in a patient underwent follow-up coronary angiography. The struts at the proximal site of stent segment were exposed similar to immediately after implantation. Blood flow was observed behind stent struts. These findings showed that struts were not covered by neointima and malapposed. On yellow plaque behind the malapposed struts, red thrombus was found

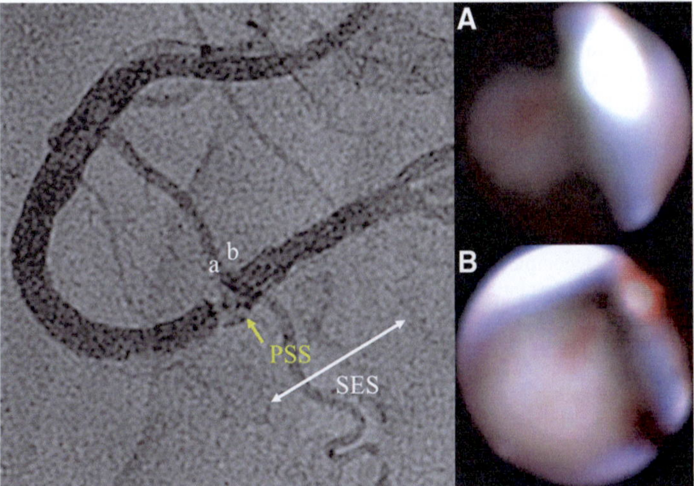

Fig. 16.5 Representative angioscopic finding at a PSS site in a patient with VLST. Emergency coronary angiography at the time of VLST showed the occlusion of proximal site of stent segment. After performing thrombus aspiration, coronary angiography showed TIMI-3 flow with contrast staining outside the proximal site of stent segment. Coronary angioscopy showed that struts were uncovered by neointima and malapposed. On yellow plaque behind the malapposed struts, red thrombus was found

PSS is not an infrequent phenomenon after the first generation of DES implantation, formed mainly by positive vessel remodeling caused by hypersensitivities and persisting inflammatory reaction. Angioscopically, PSS is associated with delayed neointimal coverage, higher grade of yellow plaque, and higher incidence of thrombus. These findings suggested that PSS may lead to the occurrence of VLST in the future. Careful medications, including dual antiplatelet therapy and intensive statin therapy, should be warranted for the prevention of LST in patients with PSS. Coronary angioscopy is a useful imaging device to assess the intimal surface after stenting and understand the pathogenesis of thrombus formation.

References

1. Moses JW, Leon MB, Popma JJ, Fitzgerald PJ, Homes DR, O'Shaughnessy C, Caputo RP, Kereakes DJ, Williams DO, Teirstein PS, Jaeger JL, Kuntz RE, SIRIUS Investigators. Sirolimus-eluting stents versus standard stents in patients with stenosis in a native coronary artery. N Engl J Med. 2003;349:1315–23.
2. Morice MC, Serruys PW, Sousa JE, Fajadet J, Hayashi EB, Perin M, Colombo A, Schuler G, Barragan P, Guagliumi G, Molnar F, Falotico R, RAVEL Study Group. A randomized comparison of a sirolimus-eluting stent with a standard stent for coronary revascularization. N Engl J Med. 2002;346:1773–80.
3. Daemen J, Wenaweser P, Tsuchida K, Abrecht L, Vaina S, Morger C, Kukreja N, Juni P, Sianos G, Hellige G, DOmburg RT, Hess OM, Boersma E, Meier B, Windecker S, et al. Early and late coronary thrombosis of sirolimus-eluting and paclitaxel-eluting stents in routine clinical practice: data from a large two-institutional cohort study. Lancet. 2007;369:667–78.
4. McFadden EP, Stabile E, Regar E, Cheneau E, Ong AT, Kinnaird T, Suddath WO, Weissman NJ, Torguson R, Kent KM, Pichard AD, Satler LF, Waksman R, Serruys PW. Late thrombosis in drug-eluting coronary stents after discontinuation of antiplatelet therapy. Lancet. 2004;364:1519–21.
5. Recalde SA, Moreno R, Barreales L, Rivero F, Galeote G, Valero JS, Calvo L, Lopez E, Sendon LJ. Risk of late-acquired incomplete stent apposition after drug-eluting stent versus bare-metal stent. A meta-analysis from 12 randomized trials. J Invasive Cardiol. 2008;20:417–22.
6. Cook S, Wenaweser P, Togni M, Billinger M, Morger C, Seiler C, Vogel R, Hess O, Meier B, Windecker S. Incomplete stent apposition and very late stent thrombosis after drug-eluting stent implantation. Circulation. 2007;115:2426–34.
7. Kon H, Sakai H, Otsubo M, Takano H, Okamoto K, Sato T, Kimura T, Inoue K. Contrast staining outside the sirolimus-eluting stent leading to coronary aneurysm formation: a case of very late stent thrombosis associated with hypersensitivity reaction. Circ Cardiovasc Interv. 2011;4:e1–3.
8. Imai M, Kadota K, Goto T, Fujii S, Yamamoto H, Fuku Y, Hosogi S, Hirono A, Tanaka H, Tada T, Morimoto T, Shiomi H, Kozuma K, Inoue K, Suzuki N, Kimura T, Mitsudo K. Incidence, risk factors, and clinical sequelae, of angiographic peri-stent contrast staining after sirolimus-eluting stent implantation. Circulation. 2011;123:2382–91.
9. Kozuma K, Costa MA, Sabate M, Serrano P, van der Giessen WJ, Ligthart JM, Coen VL, Levendag PC, Serruys PW. Late stent malapposition occurring after intracoronary beta-irradiation detected by IVUS. J Invasive Cardiol. 1999;11:651–5.
10. Mintz GS, Weissman NJ, Fitzgerald PJ. IVUS assessment of the mechanisms and results of brachytherapy. Circulation. 2001;104:1320–5.

11. Ako J, Morino Y, Honda Y, Hassan A, Sonoda S, Yock PG, Leon MB, Moses JW, Bonneau HN, Fitzgerald PJ. Late incomplete stent apposition after sirolimus-eluting stent implantation: a serial intravascular ultrasound analysis. J Am Coll Cardiol. 2005;46:1002–5.
12. Hong MK, Mintz GS, Lee CW, Park DW, Park KM, Lee BK, Kim YH, Song JM, Han KH, Kang DH, Cheong SS, Song JK, Kim JJ, Park SW, Park SJ. Late stent malapposition after drug-eluting stent implantation: an intravascular ultrasound analysis with long-term follow-up. Circulation. 2006;113:414–19.
13. Siqueira DA, Abizaid AA, Costa Jde R, Feres F, Mattos LA, Staico R, Tanajura LF, Chaves A, Centemero M, Sousa AG, Sousa JE. Late incomplete apposition after drug-eluting stent implantation: incidence and potential for adverse clinical outcomes. Eur Heart J. 2007;28:1304–9.
14. Ishihara T, Awata M, Fujita M, Watanabe T, Iida O, Ishida Y, Nanto S, Uematsu M. Angioscopic assessment of peri-stent contrast staining following drug-eluting stent implantation. Circ J. 2014;78:122–7.
15. Virmani R, Guagliumi G, Farb A, Musumeci G, Grieco N, Motta T, Mihalcsik L, Tespili M, Valsecchi O, Kolodgie FD. Localized hypersensitivity and late coronary thrombosis secondary to a sirolimus-eluting stent; should we be cautious? Circulation. 2004;109:701–5.
16. Nakazawa G, Otsuka F, Nakano M, Vorpahl M, Yazdani SK, Ladich E, et al. The pathology of neoatherosclerosis in human coronary implants bare-metal and drug-eluting stents. J Am Coll Cardiol. 2011;57:1314–22.

Chapter 17
Neoatherosclerosis

Hideo Kawakami and Hiroshi Matusoka

Abstract Today, neoatherosclerosis as atherogenic plaque formation process after stent implantation is widely recognized, but was unknown only a decade ago. In the bare-metal stent era, the neointimal proliferation in chronic phase following percutaneous coronary intervention appeared thick and white, without thrombi. Yellow neointima within the stent segment, now called "neoatherosclerosis," was firstly observed after implantation of drug-eluting stent involving sirolimus-eluting stent. Surprisingly, about half of the stents had yellow neointima 1 year after its implantation. In those days, it was understood that formation of yellow neointima is specific to sirolimus-eluting stent. However, yellow neointima developed in a few patients underwent implantation of other drug-eluting stents and bare-metal stents. Neoatherosclerosis can be detected by angioscopy and other imaging modalities such as intravascular ultrasound, optical coherence tomography, and computed tomography. Different mechanisms depending on the type of stents may be involved in neoartherosclerosis. Following drug-eluting stent implantation, incomplete or delayed reendothelialization may contribute to the atherogenesis because of an inefficient barrier against the excessive uptake of circulating lipids. Regarding bare-metal stents, neoatherosclerosis may be similar to the development of atherosclerosis in native coronary arteries. Considering these proposed mechanisms of in-stent neoatherosclerosis, statin therapy may be effective for preventing neoatherosclerosis.

Keywords Drug-eluting stent • Bare-metal stent • Yellow neointima • Delayed endothelialization • Statin

H. Kawakami, M.D., Ph.D. (✉) • H. Matusoka, M.D., Ph.D., FJCC
Department of Cardiology, Ehime Prefectural Imabari Hospital, 4-5-5, Ishii-cho, Imabari, Ehime 794-0006, Japan
e-mail: i-kawakami-h@epnh.pref.ehime.jp

© Springer Japan 2015
K. Mizuno, M. Takano (eds.), *Coronary Angioscopy*,
DOI 10.1007/978-4-431-55546-9_17

17.1 Introduction

Today, neoatherosclerosis after stent implantation is widely recognized as an atherogenic plaque formation [1], but the word was unheard-of a decade ago. In the bare-metal stent (BMS) era, 6-month follow-up angioscopy after percutaneous coronary intervention (PCI) revealed that thick, smooth, and white neointima without thrombi fully covered the stent struts; the struts were invisible even in a case of acute coronary syndrome (ACS) that has complex yellow plaque and thrombi in the culprit lesion [2, 3]. Therefore, this phenomenon was understood to be plaque sealing and stabilization and was believed to continue indefinitely (Fig. 17.1). Afterward, Yokoyama S et al. reported that neoatherosclerosis occurred several years after BMS implantation [4]. With the introduction of the first-generation drug-eluting stent (DES), the same effect of plaque stabilization was expected. However, contrary to the expectation, plaque healing after implantation of sirolimus-eluting stent (SES) was completely different from that of BMS [5, 6]. Within the segment of SES, uncovered struts, thrombi, and yellow plaque under the struts were observed. Remarkably, thin, but yellow neointima covered part of the struts [7]. Yellow neointima had not been reported prior to the DES era, and the phenomenon was unfamiliar. The yellow neointima was regarded as atherosclerotic plaque according to a previous ex vivo study [8]. Later, pathological analysis confirmed that the yellow neointima was consistent with atherosclerosis [1]. In this chapter, we describe the typical neoatherosclerosis on the basis of angioscopic findings.

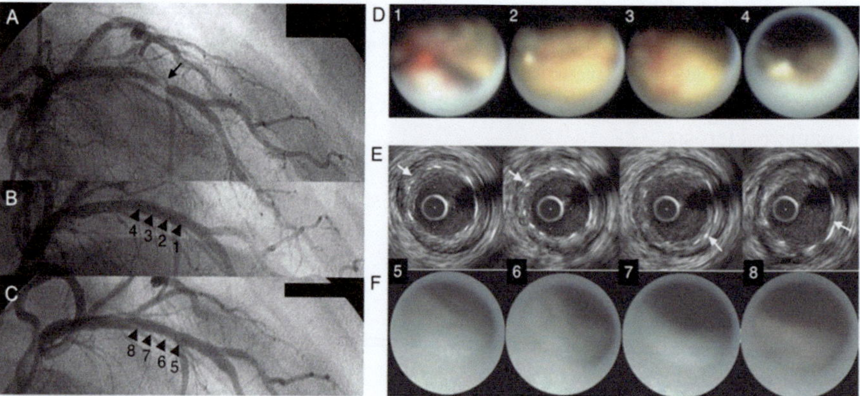

Fig. 17.1 Neointima formation after BMS implantation. This image shows a case of unstable angina in a 58-year-old-man. The *black*, *numbered arrowheads* in panel **B** and **C** correspond with the images in panels **D**, **E**, and **F**. (**A**) Coronary angiography before percutaneous coronary intervention (PCI). Significant (90 % of the diameter) stenosis is observed at midportion of the left descending artery (*black arrow* in **A**). (**B**) Immediately after PCI. The patient received a bare-metal stent (BMS) implant. (**C**) 8 months after PCI, no in-stent restenosis is apparent. (**D**) Angioscopic images immediately after PCI. The plaque behind the BMS was dense yellow with a red thrombus. (**E**) Intravascular ultrasound images 8 months after PCI. Thick neointima is seen covering the stent struts using intravascular ultrasound. (**F**) Angioscopic images 8 months after PCI. The stent struts, behind the white, thick, neointima, are not evident and the thrombus was none

17.2 First-Generation Drug-Eluting Stents

Conventional PCI including BMS deployment had an Achilles' heel; in-stent restenosis (ISR) occurred in more than 20 % of the cases [9, 10]. To overcome this Achilles' heel, a new concept of coronary stents, DESs were developed such as SES and paclitaxel-eluting stents (PES). Since their introduction, these two types of DESs have been broadly used, and the Achilles' heel associated with ISR was almost completely solved because of low frequency of the DES-ISR below 10 % [11, 12]. However, an unanticipated new problem emerged following DES use: late and very late stent thrombosis with high mortality rate [13]. Several mechanisms of the stent thrombosis have been considered to be responsible, including delayed neointimal formation [14], hypersensitivity reaction to the stent polymer [15], and neoatherosclerosis [1]. In the BMS era, 6-month follow-up angioscopy revealed that thick, smooth, and white neointima fully covered the stent struts and there were no thrombi within the BMS segment; the struts could not be seen, even after ACS that has complex yellow plaque and massive thrombi in its culprit lesion [2, 3]. Thus, this phenomenon was understood to be the effect of plaque stabilization, sealing, or whitening (*bihaku* in Japanese) [3]. Following the introduction of the first-generation DESs, similar effect of DESs on plaque stabilization was expected; however, contrary to the expectation, plaque healing of first-generation DESs was completely different from the BMS [16]. In 2006, we firstly reported the formation of yellow neointima 3 months after SES implantation [7]. In the study, we clearly demonstrated that the frequency of yellow plaque increased from 29 % immediately after stenting to 86 % of the follow-up (Fig. 17.2). Figure 17.3 shows that the white plaque had changed to yellow neointima, and we concluded that this phenomenon represented plaque destabilization by SES implantation. It was also speculated that the mechanisms of plaque destabilization involved thinning of fibrous cap as apoptosis due to a pharmacological effect of sirolimus [17] or polymer-induced inflammation of the plaque [15]. In those days, the phenomenon was not considered to be neoatherosclerosis. To investigate when yellow neointima appeared, we performed angioscopic observation at different follow-up periods. Surprisingly, a quarter of the patients had yellow neointima within 4 months and about half had that within 8 months (Fig. 17.4). Why the frequencies of yellow neointimal formation was different between the first and second reports? It was speculated that diversity of baseline patients and lesion characteristics made the differences. First report included ACS cases, whereas second report excluded ACS cases. Atherogenesis progressed in short term following SES implantation. Up to now, there is no data regarding the long-term prognosis of yellow neointima of SES. In comparison between SES and PES, yellow-plaque grade was higher in SES than in PES, as Fig. 17.5 shows [18]. This result suggested higher atherogenic potential of SES compared to PES. A recent pathological study has clarified the mechanisms of neoatherosclerosis after stent implantation (See Sect. 17.6) [1].

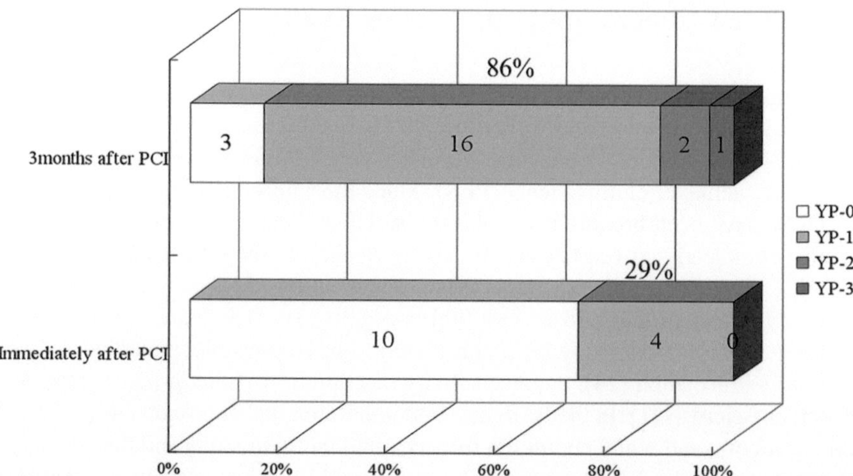

Fig. 17.2 Yellow color present at stented site, 3 months after sirolimus-eluting stent (SES) implantation. The yellow-colored grade markedly increased 3 months after SES implantation. By angioscopy, progression of atherosclerosis was demonstrated with a yellow-colored density because of thinner formation of fibrous cap. Progression of atherosclerotic plaque was assessed by a yellow-colored grade. Grade 0 was white, grade I was light yellow, grade II was normal yellow, grade III was bright yellow. YP-0, yellow-plaque grade 0; YP-1, yellow-plaque grade 1; YP-2, yellow-plaque grade 2; YP-3, yellow-plaque grade 3

17.2.1 Sirolimus-Eluting Stent (SES)

Since SES had launched into the market, this stent rose an epoch-making change in the field of PCI. In the RAVEL (RAndomized study with the sirolimus-eluting VElocity balloon-expandable stent in the treatment of patients with de novo native coronary artery Lesions) [11] and SIRIUS (a U.S. multicenter, randomized double-blind study of the sirolimus-eluting stent in de novo native coronary lesions) [12] studies showed infrequent ISR after SES implantation. Afterward, unconsidered complication in the DES era occurred, that is, late and very late stent thrombosis [13]. The Bern-Rotterdam study [19] and j-Cypher Registry [20] demonstrated that cumulative incidence of very late stent thrombosis was gradually increasing throughout several years after PCI using SES. Several mechanisms of the phenomenon were considered, and one of them is neoatherosclerosis [21]. Figure 17.6 demonstrates representative case of neoatherosclerosis after SES implantation. In this case, the newly formed yellow plaque with a red thrombus was observed 5 months after stenting. Furthermore, 403 days after PCI, the yellow neointima still remained, and it changed thicker and denser than previous observation. From the angioscopic findings, SES-induced neoatherosclerosis might be progressive. Figure 17.7 shows a case of very late stent thrombosis associated with yellow intima. A 43-year-old man, with a history of stable angina pectoris, underwent elective PCI procedure of SES implantation into the left circumflex artery. Immediately after the

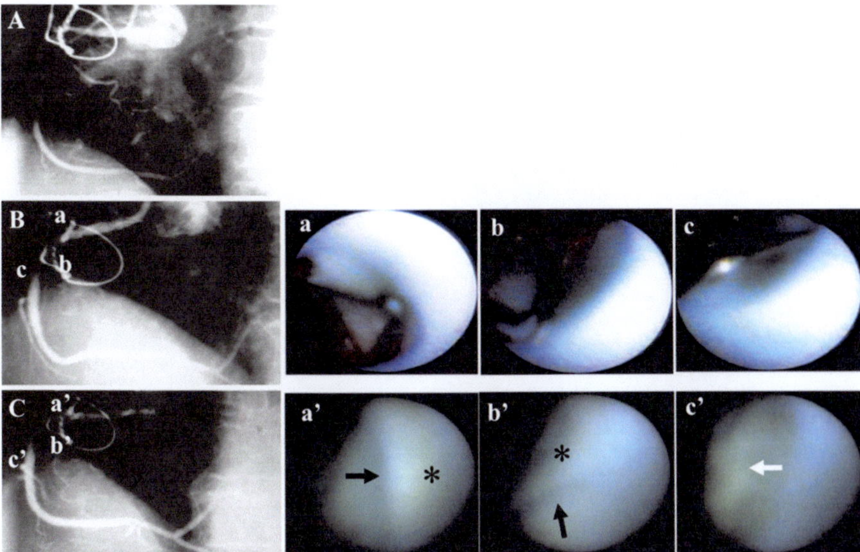

Fig. 17.3 Yellow neointima formation, 3 months after percutaneous coronary intervention (PCI) in a 70-year-old female with an old myocardial infarction. (**A**) Coronary angiography before stent implantation; 99 % diameter stenosis is evident at proximal right coronary artery. (**B**) *Left panel* shows coronary angiography immediately after stent implantation. Narrowing site was opened by sirolimus-eluting stent. *Small letters* in *left panel* correspond with the images of angioscopy. Angioscopic images (*right panels*) immediately after PCI (*a, b, c*). The stent struts are clearly seen, with sharp light reflection. Red thrombi are evident under the stent strut (*a*) and the plaque was white. (**C**) Ninety-seven days after stent implantation, in-stent restenosis is not evident at the stented site. *Small letters* in *left panel* correspond with the images of angioscopy. By angioscopy, the stent struts are visible, without light reflection (*black arrow* in *b'*, *c'*). The plaque color has changed from white to yellow (* in *a' b'*), and the white thrombus, covering the stent strut (*white arrow* in *c'*), is evident. (*a, a'*: proximal lesion of the stent; *b, b'*: midportion of the stent; *c, c'*: distal lesion of the stent)

PCI, the plaque under the stent was completely white. One year later, the color at the segment of SES changed to yellow. Very late stent thrombosis originated from the SES segment occurred 9 years later. Angioscopic observation found an intense yellow plaque with red thrombi at the culprit lesion. In this case, the cause of very late stent thrombosis was considered to be rupture of the neoatherosclerosis. Thus, yellow neointimal formation after SES implantation may be a possible risk factor of very late stent thrombosis.

17.2.2 *Paclitaxel-Eluting Stent (PES)*

PES, another type of the first-generation DES, showed a different vascular healing response than from SES. The primary characteristic of this stent type was the increased numbers of residual thrombi on the stent during in the chronic phase

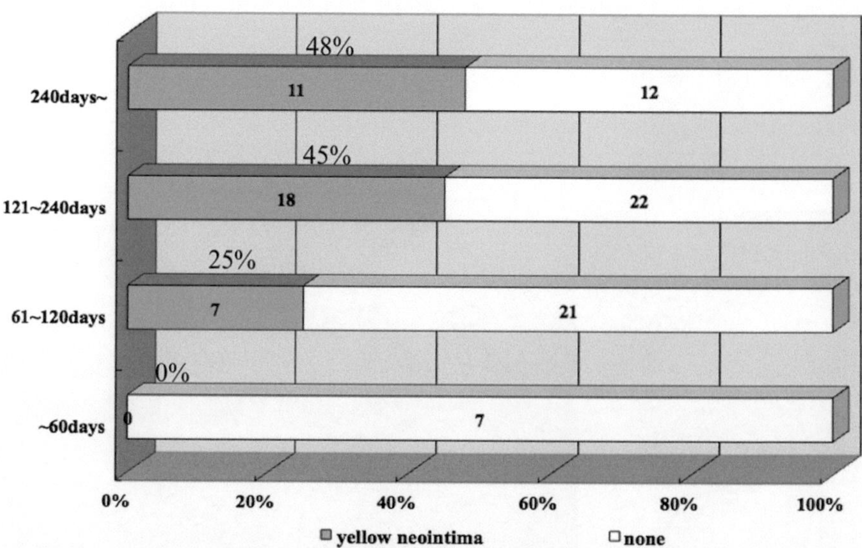

Fig. 17.4 Frequency of yellow neointima at the stent implant site after sirolimus-eluting stent implantation. There were no yellow neointima formations within 2 months. After then, the rate of yellow neointima formation gradually increased over time, after percutaneous coronary intervention

[22]. Figure 17.8 shows a case of good vascular healing after PES implantation. All of the PES struts are covered with white neointima without thrombus formation. On the other hand, yellow neointima infrequently developed as Fig. 17.9 shows. This patient suffered from angina pectoris due to BMS-ISR. He underwent PES implantation at the ISR lesion to avoid recurrent restenosis. Angioscopy demonstrated absolutely white neointima before PES implantation. One year after PES implantation, the stent segment was patent and had minimum neointimal growth on angiography. However, the newly formed neointima with yellow color was found by angioscopic observation.

17.3 Second-Generation Drug-Eluting Stents

Considering the disadvantages of the first-generation DESs, drug pharmacokinetics and drug-carrying polymers improved for the next generation of DESs. In the fast-release zotarolimus-eluting stent (E-ZES), at least 90 % of the drug releases within two weeks of its implantation. Thus, the drug release of E-ZES is earlier than the first-generation DESs. Approach of everolimus-eluting stent (EES) is different from the first-generation DES, and the DES has more biocompatible polymer. Although problems caused by stent polymer of the first-generation DESs are almost solved, some of them may remain. Figure 17.10 shows the presence of a yellow plaque in

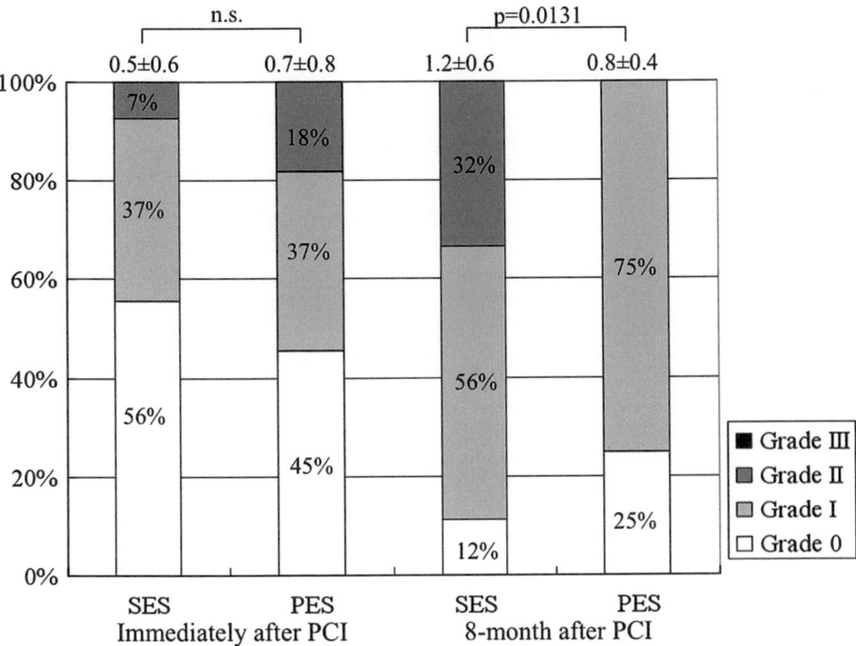

Fig. 17.5 The grades of yellow plaque immediately, and 8 months, after percutaneous coronary intervention (PCI) using first-generation drug-eluting stents. Immediately after PCI, there is no difference between the two groups, with regard to the yellow grade; 8 months after PCI, the yellow-plaque grade was significantly higher in the sirolimus-eluting stent group than in paclitaxel-eluting stent group

the segments of E-ZES and EES one year after their implantation in patients with ACS and non-ACS. The grade of yellow plaque was significantly higher in the EES group, among ACS patients, than ACS and non-ACS in E-ZES groups and non-ACS in EES group. The exact reasons for the presence of the yellow plaque are unclear. Residual yellow plaque underneath the struts may be observed through the thin neointima, or atherogenic yellow neointima may appear as well as the first-generation DESs. Whether or not, such stent segment seems to be angioscopically vulnerable lesion [23].

17.3.1 Fast-Release Zotarolimus-Eluting Stent (E-ZES)

In E-ZES, 90 % of the drug is released within 2 weeks after the implantation. Therefore, vascular healing response of E-ZES is earlier than other DESs and mimics that of BMS. In E-ZES, rather thicker neointima covers the stent struts compared with first-generation DESs [24]. Formation of yellow neointima was rare one year after E-ZES implantation. Figure 17.11 shows typical angioscopic images

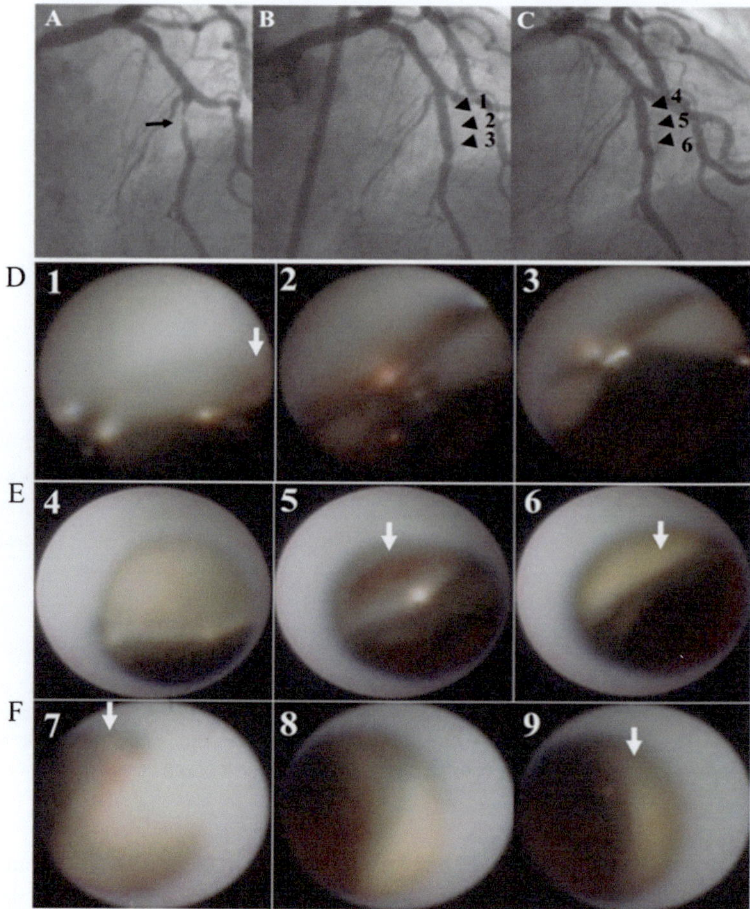

Fig. 17.6 Yellow neointima formation after sirolimus-eluting stent implantation. Angiograms and angioscopic images of a 73-year-old female, with old myocardial infarction. The *black, numbered arrowheads* in panels **B** and **C** correspond to the images in panels **D** and **E**. (**A**) In the pre-percutaneous coronary intervention (PCI) angiogram, 90 % diameter stenosis can be seen in midsegment of left anterior descending artery. (*black arrow* in **A**). (**B**) In the angiogram taken immediately after PCI, the newly implanted sirolimus-eluting stent is evident. (**C**) The angiogram taken 162 days after PCI shows no in-stent restenosis of the stented site. (**D**) The angioscopic images taken immediately after PCI show the presence of white plaque, with a small red thrombus (*white arrow* in *D1*). (**E**) The angioscopic images taken 162 days after PCI show the presence of a red thrombus near the stent struts (*white arrow* in *E5*). Yellow neointima is seen covering the stent struts (*white arrow* in *E6*). (**F**) The angioscopic images taken 403 days after PCI show that the red thrombus (*white arrow* in *F7*) is still evident. Yellow neointima is seen covering the stent struts. The yellow neointima is thicker and denser than before

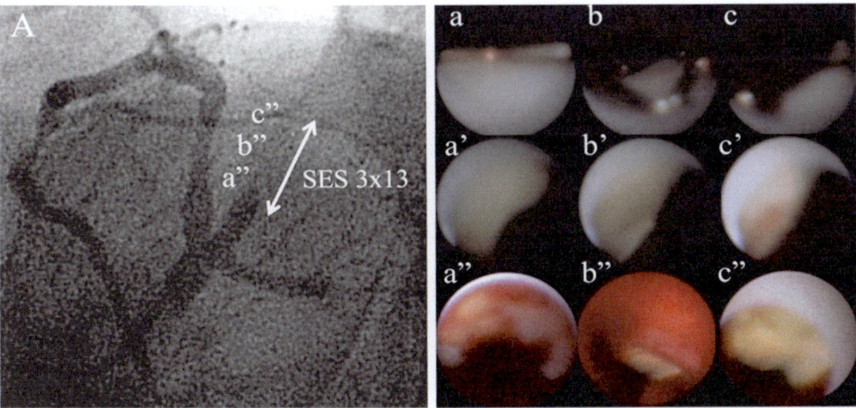

Fig. 17.7 A case of very late stent thrombosis. A 43-year-old man with stable angina pectoris received a sirolimus-eluting stent (SES), electively, in the left circumflex artery. (**A**) Left coronary angiogram (spider view). *a*, *b*, *c* Angioscopic images immediately after percutaneous coronary intervention (PCI). The plaque color under the stent is completely white. *a'*, *b'*, *c'* Angioscopic images one year after PCI. The neointima color at the SES implant site is yellow with red thrombus (*c'*). *a''*, *b''*, *c''* Angioscopic images at the site of the very late stent thrombosis. Angioscopy reveals dense, yellow, plaque with massive red thrombi

of E-ZES implantation for ACS patient. There was a light yellow plaque in the acute phase and in the chronic phase. The stent struts were invisible, and they were completely covered with thick and white neointima at follow-up. E-ZES may have sufficient effects of plaque sealing as well as BMS.

17.3.2 Everolimus-Eluting Stent (EES)

Several sorts of DESs are now available; EES is thought to be the most balanced DESs in reduction of ISR and stent thrombosis. Recent reports have demonstrated that incidence of very late stent thrombosis was significantly lower than first-generation DESs [25]. In addition, possibility of discontinuation of dual antiplatelet therapy within three months is suggested [26]. In EES, the atherogenic potential of neointima seemed to be decreased due to its biocompatible polymer. These conclusions were based on meta-analysis and retrospective analysis. However, there are some cases showing that EESs do not initiate favorable healing, but formed yellow intima. Figure 17.12 clearly demonstrates the presence of yellow neointima after stenting of EES. The patient underwent hybrid stenting at the proximal of the right coronary artery using E-ZES and EES distal to the E-ZES. One year later, thick and white neointima covered the E-ZES, while yellow neointima was found at the EES segment by angioscopy suggesting difference of healing response between the two DESs and neoatherosclerosis of EES.

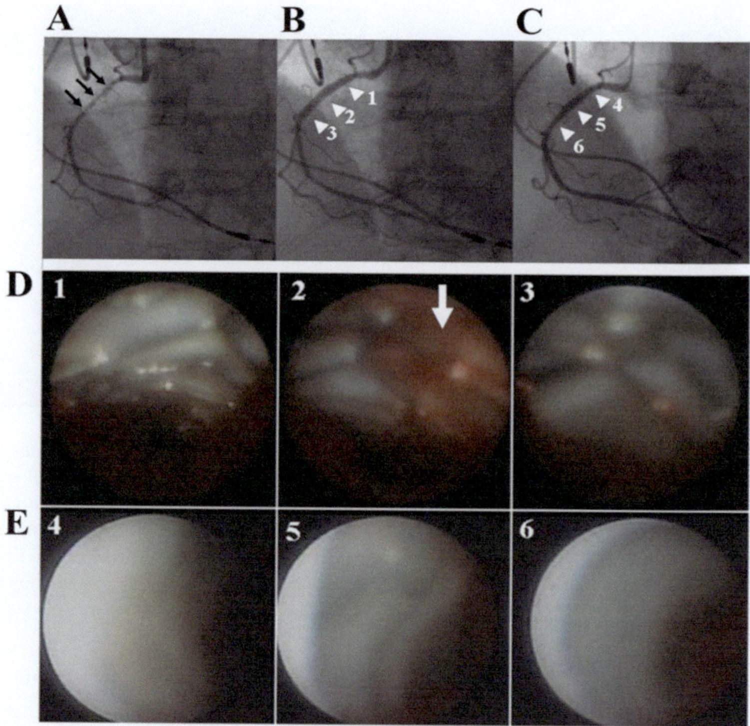

Fig. 17.8 A case involving paclitaxel-eluting stent (PES) implantation. (**A**) Before percutaneous coronary intervention (PCI), severe stenosis is evident at the proximal right coronary artery. (**B**) The PES is shown after implantation. (**C**) One year after implantation, there is no evidence of in-stent restenosis. (**D**) Angioscopic images immediately after PCI show a white plaque with a red thrombus (*white arrow* in *D-2*). (**E**) Angioscopic images one year after PCI show the white neoinitma, fully covering the stent struts; neoatherosclerosis is not evident

17.3.3   Other Second-Generation Drug-Eluting Stents

Slow-release zotarolimus-eluting stent (R-ZES) and biolimus A9-eluting stents (BES) are the other second-generation DESs. At the present, we have no enough data on vascular healing response regarding these two new stents. According to recent papers, BES has an abluminal bioabsorbable polymer and R-ZES has a highly biocompatible polymer. In fact, Awata M et al. [27] clearly demonstrated by angioscopy that BES induced better healing having more homogeneous neointima as compared with SES implantation; however, atherogenic potential has been uncertain.

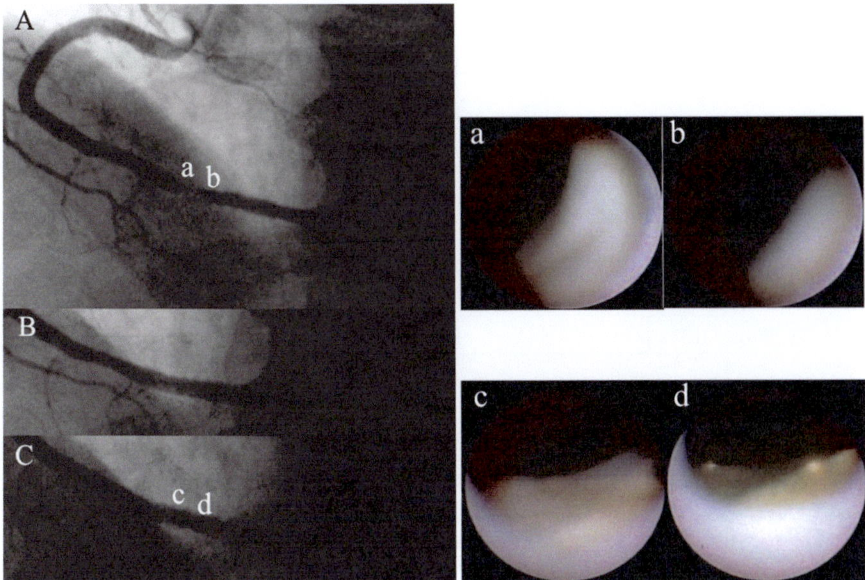

Fig. 17.9 A case of paclitaxel-eluting stent (PES) implantation after bare-metal stent in-stent restenosis. (**A**) Before percutaneous coronary intervention (PCI), severe restenosis is evident in distal right coronary artery. (**B**) The PES is implanted. (**C**) One year later, there is no evidence of in-stent restenosis. *a*, *b* Angioscopic images before PCI show white neointima, which is thought to be proliferation of smooth muscle. *c*, *d* Angioscopic images one year after PCI show the presence of yellow neoinitma; neoatherosclerosis occurred

17.4 Bare-Metal Stent (BMS)

As mentioned in the previous chapter, BMS segments escaped from ISR were considered favorable healing continue within a couple of years because the segments are covered with thick and white neointima and that completely seals vulnerable plaque under the stents in chronic phase. According to an angioscopic follow-up examination in long-term period, the neointima becomes thinner and transparent 3 years after BMS implantation [28]. Recent analyses show that very late stent thrombosis originated from BMS segment occurs as well as DESs. The mechanism of very late stent thrombosis is rupture of atheromatous lesion within the BMS segment [1]. Figure 17.13 shows angioscopic images of a patient with unstable angina. The patient underwent BMS implantation in the left circumflex artery 9 years before the onset. Angioscopic observation revealed the presence of dense yellow plaque and white thrombi. These findings indicated that neoatherosclerosis of BMS and following its disruption caused ACS. In such cases, at least optimal medical therapy seems to be important after stent implantation.

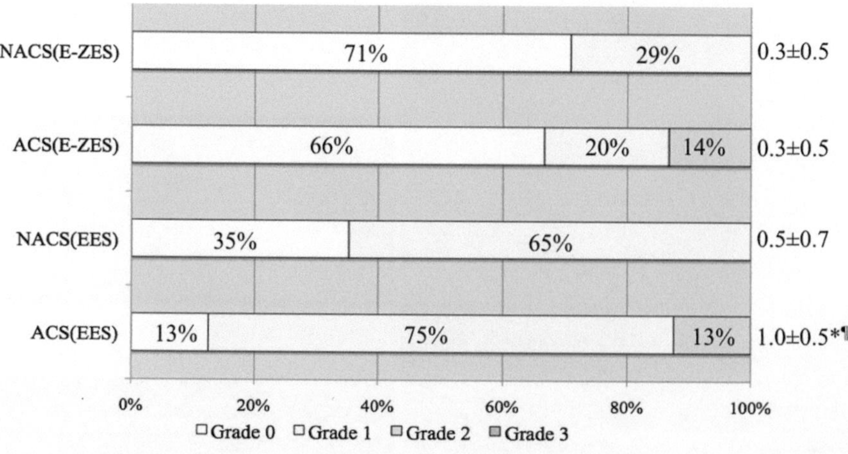

Fig. 17.10 Yellow-plaque grades after the implantation of second-generation drug-eluting stents. The existence of residual or newly formed yellow plaque is lower in the fast-release zotarolimus-eluting stent group compared with the everolimus-eluting stent group, especially among ACS patients. NACS, non-acute coronary syndrome; ACS, acute coronary syndrome

17.5 Other Imaging Modalities for Detection of Neoatherosclerosis

Angioscopy has played an important role in validation of neoatherosclerosis after stent implantation. However, other modalities can also detect the neoatherosclerosis. In this section, several cases of neoatherosclerosis detected by intravascular ultrasound (IVUS), optical coherence tomography (OCT), and computed tomography (CT) will be presented.

17.5.1 Intravascular Ultrasound (IVUS)

IVUS was the first modality used to observe the intravascular structure in living patients [29]. IVUS has played an important role in the assessment of vessel structure including atherosclerosis. Furthermore, recent IVUS techniques have also permitted tissue characterization of the vessel wall [30, 31]. In-stent neoatheroma may be also analyzed by recent IVUS images. However, the resolution of IVUS is 100 μm, and it has limitation of detecting thin neointima. IVUS analysis is suitable for detection of thick neointima and ISR lesions. Figure 17.14 shows an ISR lesion of SES in midportion of right coronary artery. Angioscopy revealed that the neointimal tissue was a yellow, so-called neoatherosclerosis. Integrated backscatter

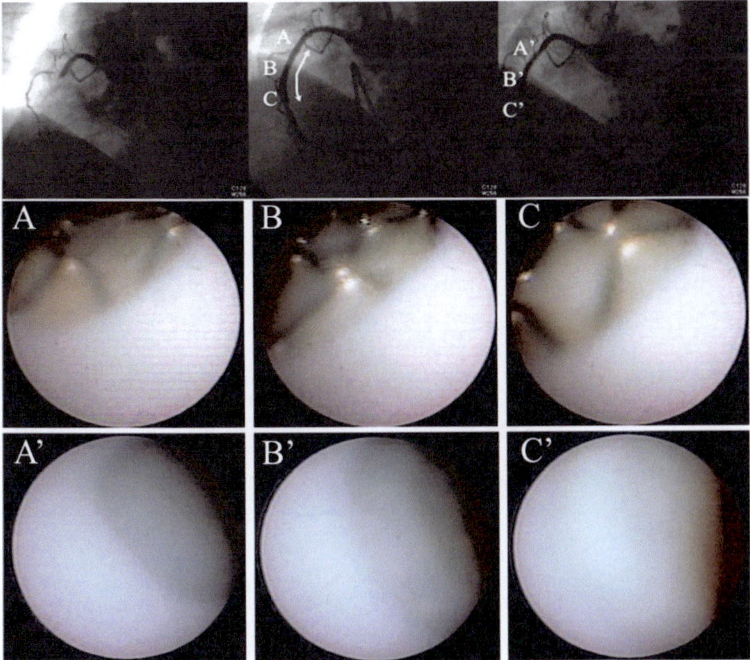

Fig. 17.11 An acute coronary syndrome patient showing typical angioscopic images after fast-release zotarolimus-eluting stent (E-ZES) implantation. *Upper left panel* Right coronary angiogram before percutaneous coronary intervention (PCI). *Upper middle panel* Right coronary angiogram immediately after PCI. *Upper right panel* Right coronary angiogram one year after PCI. There is no in-stent restenosis evident after the PCI. (**A, B, C**) An E-ZES is shown in the proximal right coronary artery with light yellow plaque during the acute phase. (A', B', C') One year later, the stent struts are not visible due to the thick, white neointima

IVUS clearly indicated the presence of lipid-rich tissue in the ISR lesion. The lesion was treated by BMS, for the expectation of sealing effect of the BMS. Our attempt was successful; thick and white neointima covered the ISR lesion without recurrence of restenosis at follow-up study [32]. Thus, integrated backscatter IVUS is also useful for characterization of neointimal tissue in thick ISR lesion.

17.5.2 *Optical Coherence Tomography (OCT)*

OCT is a recent intravascular imaging technique and its resolution is about 10 μm, enabling detection of the thin fibrous cap of atheroma and thin neointima of DESs segment [33]. Thus, OCT became gold standard for assessment of in-stent neointima [34]. In addition, OCT provides accurate tissue characteristics, such as lipid pool, calcification, and thrombi [35]. Furthermore, OCT can detect

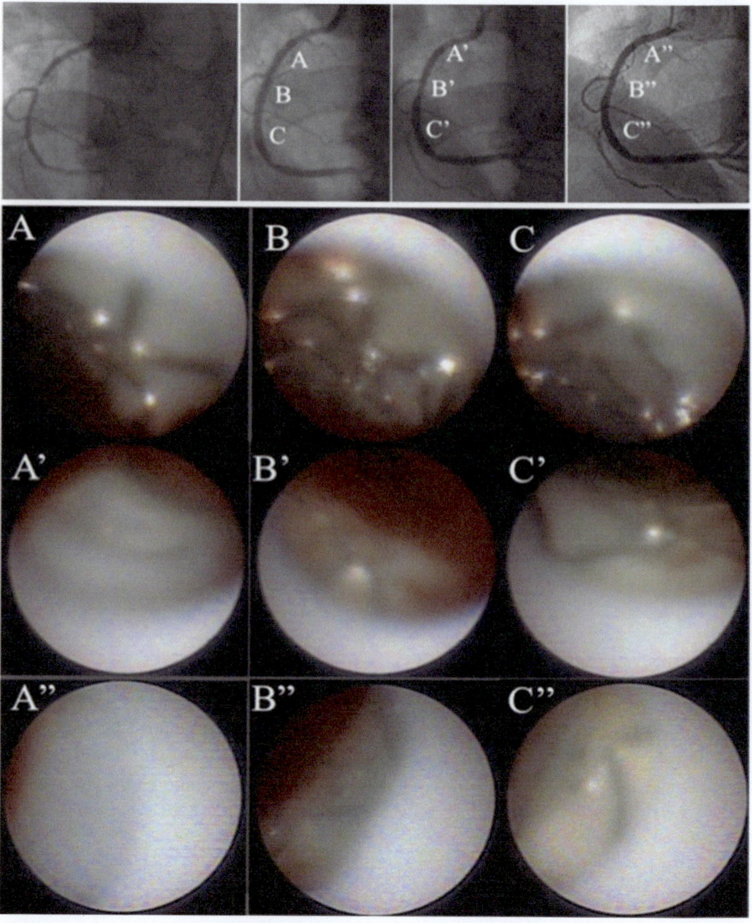

Fig. 17.12 A patient with hybrid stenting involving an everolimus-eluting stent (EES) in segment 2 and a fast-release zotarolimus-eluting stent (E-ZES) in segment 1. The *upper panel* from the *left* shows coronary angiograms before percutaneous coronary intervention (PCI), immediately after PCI, 3 months after PCI, and 1 year after PCI. There is no in-stent restenosis evident after the PCI. (**A**) Immediately after PCI, at E-ZES implantation site. (**B**) Immediately after PCI, at Overlapping site. (**C**) Immediately after PCI, at EES implantation site. The two stents are implanted on the white plaque. (*A'*) Three months after PCI, at the E-ZES site. The stent struts are covered with thick, white neointima. (*B'*) Three months after PCI, at the overlapping site. The stent struts are covered with thin neointima. (*C'*) Three months after PCI, at the EES site. The stent struts are covered with a thin neointima. (*A''*) One year after PCI, at the E-ZES site. The stent struts are covered with a thick, white neointima. (*B''*) One year after PCI, at the overlapping site. The stent struts are covered with thin neointima. (*C''*) One year after PCI, at the EES site. The stent struts are covered with thin neointima. The neointima color appears to be yellowish

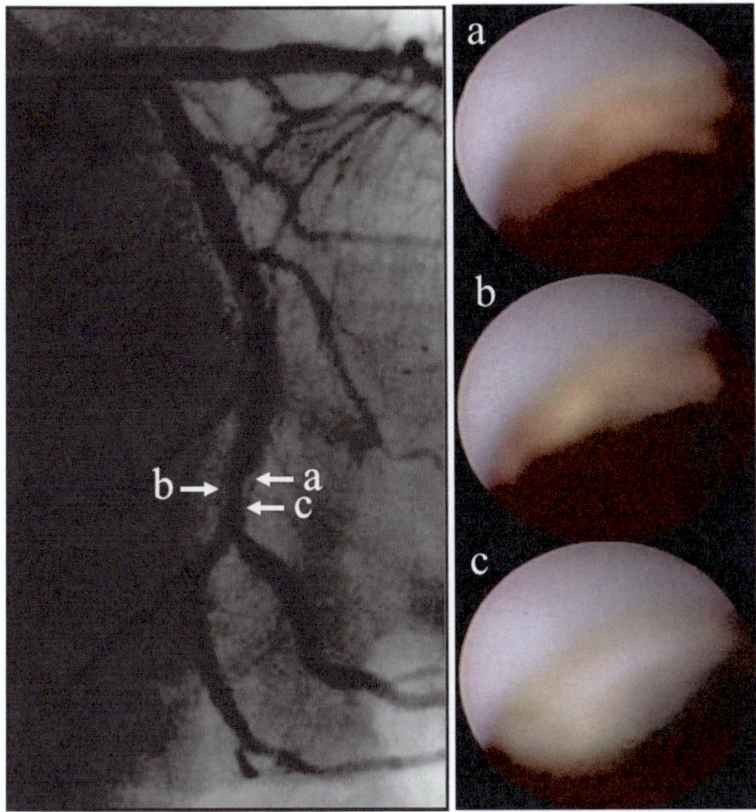

Fig. 17.13 Bare-metal stent (BMS) neoatherosclerosis. The *left panel* shows the results of a coronary angiogram. Severe stenosis is evident in the distal left circumflex artery. This patient received a BMS in segment 13, 9 years earlier. (*a, b, c*) Angioscopy reveals dense, yellow plaque, with white thrombi

macrophage recruitment in the plaque indicative of inflammation [36]. Figure 17.15 shows angioscopically yellow neointima of SES segment. In this segment, lipid-rich neointima and macrophage infiltration were found by OCT [37].

17.5.3 Computed Tomography (CT)

A recent trend for the diagnosis of coronary artery disease is initially performed CT angiography [38]. CT angiography is valuable for understanding plaque characteristics in a noninvasive way [39]. CT may be valuable for detecting ISR after stenting. Figure 17.16 shows a case of ISR occurred 5 years after SES implantation. Not only

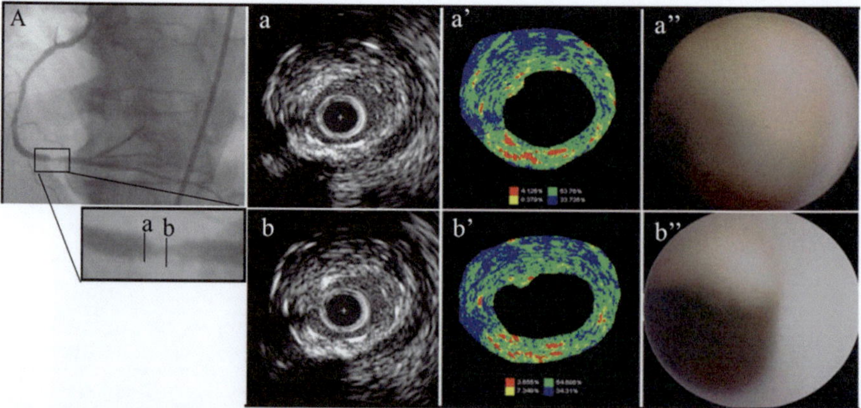

Fig. 17.14 A case of in-stent restenosis after the implantation of a sirolimus-eluting stent. (**A**) Coronary angiogram showing severe stenosis in distal right coronary artery. (*a*, *b*) Gray scale intravascular ultrasound images showing thick neointima developing in the stent. (*a'*, *b'*) Integrated backscatter-intravascular ultrasound images showing a *blue color* predominating in the thick neointima, indicating a lipid-rich neointima. (*a"*, *b"*) Angioscopy revealing yellow neointima tissue (lipid-rich plaque)

coronary angiography but also CT clearly detects the ISR lesion. Angioscopic color of the ISR lesion was yellow. In quantitative CT analysis of the lesion, CT value was 24 HU, indicating lipid-dominant tissue. Also, CT may be useful for the analysis of tissue components in ISR lesion.

17.6   Mechanisms of In-Stent Neoatherosclerosis

Nakazawa et al.[1] reported that in-stent neoatherosclerosis occurs in both BMSs and DESs. However, neoatherosclerosis of DESs is observed more frequently and at earlier time points (median, 420 days) compared with BMSs (median, 2,160 days). Moreover, neoatherosclerosis associated with DESs is associated with unstable symptoms within 2 years after their implantation, whereas similar features occur at a late phase (average time to implant, 6 years) following BMS implantation. These results indicate that different mechanisms are responsible for neoatherosclerosis between DES and BMS. Following DES implantation, incomplete endothelialization, and the inability to maintain a fully functional, endothelialized luminal surface within the stented segment appears to induce permeability of inflammatory cells and/or lipid and subsequent neoatherosclerosis. Normal endothelium commonly works as an efficient barrier against the excessive uptake of circulating lipid regardless of the segment of DESs and BMSs. The incomplete or delayed endothelial regrowth in DESs may contribute to atherogenesis due to the inefficient barrier

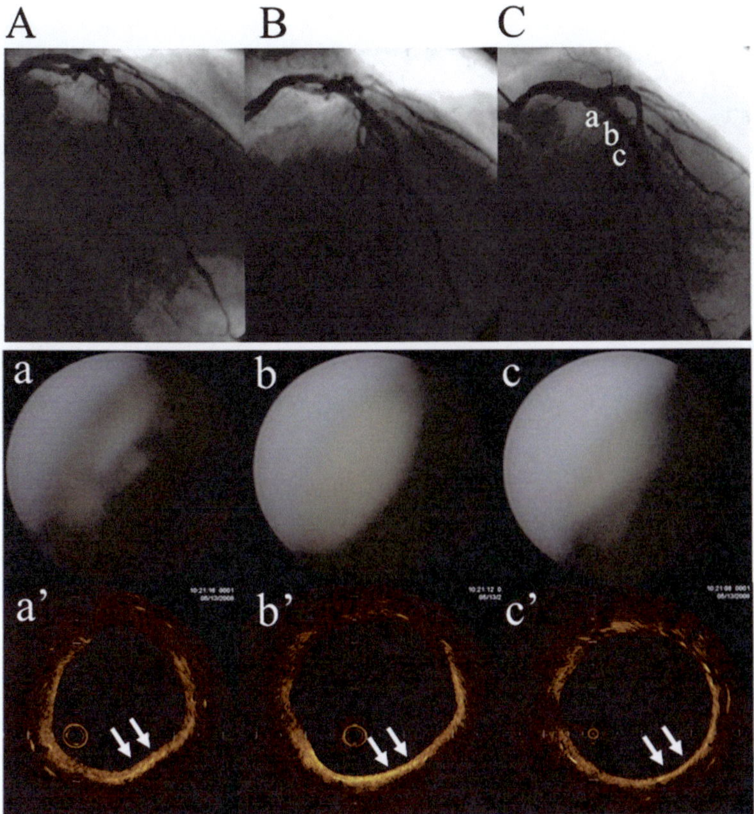

Fig. 17.15 A case of in-stent yellow neointima after sirolimus-eluting stent implantation. (**A**) Coronary angiogram before percutaneous coronary intervention (PCI) showing severe stenosis in segment 7. (**B**) Coronary angiogram immediately after PCI. (**C**) Coronary angiogram 1 year after PCI. Angioscopic images show yellow neointima (*a*, *b*, *c*). Using optical coherence tomography, high intensity neointima, without backscatter (*white arrows*), is shown to cover the stent struts, indicating lipid-rich neointima

effect. In the segment of BMSs with complete endothelialization, neoartherosclerosis may occur in a manner similar to the development of atherosclerosis in native coronary arteries. Regarding the potential mechanisms of atherosclerotic transformation inside the BMS segment, so far few interpretations have arisen. One is that stainless steel of the BMS evokes a remarkable foreign-body inflammatory reaction to the metal, and peri-stent chronic inflammatory cells may accelerate new atherosclerotic changes [40].

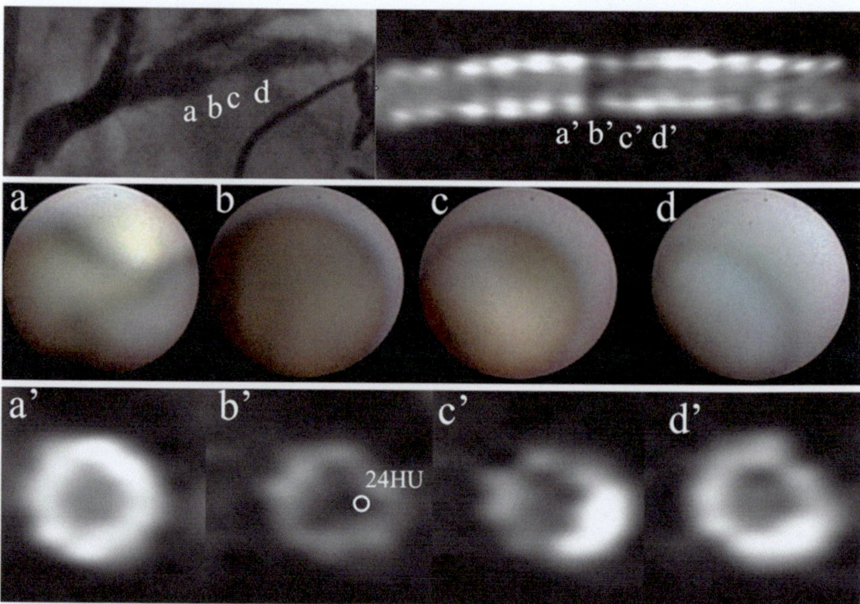

Fig. 17.16 A case of in-stent restenosis after sirolimus-eluting stent implantation. *Upper left panel*: A coronary angiogram shows severe stenosis in proximal left discending coronary artery. *Upper right panel*: A computed tomography (CT) coronary angiogram shows a low-intensity plaque in the proximal left descending coronary artery. Angioscopic images show yellow plaque at the site of severe stenosis (*b*, *c*). CT analysis reveals that the CT value of the in-stent restenosis site was 24 Hounsfield Unit, indicating lipid-rich plaque

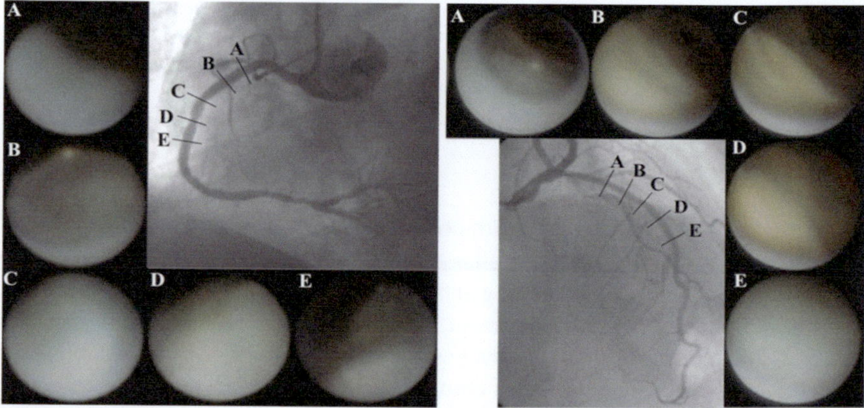

Fig. 17.17 Effect of statin therapy. The right panel shows angioscopic images, after SES implantation, in conjunction with statin therapy (LDL-C concentration, 76 mg/dL). There was no yellow neointima, 1 year after PCI. The *left panel* shows angioscopic images after SES implantation in the absence of statin therapy (LDL-C concentration, 147 mg/dL); yellow neointima formation was evident 1 year after PCI

17.7 Prevention of In-Stent Neoatherosclerosis

Considering the mechanisms of in-stent neoatherosclerosis, statin therapy may prevent neoatherosclerosis. Kanai et al. reported [41] the development of yellow plaque under implanted SES. In aggressive lowering of low-density lipoprotein-cholesterol (LDL-C) group, angioscopic grade of yellow plaque, within the SES segment, was significantly decreased from 9 to14 months of follow-ups compared to baseline. They concluded that the adequate lowering of LDL-C using a statin might prevent the biochemical action and development of atherosclerosis associated with SES implantation. Figure 17.17 shows presence and absence of neoatherosclerosis after SES implantation in different levels of LDL-C. With statin treatment, white neointima is present one year after PCI. Without statin, yellow neointima formation occurred within one year after PCI. These observations indicated that optimal medical therapy, using statins, may prevent neoatherosclerosis after implantation of either DESs or BMSs.

17.8 Conclusion

In this chapter, we have explained the new concept of "neoatherosclerosis" on the basis of angioscopic images. Today, neoatherosclerosis after stent implantation is prevalently accepted, and angioscopy plays an important role in the discovery of this phenomenon. Since seeing is believing, continuing to clarify changes of the coronary lumen by angioscopy may be required.

References

1. Nakazawa G, Otsuka F, Nakano M, et al. The pathology of neoatherosclerosis in human coronary implants bare-metal and drug-eluting stents. J Am Coll Cardiol. 2011;57:1314–22. doi:10.1016/j.jacc.2011.01.011.
2. Ueda Y, Asakura M, Hirayama A, et al. Intracoronary morphology of culprit lesions after reperfusion in acute myocardial infarction: serial angioscopic observations. J Am Coll Cardiol. 1996;27:606–10. doi:10.1016/0735-1097(95)00534-X.
3. Sakai S, Mizuno K, Yokoyama S, et al. Morphologic changes in infarct-related plaque after coronary stent placement: a serial angioscopy study. J Am Coll Cardiol. 2003;42:1558–65. doi:10.1016/j.jacc.2003.06.003.
4. Yokoyama S, Takano M, Yamamoto M, et al. Extended follow-up by serial angioscopic observation for bare-metal stents in native coronary arteries: from healing response to atherosclerotic transformation of neointima. Circ Cardiovasc Interv. 2009;2:205–12. doi:10.1161/CIRCINTERVENTIONS.109.854679.
5. Kotani J, Awata M, Nanto S, et al. Incomplete neointimal coverage of sirolimus-eluting stents: angioscopic findings. J Am Coll Cardiol. 2006;47:2108–11. doi:10.1016/j.jacc.2005.11.092.
6. Dai K, Ishihara M, Inoue I, et al. Coronary angioscopic findings eight months after sirolimus-eluting stent implantation: a comparison between ST-elevation myocardial infarction and stable angina pectoris. EuroIntervention. 2010;6:251–6. doi:10.4244/.

7. Kawakami H, Matsuoka H, Nakamura M, et al. Angioscopic observation three months after sirolimus-eluting stent implantation: can we stop strong anti-platelet therapy after three months? Jpn J Interv Cardiol. 2006;21:409–16.
8. Miyamoto A, Abera GS, Mizuno K. Vulnerable plaques assessed by quantitative colorimetric analysis during angioscopy. J Jpn Coll Angiol. 1999;39:747–51.
9. Serruys PW, de Jaegere P, Kiemeneij F, et al. A comparison of balloon-expandable-stent implantation with balloon angioplasty in patients with coronary artery disease. Benestent Study Group. N Engl J Med. 1994;331:489–95.
10. Fischman DL, Leon MB, Baim DS, et al. A randomized comparison of coronary-stent placement and balloon angioplasty in the treatment of coronary artery disease. Stent Restenosis Study Investigators. N Engl J Med. 1994;331:496–501.
11. Morice MC, Serruys PW, Sousa JE, et al. A randomized comparison of a sirolimus-eluting stent with a standard stent for coronary revascularization. N Engl J Med. 2002;346:1773–80.
12. Moses JW, Leon MB, Popma JJ, et al. Sirolimus-eluting stents versus standard stents in patients with stenosis in a native coronary artery. N Engl J Med. 2003;349:1315–23.
13. McFadden EP, Stabile E, Regar E, et al. Late thrombosis in drug-eluting coronary stents after discontinuation of antiplatelet therapy. Lancet. 2004;364:1519–21. doi:10.1016/S0140-6736(04)17275-9.
14. Finn AV, Kolodgie FD, Harnek J, et al. Differential response of delayed healing and persistent inflammation at sites of overlapping sirolimus- or paclitaxel-eluting stents. Circulation. 2005;112:270–8. doi:10.1161/CIRCULATIONAHA.104.508937.
15. Virmani R, Guagliumi G, Farb A, et al. Localized hypersensitivity and late coronary thrombosis secondary to a sirolimus-eluting stent: should we be cautious? Circulation. 2004;109:701–5. doi:10.1161/01.CIR.0000116202.41966.D4.
16. Kawakami H, Matsuoka H, Oshita A, et al. A case of a newly developed yellow neointima at stent implanted site 1 year after sirolimus-eluting stent placement: angioscopic findings. J Cardiol. 2009;54:153–7. doi:10.1016/j.jjcc.2008.10.010.
17. Huang S, Shu L, Dilling MB, et al. Sustained activation of the JNK cascade and rapamycin-induced apoptosis are suppressed by p53/p21(Cip1). Mol Cell. 2003;11:1491–501. doi.org/10.1016/S1097-2765(03)00180-1.
18. Kawakami H, Matsuoka H, Oshita A, et al. Angioscopic findings 8 months after drug-eluting stent implantation. -sirolimus-eluting stent vs paclitaxel-eluting stent-. Jpn J Endovasc Interv. 2009;1:22–8.
19. Wenaweser P, Daemen J, Zwahlen M, et al. Incidence and correlates of drug-eluting stent thrombosis in routine clinical practice. J Am Coll Cardiol. 2008;52:1134–40.
20. Kimura T, Morimoto T, Nakagawa Y, et al. Very late stent thrombosis and late target lesion revascularization after sirolimus-eluting stent implantation: five-year outcome of the j-Cypher Registry. Circulation. 2012;125:584–91. doi:10.1161/CIRCULATIONAHA.111.046599.
21. Higo T, Ueda Y, Oyabu J, et al. Atherosclerotic and thrombogenic neointima formed over sirolimus drug-eluting stent: an angioscopic study. J Am Coll Cardiol Img. 2009;2:616–24. doi:10.1016/j.jcmg.2008.12.026.
22. Takano M, Yamamoto M, Murakami D, et al. Lack of association between large angiographic late loss and low risk of in-stent thrombus: angioscopic comparison between paclitaxel- and sirolimus-eluting stents. Circ Cardiovasc Interv. 2008;1:20–7. doi:10.1161/CIRCINTERVENTIONS.108.769448.
23. Kawakami H, Namiguchi K, Seike F, et al. Angioscopic and optical coherence tomographic analysis in patients with acute coronary syndrome after bare metal stent, zotarolimus and everolimus-eluting stent implantation. Shinzo. 2014;46:861–72.
24. Awata M, Nanto S, Uematsu M, et al. Angioscopic comparison of neointimal coverage between zotarolimus- and sirolimus-eluting stents. J Am Coll Cardiol. 2008;52:789–90. doi:10.1016/j.jacc.2008.07.007.
25. Palmerini T, Biondi-Zoccai G, Della Riva D, et al. Clinical outcomes with bioabsorbable polymer- versus durable polymer-based drug-eluting and bare-metal stents: evidence from a comprehensive network meta-analysis. J Am Coll Cardiol. 2014;63(2):99–307. doi:10.1016/j.jacc.2013.09.061.

26. Loh JP, Torguson R, Pendyala LK, et al. Impact of early versus late clopidogrel discontinuation on stent thrombosis following percutaneous coronary intervention with first- and second-generation drug-eluting stents. Am J Cardiol. 2014;113:1968–76. doi:10.1016/j.amjcard.2014.03.041.
27. Awata M, Uematsu M, Sera F, et al. Angioscopic assessment of arterial repair following biodegradable polymer-coated biolimus A9-eluting stent implantation. – comparison with durable polymer-coated sirolimus-eluting stent-. Circ J. 2011;75:1113–19. doi:10.1253/circj.CJ-10-0776.
28. Asakura M, Ueda Y, Nanto S, et al. Remodeling of in-stent neointima, which became thinner and transparent over 3 years: serial angiographic and angioscopic follow-up. Circulation. 1998;97:2003–6. doi:10.1161/01.CIR.97.20.2003.
29. Moriuchi M, Saito S, Honye J, et al. Intravascular ultrasound imaging in human peripheral and coronary arteries in vivo. Jpn Circ J. 1992;56:578–85.
30. Nair A, Kuban BD, Tuzcu EM, et al. Coronary plaque classification with intravascular ultrasound radiofrequency data analysis. Circulation. 2002;106:2200–6. doi:10.1161/01.CIR.0000035654.18341.5E.
31. Kawasaki M, Takatsu H, Noda T, et al. In vivo quantitative tissue characterization of human coronary arterial plaques by use of integrated backscatter intravascular ultrasound and comparison with angioscopic findings. Circulation. 2002;105:2487–92. doi:10.1161/01.CIR.0000017200.47342.10.
32. Matsuoka H, Kawakami H, Ohshita A, et al. Bare metal stent implantation for in-stent restenosis with a drug-eluting stent. J Cardiol. 2010;55:135–8. doi:10.1016/j.jjcc.
33. Kubo T, Imanishi T, Takarada S, et al. Implication of plaque color classification for assessing plaque vulnerability: a coronary angioscopy and optical coherence tomography investigation. JACC Cardiovasc Interv. 2008;1:74–80. doi:10.1016/j.jcin.2007.11.001.
34. Matsumoto D, Shite J, Shinke T, et al. Neointimal coverage of sirolimus-eluting stents at 6-month follow-up: evaluated by optical coherence tomography. Eur Heart J. 2007;28:961–7. doi:10.1093/eurheartj/ehl413.
35. Kume T, Akasaka T, Kawamoto T, et al. Assessment of coronary arterial thrombus by optical coherence tomography. Am J Cardiol. 2006;15(97):1713–17. doi:10.1016/j.amjcard.2006.01.031.
36. Tearney GJ, Yabushita H, Houser SL, et al. Quantification of macrophage content in atherosclerotic plaques by optical coherence tomography. Circulation. 2003;107:113–19. doi:10.1161/01.CIR.0000044384.41037.43.
37. Takano M, Yamamoto M, Inami S, et al. Appearance of lipid-laden intima and neovascularization after implantation of bare-metal stents. Extended late-phase observation by intracoronary optical coherence tomography. J Am Coll Cardiol. 2010;55:26–32. doi:10.1016/j.jacc.2009.08.032.
38. Achenbach S, Giesler T, Ropers D, et al. Detection of coronary artery stenoses by contrast-enhanced, retrospectively electrocardiographically-gated, multislice spiral computed tomography. Circulation. 2001;103:2535–8. doi:10.1161/01.CIR.103.21.2535.
39. Inoue F, Sato Y, Matsumoto N, et al. Evaluation of plaque texture by means of multislice computed tomography in patients with acute coronary syndrome and stable angina. Circ J. 2004;68:840–4. doi.org/10.1253/circj.68.840.
40. Inoue K, Abe K, Ando K, et al. Pathological analyses of long-term intracoronary Palmaz-Schatz stenting: is its efficacy permanent? Cardiovasc Pathol. 2004;13:109–15.
41. Kanai T, Hiro T, Takayama T, et al. Serial change and its determinants of residual plaque characteristics under sirolimus-eluting stent: a coronary angioscopic study. J Cardiol. 2012;60:270–6. doi:10.1016/j.jjcc.2012.06.002.

Chapter 18
Angioscopic Evaluation of In-Stent Restenosis

Masami Nishino

Abstract Although drug-eluting stents (DESs) have greatly reduced the incidence of in-stent restenosis (ISR), the management of patients with ISR remains an important clinical problem. The use of DESs can reduce one of the main factors for ISR, neointimal hyperplasia, but recent data have revealed that neoatherosclerosis may also play an important role in ISR, especially in DES cases. ISR shows two patterns: early ISR (<1 year) especially for bare-metal stents (BMSs) and late ISR (≥1 year) especially for DESs. Angioscopy is the only image modality that can directly visualize the coronary artery lumen. In the early ISR phase, if white plaques on the stent and complete neointimal coverage are found by angioscopy, the neointimal condition is considered stable, but clinicians should carefully evaluate whether the neointimal condition can cause myocardial ischemia at this phase. In the late ISR phase, if yellow plaques in the stent segments are found angioscopically, the potential for neoatherosclerosis in ISR tissue should be considered. Angioscopy can provide original and important information about the neointima at early and late phases of ISR.

Keywords In-stent restenosis • Neoatherosclerosis • Yellow plaque • Thrombus • Bare meal stent drug-eluting stent

18.1 Introduction

The major clinical problem in the use of balloon angioplasty is the occurrence of restenosis, which has been observed in approximately 30–40 % of patients [1]. Restenosis is characterized by the following three major factors: (1) acute elastic recoil, (2) chronic elastic recoil (negative remodeling), and (3) neointimal proliferation. To resolve the elastic recoil problem, bare-metal stents (BMSs) were

M. Nishino, M.D., Ph.D., FACC (✉)
Division of Cardiology, Osaka Rosai Hospital, 1179-3, Nagasone-cho, Kita-ku, Sakai, Osaka 591-8025, Japan
e-mail: mnishino@orh.go.jp

© Springer Japan 2015
K. Mizuno, M. Takano (eds.), *Coronary Angioscopy*,
DOI 10.1007/978-4-431-55546-9_18

developed [2]. BMS implantation resulted in a decline of the restenosis rate to 20–30 % [3], but the use of a BMS does not resolve another of the major factors for restenosis: neointimal proliferation.

Drug-eluting stents (DESs) were developed to address neointimal proliferation. Drugs that inhibit neointimal proliferation, with a stent as a local delivery platform, have been found to be a highly promising method for preventing in-stent restenosis (ISR). The use of DESs has achieved markedly reduced ISR, at approximately 12 % [4], but ISR remains a major clinical problem even in the DES era because a completely effective strategy for preventing ISR has not yet been established [5, 6]. In addition, a recent pathological study showed that neoatherosclerosis represents a common substrate in patients with late stent failure, including late ISR [7].

Early ISR (<1 year) was found to be greatly reduced with the use of DESs, but DES cases also demonstrated evidence of continuous neointimal growth during long-term follow-up, which was designated the "late catch-up phenomenon," including late ISR [8]. Therefore, at present, both early and late ISR should be considered when we evaluate ISR lesions.

18.2 Angioscopic Evaluation for Early ISR (<1 Year)

Angioscopy can only visualize the surface of the coronary artery lumen; it cannot evaluate the cross-sectional components of in-stent tissue characteristics, as can intravascular ultrasound (IVUS) and optical coherence tomography (OCT). However, angioscopy is the only imaging modality that can directly evaluate the color of plaques and the existence of thrombi on the surface of the coronary artery lumen. Intimal hyperplasia after BMS implantation was found to peak early, between 6 months and 1 year, followed by intimal regression with luminal enlargement [9]. These phenomena are supported by histological research [10].

A serial angioscopy study demonstrated luminal changes in early restenosis phase after BMS stent implantation. The BMSs <1 month after implantation were often not completely covered by neointima and were accompanied by a thrombus, but BMSs at approximately 6 months were completely covered by white neointima [11]. The neointima over a BMS usually completely covers the stent, yellow plaques under the stent, and any thrombus [11–13].

In cases of early ISR (which frequently occurs after BMS implantation), angioscopy can provide images of the complete neointima coverage (Fig. 18.1). Compared to early ISR after BMS implantation, DES tended to show focal pattern, often affecting the stent edges, that may be occurred by geographic-miss phenomenon or strut fractures [14]. The clinical impact using angioscopy for these cases is usually weak. IVUS or OCT may be more useful to evaluate early ISR cases, especially for clinical decision-making regarding the strategy for intervention therapy. However, several studies of the clinical impact of angioscopy at 6–8 months after implantation among patients with a DES have been informative. For example, Awata et al. reported that angioscopic findings at approximately 8 months' follow-

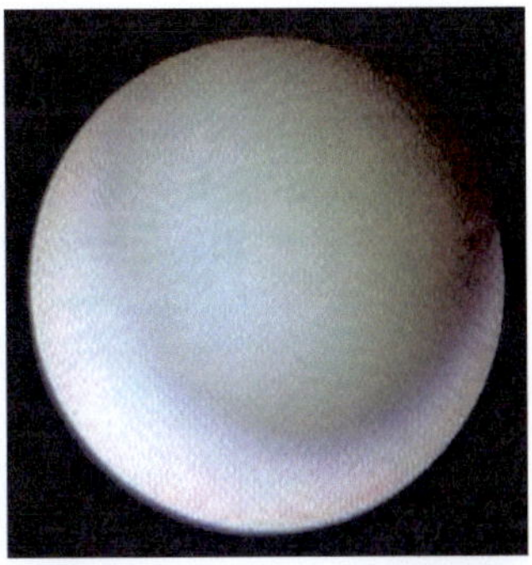

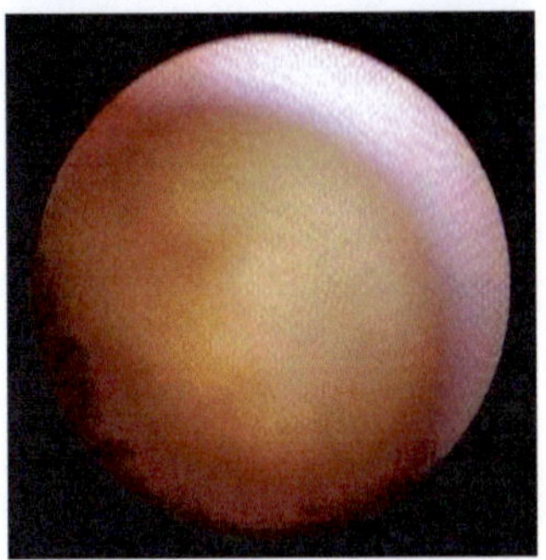

Fig. 18.1 A case of early in-stent restenosis who received bare-metal stent. Angioscopy revealed complete coverage with white plaque

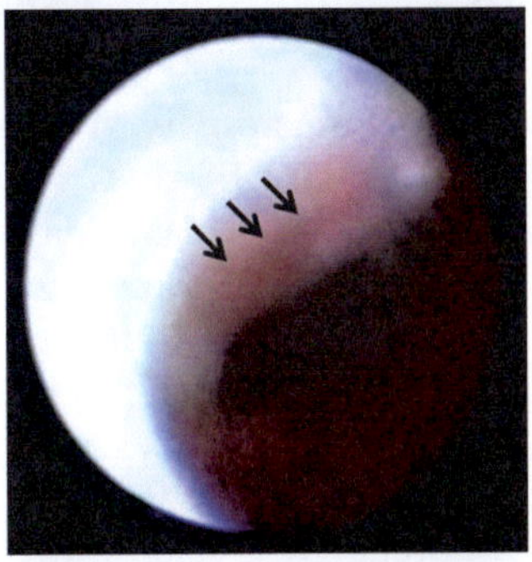

Fig. 18.2 Red thrombus (*arrows*) around stent struts

Fig. 18.3 A case of late in-stent restenosis who received drug-eluting stent. New formation of yellow plaque on stent was found by an angioscopy

up showed a lower grade of neointimal coverage and a higher incidence of the presence of a subclinical thrombus (Fig. 18.2) and yellow plaque (Fig. 18.3) in DES cases (sirolimus-eluting stents) compared to BMS cases [15]. In this study, serial angioscopy showed only persistent yellow plaques underneath the stent struts, and there were no new formation of yellow plaques which were considered as neoatherosclerosis.

However, these angioscopic findings (including the existence of angioscopic [subclinical] thrombi) had no direct link to major cardiac events including thrombotic clinical events and ISR. We have also shown that the lower minimum grade and more heterogeneous properties of neointimal coverage and thrombi in DES cases compared to BMS cases at 8 months' angioscopic evaluation did not correlate with cardiac events (including ISR) over a period of 3 years [16]. Other studies demonstrated that yellow plaques (which can be visualized only by angioscopy) may be correlated with advanced atherosclerotic degeneration ruptures and may lead to neointimal progression including ISR in both BMS and DES cases [12, 17]. We thus believe that the angioscopic findings, especially those of yellow plaque, at an 8-month follow-up can be used as a marker to predict future cardiac events, including ISR.

18.3   Angioscopic Evaluation for Late ISR (≥1 Year)

Neoatherosclerosis is an important indicator of late ISR in both BMS and DES cases [18]. In DES cases, neoatherosclerosis occurred in >40 % of the patients by 9 months after implantation, whereas in BMS cases, it did not begin to appear until 2 years and remained a rare finding until 4 years [19]. Moreover, it was reported that DESs promoted the new formation of yellow neointima at 10 months after implantation [16] and that neoatherosclerosis occurred earlier in DES compared to BMS [18, 20, 21]. Thus, it is even more important to evaluate neoatherosclerosis in DES than in BMS.

Several OCT studies revealed that its findings of neoatherosclerosis involved the presence of neointimal disruption, lipid-laden neointima, lipid pools, thin-cap fibroatheromas (TCFAs) and macrophage accumulation [22, 23]. It was also shown that TCFA findings (Fig. 18.4) by OCT were well correlated with angioscopic yellow plaques, supported by a virtual histology-IVUS study [24] and a histological study [25]. Angioscopic evaluations may be useful to evaluate and predict late ISR correlated with neoatherosclerosis. If yellow plaque is detected in the late phase (≥1 year) after BMS or DES implantation, clinicians should pay close attention to the possibility of neoatherosclerosis, which may lead to late ISR.

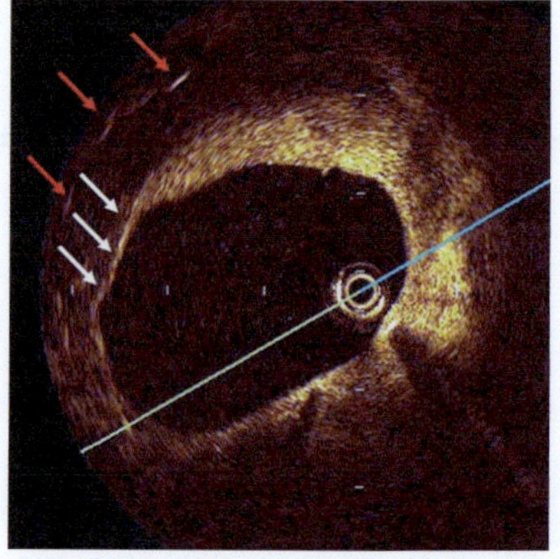

Fig. 18.4 *White arrows*: thin-cap fibroatheromas (TCFA) in in-stent tissue detected by optical coherence tomography (OCT). *Red arrows*: the stent strut

18.4 Summary

Angioscopy is the only modality that directly visualizes the surface of the coronary artery lumen. In the early ISR phase, angioscopic findings of complete coverage by white neointima are well correlated with stable condition after stent implantation. However, if a patient shows ischemic findings due to narrowing of the coronary lumen, repeated intervention therapy should be performed. In the late ISR phase, angioscopic findings of yellow plaque may be correlated with neoatherosclerosis. When yellow plaque is angioscopically identified in this phase, careful follow-up should be conducted to examine the multifaceted and elusive condition causing both ISR and stent thrombosis.

References

1. Landau C, Lange RA, Hillis LD. Percutaneous transluminal coronary angioplasty. N Engl J Med. 1994;330:981–93.
2. Mintz GS, Popma JJ, Pichard AD, Kent KM, Satler LF, Wong C, Hong MK, Kovach JA, Leon MB. Arterial remodeling after coronary angioplasty: a serial intravascular ultrasound study. Circulation. 1996;94:35–43.
3. Lowe HC, Oesterle SN, Khachigian LM. Coronary in-stent restenosis: current status and future strategies. J Am Coll Cardiol. 2002;39:183–93.
4. Cassese S, Byrne RA, Tada T, Pinieck S, Joner M, Ibrahim T, King LA, Fusaro M, Laugwitz KL, Kastrati A. Incidence and predictors of restenosis after coronary stenting in 10 004 patients with surveillance angiography. Heart. 2014;100:153–9.
5. Dibra A, Kastrati A, Alfonso F, Seyfarth M, Perez-Vizcayno MJ, Mehilli J, Schomig A. Effectiveness of drug-eluting stents in patients with bare-metal in-stent restenosis: meta-analysis of randomized trials. J Am Coll Cardiol. 2007;49:616–23.
6. Kastrati A, Dibra A, Spaulding C, Laarman GJ, Menichelli M, Valgimigli M, Di Lorenzo E, Kaiser C, Tierala I, Mehilli J, Seyfarth M, Varenne O, Dirksen MT, Percoco G, Varricchio A, Pittl U, Syvanne M, Suttorp MJ, Violini R, Schomig A. Meta-analysis of randomized trials on drug-eluting stents vs. bare-metal stents in patients with acute myocardial infarction. Eur Heart J. 2007;28:2706–13.
7. Nakazawa G, Finn AV, Vorpahl M, Ladich ER, Kolodgie FD, Virmani R. Coronary responses and differential mechanisms of late stent thrombosis attributed to first-generation sirolimus- and paclitaxel-eluting stents. J Am Coll Cardiol. 2011;57:390–8.
8. Grube E, Dawkins K, Guagliumi G, Banning A, Zmudka K, Colombo A, Thuesen L, Hauptman K, Marco J, Wijns W, Joshi A, Mascioli S. TAXUS VI final 5-year results: a multicentre, randomised trial comparing polymer-based moderate-release paclitaxel-eluting stent with a bare metal stent for treatment of long, complex coronary artery lesions. EuroIntervention. 2009;4:572–7.
9. Kimura T, Yokoi H, Nakagawa Y, Tamura T, Kaburagi S, Sawada Y, Sato Y, Yokoi H, Hamasaki N, Nosaka H, et al. Three-year follow-up after implantation of metallic coronary-artery stents. N Engl J Med. 1996;334:561–6.
10. Nobuyoshi M, Kimura T, Ohishi H, Horiuchi H, Nosaka H, Hamasaki N, Yokoi H, Kim K. Restenosis after percutaneous transluminal coronary angioplasty: pathologic observations in 20 patients. J Am Coll Cardiol. 1991;17:433–9.
11. Ueda Y, Nanto S, Komamura K, Kodama K. Neointimal coverage of stents in human coronary arteries observed by angioscopy. J Am Coll Cardiol. 1994;23:341–6.

12. Yokoyama S, Takano M, Yamamoto M, Inami S, Sakai S, Okamatsu K, Okuni S, Seimiya K, Murakami D, Ohba T, Uemura R, Seino Y, Hata N, Mizuno K. Extended follow-up by serial angioscopic observation for bare-metal stents in native coronary arteries: from healing response to atherosclerotic transformation of neointima. Circ Cardiovasc Interv. 2009;2:205–12.

13. Ueda Y, Asakura M, Yamaguchi O, Hirayama A, Hori M, Kodama K. The healing process of infarct-related plaques. Insights from 18 months of serial angioscopic follow-up. J Am Coll Cardiol. 2001;38:1916–22.

14. Alfonso F. Treatment of drug-eluting stent restenosis the new pilgrimage: quo vadis? J Am Coll Cardiol. 2010;55:2717–20.

15. Awata M, Kotani J, Uematsu M, Morozumi T, Watanabe T, Onishi T, Iida O, Sera F, Nanto S, Hori M, Nagata S. Serial angioscopic evidence of incomplete neointimal coverage after sirolimus-eluting stent implantation: comparison with bare-metal stents. Circulation. 2007;116:910–16.

16. Nishino M, Yoshimura T, Nakamura D, Lee Y, Taniike M, Makino N, Kato H, Egami Y, Shutta R, Tanouchi J, Yamada Y. Comparison of angioscopic findings and three-year cardiac events between sirolimus-eluting stent and bare-metal stent in acute myocardial infarction. Am J Cardiol. 2011;108:1238–43.

17. Higo T, Ueda Y, Oyabu J, Okada K, Nishio M, Hirata A, Kashiwase K, Ogasawara N, Hirotani S, Kodama K. Atherosclerotic and thrombogenic neointima formed over sirolimus drug-eluting stent: an angioscopic study. JACC Cardiovasc Imaging. 2009;2:616–24.

18. Nakazawa G, Otsuka F, Nakano M, Vorpahl M, Yazdani SK, Ladich E, Kolodgie FD, Finn AV, Virmani R. The pathology of neoatherosclerosis in human coronary implants bare-metal and drug-eluting stents. J Am Coll Cardiol. 2011;57:1314–22.

19. Park SJ, Kang SJ, Virmani R, Nakano M, Ueda Y. In-stent neoatherosclerosis: a final common pathway of late stent failure. J Am Coll Cardiol. 2012;59:2051–7.

20. Gonzalo N, Serruys PW, Okamura T, van Beusekom HM, Garcia-Garcia HM, van Soest G, van der Giessen W, Regar E. Optical coherence tomography patterns of stent restenosis. Am Heart J. 2009;158:284–93.

21. Takano M, Yamamoto M, Inami S, Murakami D, Ohba T, Seino Y, Mizuno K. Appearance of lipid-laden intima and neovascularization after implantation of bare-metal stents extended late-phase observation by intracoronary optical coherence tomography. J Am Coll Cardiol. 2009;55:26–32.

22. Kang SJ, Mintz GS, Akasaka T, Park DW, Lee JY, Kim WJ, Lee SW, Kim YH, Whan Lee C, Park SW, Park SJ. Optical coherence tomographic analysis of in-stent neoatherosclerosis after drug-eluting stent implantation. Circulation. 2011;123:2954–63.

23. Lee SY, Shin DH, Mintz GS, Kim JS, Kim BK, Ko YG, Choi D, Jang Y, Hong MK. Optical coherence tomography-based evaluation of in-stent neoatherosclerosis in lesions with more than 50 % neointimal cross-sectional area stenosis. EuroIntervention. 2013;9:945–51.

24. Yamamoto M, Takano M, Okamatsu K, Murakami D, Inami S, Xie Y, Seimiya K, Ohba T, Seino Y, Mizuno K. Relationship between thin cap fibroatheroma identified by virtual histology and angioscopic yellow plaque in quantitative analysis with colorimetry. Circ J. 2009;73:497–502.

25. Fujii K, Hao H, Imanaka T, Kawano T, Takayama T, Hirayama A, Yamada T, Ishibashi-Ueda H, Hirota S, Masuyama T. In-stent thin-cap fibroatheroma after drug-eluting stent implantation: ex-vivo evaluation of optical coherence tomography and intracoronary angioscopy. JACC Cardiovasc Interv. 2014;7:446–7.

Chapter 19
Pharmacological Intervention

Masamichi Takano

Abstract Ischemic heart disease is a life-threatening disorder; especially acute coronary syndrome (ACS) is a major cause of death in the world. Coronary arteries of angiographic significant stenosis with patients' symptoms or certified myocardial ischemia are generally administered by revascularization therapies, such as coronary artery bypass surgery and percutaneous coronary intervention using balloon angioplasty or metallic stent deployment. However, ACS often arises from mild to moderate stenosis without the evidence of myocardial ischemia in a brief period. Accurate prospect of ACS is therefore complicated at the present, and pharmacological intervention as preventive insurance is extremely important. Among medical treatment for coronary risk factors, lipid-lowering therapy represented by administration of HMG-CoA reductase inhibitor (statin) is the most powerful, practical, and established way to prevent against ACS. From an angioscopic point of view, morphological changes in atherosclerotic coronary plaque focused on lipid-lowering intervention are reviewed in this chapter.

Keywords Vulnerable plaque • TCFA • Yellow plaque and statin

19.1 Pathogenesis of Acute Coronary Syndrome

In the clinical settings, ischemic heart disease is roughly classified into stable condition and unstable one. The former shows stable angina pectoris (stable coronary syndrome) and the later indicates acute coronary syndrome (ACS) including unstable angina pectoris, acute myocardial infarction, and sudden coronary death. Although they have severe lumen narrowing or complete occlusion of epicardial artery in common, their pathogenesis is decisively difficult according to previous histological investigations [1]. The remarkable findings in most ACS cases are the presence of atherosclerotic plaque disruption and massive thrombus at the culprit lesion. They are unusually found in stable coronary syndrome. Therefore, it is under-

M. Takano, M.D., Ph.D. (✉)
Cardiovascular Center, Nippon Medical School Chiba Hokusoh Hospital, 1715 Kamakari, Inzai, Chiba 270-1694, Japan
e-mail: takanom@nms.ac.jp

© Springer Japan 2015
K. Mizuno, M. Takano (eds.), *Coronary Angioscopy*,
DOI 10.1007/978-4-431-55546-9_19

stood that plaque disruption and subsequent formation of flow-limiting thrombus is the principal pathogenesis of ACS [2]. Plaque disruption is pathologically divided into its rupture and superficial intimal injury, so-called erosion [3]. In addition, ruptured plaque has large lipid core under a thin fibrous cap, and infiltration of inflammatory cells, such as monocyte, macrophage, and lymphocyte [4]. Lipid-rich plaque of the fibrous cap thickness <65 μm is specially designated thin-cap fibroatheroma (TCFA). Rupture of TCFA and plaque erosion approximately account for two thirds and one third of ACS, respectively. Other minority is shallow-calcified nodule with denudated endothelium [5].

19.2 Vulnerable Plaque

There is terminology of vulnerable plaque that is defined as a plaque to provoking its disruption or a high-risk plaque of future disruption in a narrow sense [6]. According to angiographic findings previous to the ACS event, ACS often arises from mild to moderate stenosis that invites neither chest symptoms nor myocardial ischemia on stress test [7], despite the fact that sever stenosis is one of the factors in plaque vulnerability. Expecting the time and site of plaque disruption as the motivating step toward the onset of ACS and rapid growth of thrombus as the final step is certainly complicated. Therefore, vulnerable features have been investigated fragmentarily applying the culprit plaque that had already caused ACS.

The characteristics of vulnerable plaque based on pathological analysis and clinical examinations by use of coronary imaging devices are shown in Table 19.1. The presence of TCFA and the absolute volume of atheroma play a key role in plaque vulnerability and that is demonstrated by a recent prospective study of virtual histology intravascular ultrasound (IVUS), PROSPECT trial [8]. Taken together with the pathogenesis of ACS and the frequency of TCFA in the culprit lesion, TCFA is unmistakably representative of vulnerable plaque. Great energy of researchers has been invested into detection of TCFA instead of identifying true vulnerable plaque [9].

19.3 Atherosclerotic Plaque Through Coronary Angioscopy

19.3.1 Coronary Angioscopy

Coronary angiogram is still gold standard for diagnosis of ischemic heart disease. However, this method is just luminology and powerless to estimate the quality of the vessel wall. To date several sorts of intracoronary imaging devices (e.g., conventional gray-scale IVUS, virtual histology IVUS, integrated backscatter IVUS, optical coherence tomography [OCT], near-infrared spectroscopy [NIRS])

Table 19.1 Characteristics of vulnerable plaque

Macro-morphological aspect
Thin cap with large lipid core (Thin-cap fibroatheroma: TCFA)
Positive remodeling
Glistening or intense yellow plaque
Fissured plaque
Superficial calcified nodule
Spotty calcification
Intraplaque hemorrhage
Severe stenosis
Micromorphological aspect
Infiltration of inflammatory cells
Endothelial denudation
Physiological or functional aspect
Endothelial dysfunction

have been developed, and they are available for evaluation of plaque composition [10–13]. Coronary angioscopy is a unique imaging system that provides direct visualization of vessel lumen. Information about forward-looking angioscopic image, such as color, three-dimensional, and detailed configuration of lumen surface, is capable of diagnosing macro-morphology of atherosclerotic plaque, thrombus, and proliferating neointima in coronary bare-metal and drug-eluting stents [14–21].

Atherosclerotic plaque is broadly divided into white plaque and yellow one according to its surface color. Similarly, intracoronary thrombus is classified into white, red, mixed (white and red), and pinkish thrombus [22, 23]. On the basis of superficial form of the plaque, that is also categorized into simple plaque with smooth surface and complex one of irregularity. Findings of complex plaque include intimal flap, dissection, fissuring, ulceration, and disruption.

It is noticeable that coronary angioscopy can sensitively detect a tiny thrombus in comparison with other imaging [24]. Although thrombus transformed digital signals on the other imaging may be missed, visual color on the angioscopy simplifies diagnosis of the thrombus. By contrast, there is some weakness in angioscopic evaluation; quantification of distance or volume is impossible and its diagnosis is limited only to the lumen surface. They are compensated by cross-sectional IVUS or OCT images.

19.3.2 Angioscopic Findings of Plaque Vulnerability

Disrupted plaque in the culprit lesion of ACS is no longer vulnerable in the narrowest sense. Nevertheless, observation of the culprit plaque surely makes us understand plaque vulnerability before the conclusive event. At angioscopic

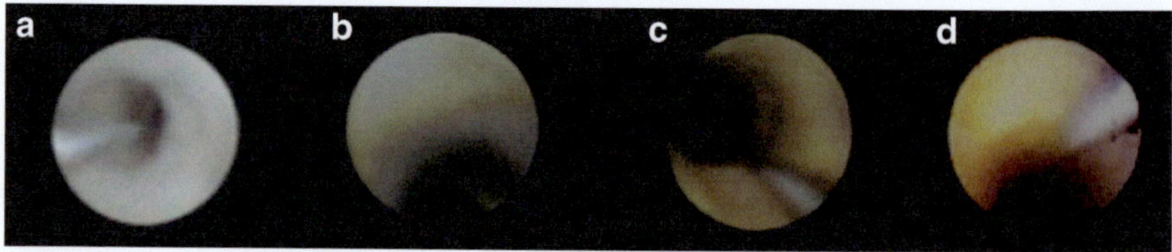

Fig. 19.1 Color of atherosclerotic coronary plaque. Semiquantitative color classification of coronary plaque is shown. Intense yellow plaque sometimes has glisten in the lumen. (**a**) White plaque (grade 0). (**b**) Light yellow plaque (grade 1). (**c**) Medium yellow plaque (grade 2). (**d**) Intense yellow plaque (grade 3)

examination in the case of ACS, massive thrombus covering disrupted plaque is commonly found as pathological reports have proved [25]. The plaque usually has yellow surface, and so yellow plaque is considered to be vulnerable. The degree of yellow color is really various, and its grading or scoring system is often used for semiquantitative analysis as the following: grade 1 = light yellow, grade 2 = medium yellow, grade 3 = intense or dark yellow, and grade 0 = no yellow (white) [26, 27] (Fig. 19.1).

In pathological validation, angioscopically yellow plaque corresponds with fibro-lipidic atheroma [28]. Integrated backscatter IVUS, virtual histology IVUS, and OCT demonstrate that the majority of yellow plaques are composed of lipid-laden elements including necrotic core [11, 29–32]. Also, yellow plaque is relevant to positive vessel remodeling on IVUS images [33]. The yellow plaque with positive remodeling has large plaque burden, and that probably contributes to local vulnerability. Thickness of fibrous tissue covering lipidic content is determinant of the plaque color, and yellow grade is conversely correlated with the fibrous cap thickness (Fig. 19.2) [31, 32]. These data suggest that intense yellow plaque is identical with TCFA of pathological definition. In contrast, white plaque is a lipidic plaque with thick fibrous cap (thick-cap fibroatheroma) or a complete fibrous plaque without lipid. With regard to thrombogenicity, the frequency of thrombus adhesion gradually increases according to the yellow grade [34]. Some intense yellow-plaque, angioscopy-derived TCFA is located in the segment of a large lumen area measured by OCT [32]. The phenomenon implies that vulnerable plaque may hide in the lesion of nonsignificant stenosis. Few small-scale prospective researches exhibit that the incidence of ACS is higher in patients having glistening yellow plaque or plural yellow plaques than in patients without those [35, 36]. Hence, it is generally believed that white plaque achieves clinically stable condition and intense yellow plaque may have potential for its disruption and thrombus formation in the future.

Complex plaque features, intimal injury recognized by the naked eye through angioscopy, reflect microscopic endothelial denudation, and they are often accompanied with attachment of mural thrombus [37, 38]. Therefore, complexity is regarded as a factor of plaque vulnerability as well as color of the high-intense yellow.

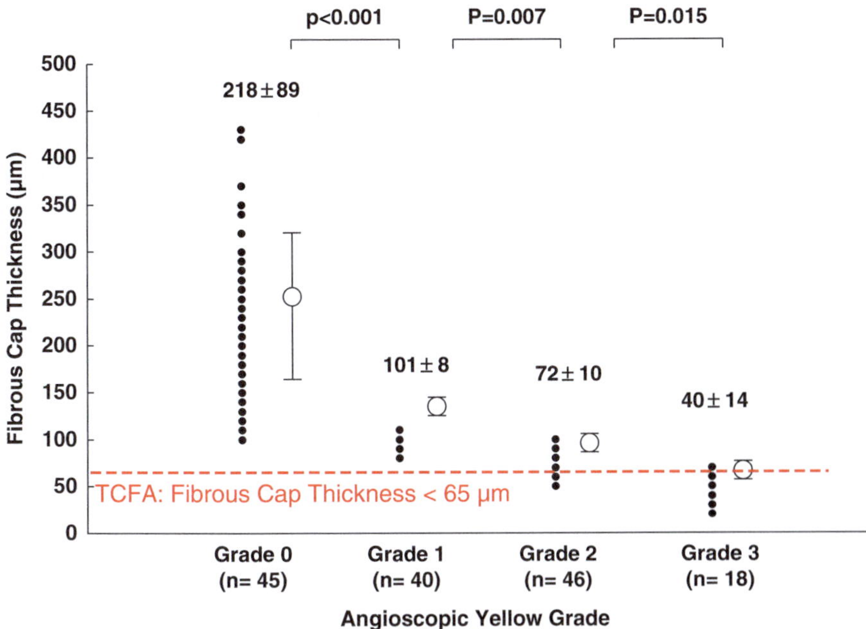

Fig. 19.2 The relationship between angioscopic yellow grade and fibrous cap thickness measured by OCT. Yellow grade of the plaque is conversely correlated with its fibrous cap thickness. Pathological thin-cap fibroatheroma (TCFA) is identical with intense yellow plaque on coronary angioscopy

19.4   Lipid-Lowering Therapy by Statin

Numerous researches of epidemiology conducted several coronary risk factors promoting atherosclerosis of systemic arteries including ischemic heart disease. Diabetes mellitus, hypertension, dyslipidemia, family history, and cigarette smoking are well known as conventional risk factors. From standpoint of preventive medicine, control of each factor and risk factor reduction are performed for primary and secondary prevention of cardiovascular disease.

Since HMG-CoA reductase inhibitor (statin) has been utilized for the treatment of dyslipidemia, serum level of low-density lipoprotein cholesterol (LDL-C) is reduced absolutely. According to basic researches, macrophage takes in oxidized LDL through scavenger receptor and changes into foam cell [39]. The cells themselves constitute lipid-rich plaque and they secrete various inflammatory cytokines advancing atheroma to inflamed condition. Activated macrophage also releases metalloproteinase and collagenase, and these proteinases thin down and weaken fibrous cap [40]. Statin displays not only direct effect on LDL-C lowering but also pleiotoropic effects, such as improving endothelial function, decreasing oxidative stress and inflammation, and inhibiting thrombogenic response [41]. Consequently, statin helps to suppress formation and development of atherosclerosis.

Large-scale clinical researches revealed that statin therapy dramatically reduces cardiovascular events including ACS [42, 43]. Considering pharmacological effects of statin, the phenomenon is reasonable. However, findings of coronary angiography disappointedly showed the minimum regression of stenosis in atherosclerotic lesion [44]. Angiogram as lumen silhouette thus failed to declare alternation of the plaque quantity and quality resulting from statin therapy.

19.5 Angioscopic Changes in Coronary Plaque After Pharmacological Intervention

The culprit plaque of ACS, stable angina pectoris, and silent myocardial ischemia usually undergoes invasive therapy such as percutaneous coronary intervention. Disrupted, thrombotic, and/or yellow plaque is sometimes located in the non-culprit lesion without significant stenosis [32, 45, 46]. In such case, pharmacological therapy is chosen even though plaque seems to be vulnerable, because the lesion has no indication of invasive intervention. Therefore, angioscopy targets on the plaque with vulnerable features for the analysis of pharmacological intervention.

The first angioscopic study of pharmacological intervention was reported in 2003 [27]. Administration of atorvastatin for 12 months significantly reduces the above yellow score (or grade) of the non-culprit plaque from 2.03 to 1.13. The change in yellow score has good correlation with the change in LDL-C level. Complexity (or disrupted) score (defined as $0 =$ smooth surface or $1 =$ irregular surface, and $0 =$ without thrombus or $1 =$ with thrombus) also decreases from 0.23 to 0.10. In the comparison group receiving diet therapy, both scores change from 1.67 to 1.99 and from 0.31 to 0.44, respectively (Fig. 19.3). The score gain of the comparison group suggests gradual progression of atherosclerosis during natural history. Other investigators later concluded resemble alternation of the plaque character [47, 48]. Another class of antihyperlipidemic drug, bezafibrate, for 6-month administration invites similar vascular response to statin [49].

The mechanisms of reduction of the yellow grade are speculated that stain increases collagen fiber in the fibrous cap of which thickness closely affects plaque color and decreases lipidic tissue of the plaque [50]. Actually, thickening of the fibrous cap due to statin therapy is confirmed by the measurement of OCT [51]. As numbers of examinations using gray-scale IVUS show, stain decreases plaque volume and acts on quantitative regression of atheroma [52–55]. However, gray-scale IVUS has inability to approve loss of lipid content. Instead, integrated backscatter IVUS, virtual histology IVUS, and NIRS verify lipid-core reduction after intervention of statin [56–58]. Decline of the complexity score means trend toward plaque healing. Therefore, statin can advance healing process of the

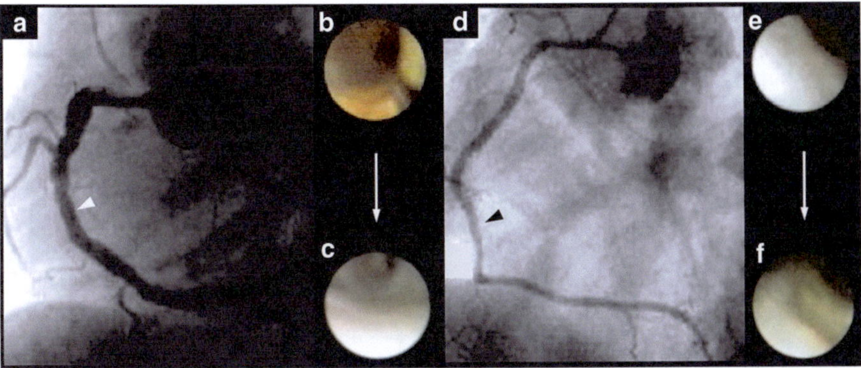

Fig. 19.3 Serial changes in plaque color. Representative angiographic and angioscopic findings of statin therapy (*left panels*; **a** to **c**) and diet therapy (*right panels*; **d** to **f**) are shown. (**a**) Angiography showed no severe stenosis in the right coronary artery (RCA). (**b**) Angioscopy found intense yellow plaque hidden in mild stenosis in the mid RCA (white arrowhead in panel **a**). (**c**) Yellow grade of the plaque markedly regressed 12 months later of aggressive lipid-lowering therapy with atorvastatin. (**d**) There was no significant stenosis in the RCA. (**e**) Almost white plaque with smooth surface was seen in normal segment the mid RCA (*black arrowhead* in panel **d**). (**f**) After 12 months of diet therapy, the previous white plaque appeared light yellow, and its surface had irregularity

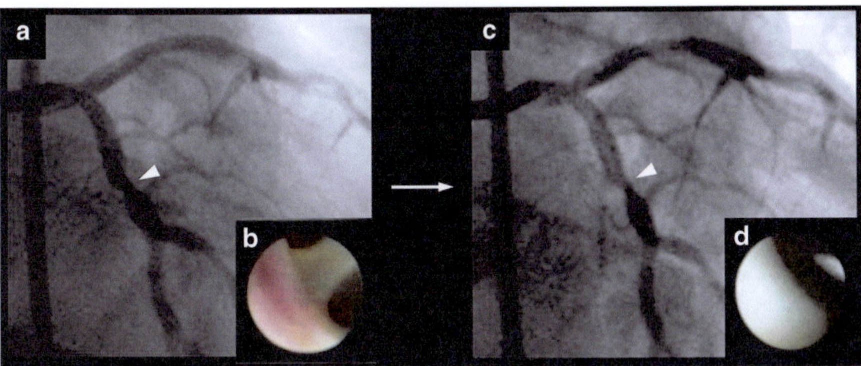

Fig. 19.4 Plaque healing caused by statin. Angiographic and angioscopic findings of plaque healing are shown. (**a**) Moderate stenosis was seen in the left circumflex artery (*white arrowhead*). (**b**) Disrupted plaque covered by pinkish thrombus was found at the lesion corresponding to angiographic moderate stenosis. (**c**) Angiographic change in lumen stenosis was slight after 12 months of atorvastatin treatment (*white arrowhead*). (**d**) Thrombotic plaque disappeared and the lumen surface was replaced by white intima. Statin completely healed up disrupted plaque

disrupted plaque (Fig. 19.4) [46]. The above angioscopic serial changes in plaque features indicate that statin dynamically changes quality of the plaque and results in plaque stabilization.

Although volumetric analysis by use of gray-scale IVUS shows both of amlodipine (antihypertensive drug) and pioglitazone (hypoglycemic drug) inhibit increase in the coronary-plaque volume [59, 60], there is no angioscopic evidence for plaque changes by these drugs. Lipidic yellow plaque is found not only in native coronary artery but also on proliferated neointima in the stent segment [61–63]. Appearance of the yellow plaque inside metallic stent is named neoatherosclerosis [64], and the lesion has possibility of the origin in acute thrombotic occlusion as well as the yellow plaque in native vessel [65]. Efficiency of pharmacological intervention for the lesion of neoatherosclerosis has been unknown.

19.6 Summary

Aggressive lipid-lowering therapy with strong statin leads regression of yellow grade and improvement of complexity of the plaque. It is understood that the angioscopic changes in plaque morphology represent qualitative transition of the plaque from vulnerable to stable. A number of new medicines inhibiting atherosclerosis have been developed and part of them are now available for the treatment and management of cardiovascular disease. Accumulation of new findings in the field of pharmacological intervention is heartily expected in the future.

References

1. Falk E, Shah PK, Fuster V. Coronary plaque disruption. Circulation. 1999;92:657–71.
2. Libby P. Current concepts of the pathogenesis of the acute coronary syndromes. Circulation. 2001;1004:365–72.
3. Farb A, Burke AP, Tang AL, et al. Coronary plaque erosion without rupture into a lipid core. A frequent cause of coronary thrombosis in sudden coronary death. Circulation. 1996;93:1354–63.
4. Naghavi M, Libby P, Falk E, et al. From vulnerable plaque to vulnerable patient: a call for new definitions and risk assessment strategies: Part I. Circulation. 2003;108:1664–72.
5. Kolodgie FD, Virmani R, Burke AP, et al. Pathologic assessment of the vulnerable human coronary plaque. Heart. 2004;90:1385–91.
6. Schaar JA, Muller JE, Falk E, et al. Terminology of high-risk and vulnerable coronary artery plaques. Report of a meeting on the vulnerable plaque, June 17 and 18, Santorini, Greece. Eur Heart J. 2004;25:1077–82.
7. Fuster V, Stein B, Ambrose JA, et al. Atherosclerotic plaque rupture and thrombosis: evolving concepts. Circulation. 1990;82:II30–42.
8. Stone GW, Maehara A, Lansky AJ, et al. A prospective natural history study of coronary atherosclerosis. N Engl J Med. 2011;364:226–35.
9. Honda Y, Fitzgerald PJ. Frontiers in intravascular imaging technologies. Circulation. 2008;117:2024–37.
10. Nair A, Kuban BD, Tuzcu EM, et al. Coronary plaque classification with intravascular ultrasound radiofrequency data analysis. Circulation. 2002;106:2200–6.
11. Kawasaki M, Takatsu H, Noda T, et al. In vivo quantitative tissue characterization of human coronary arterial plaques by use of integrated backscatter intravascular ultrasound and comparison with angioscopic findings. Circulation. 2002;105:2487–92.

12. Yabushita H, Bouma BE, Houser SL, et al. Characterization of human atherosclerosis by optical coherence tomography. Circulation. 2002;106:1640–5.
13. Moreno PR, Lodder RA, Purushothaman KR, et al. Detection of lipid pool, thin cap, and inflammatory cells in human aortic atherosclerotic plaques by near-infrared spectroscopy. Circulation. 2002;105:923–7.
14. Asakura M, Ueda Y, Nanto S, et al. Remodeling of in-stent neointima, which become thinner and transparent over 3 years: serial angiographic and angioscopic follow-up. Circulation. 1998;97:2003–6.
15. Sakai S, Mizuno K, Yokoyama S, et al. Morphological changes in infarct-related plaque after coronary stent placement: a serial angioscopy study. J Am Coll Cardiol. 2003;42:1558–65.
16. Kotani J, Awata M, Nanto S, et al. Incomplete neointimal coverage of sirolimus-eluting stents: angioscopic findings. J Am Coll Cardiol. 2006;47:2108–11.
17. Takano M, Ohba T, Inami S, et al. Angioscopic differences in neointimal coverage and in persistence of thrombus between sirolimus-eluting stents and bare metal stents after a 6-month implantation. Eur Heart J. 2006;27:2189–95.
18. Awata M, Kotani J, Uematsu M, et al. Serial angioscopic evidence of incomplete neointimal coverage after sirolimus-eluting stent implantation: comparison with bare-metal stent. Circulation. 2007;116:910–16.
19. Takano M, Yamamoto M, Xie Y, et al. Serial long-term evaluation of neointimal stent coverage and thrombus after sirolimus-eluting stent implantation by use of coronary angioscopy. Heart. 2007;93:1353–6.
20. Takano M, Yamamoto M, Murakami D, et al. Lack of association large angiographic late loss and low risk of in-stent thrombus: angioscopic comparison between paclitaxel- and sirolimus-eluting stent. Circ Cardiovasc Interv. 2008;1:20–7.
21. Takano M, Mizuno K. Coronary angioscopic evaluation for serial changes of luminal appearance after pharmacological and catheter interventions. Circ J. 2010;74:240–5.
22. Mizuno K, Satomura K, Miyamoto A, et al. Angioscopic evaluation of coronary-artery thrombi in acute coronary syndromes. N Engl J Med. 1992;326:287–91.
23. Okamatsu K, Takano M, Sakai S, et al. Elevated troponin T levels and lesion characteristics in non-ST elevation acute coronary syndromes. Circulation. 2004;109:465–70.
24. MacNeill BD, Lowe HC, Takano M, et al. Intravascular modalities for detection of vulnerable plaque: current status. Arterioscler Thromb Vasc Biol. 2003;23:1333–42.
25. Mizuno K, Miyamoto A, Satomura K, et al. Angioscopic morphology in patients with acute coronary disorders. Lancet. 1991;337:809–12.
26. Ueda Y, Asakura M, Yamaguchi O, et al. The healing process of infarct-related plaques. Insights from 18 months of serial angioscopic follow-up. J Am Coll Cardiol. 2001;38:1916–22.
27. Takano M, Mizuno K, Yokoyama S, et al. Changes in coronary plaque color and morphology by lipid-lowering therapy with atorvastatin: serial evaluation by coronary angioscopy. J Am Coll Cardiol. 2003;42:680–6.
28. Ishibashi F, Yokoyama S, Miyahara K, et al. Quantitative colorimetry of atherosclerotic plaque using the L*a*b* color space during angioscopy for the detection of lipid cores underneath thin fibrous cap. Int J Cardiovasc Imaging. 2007;6:679–91.
29. Kawano T, Honye J, Takayama T, et al. Compositional analysis of angioscopic yellow plaques with intravascular ultrasound radiofrequency data. Int J Cardiol. 2008;125:74–8.
30. Yamamoto M, Takano M, Okamatsu K, et al. Relationship between thin cap fibroatheroma identified by virtual histology and angioscopic yellow plaque in quantitative analysis with colorimetry. Circ J. 2009;73:497–502.
31. Kubo T, Imanishi T, Takarada S, et al. Implication of plaque color classification for assessing plaque vulnerability: a coronary angioscopy and optical coherence tomography investigation. JACC Cardiovasc Interv. 2008;1:74–80.
32. Takano M, Jang IK, Inami S, et al. In vivo comparison of optical coherence tomography and angioscopy for the evaluation of coronary plaque characteristics. Am J Cardiol. 2008;101:471–6.

33. Takano M, Mizuno K, Okamatsu K, et al. Mechanical and structural characteristics of vulnerable plaques: analysis by coronary angioscopy and intravascular ultrasound. J Am Coll Cardiol. 2001;38:99–104.
34. Ueda Y, Ohtani T, Shimizu M, et al. Assessment of plaque vulnerability by angioscopic classification of plaque color. Am Heart J. 2004;148:333–5.
35. Uchida Y, Nakamura F, Tomaru T, et al. Prediction of acute coronary syndromes by percutaneous coronary angioscopy in patients with stable angina. Am Heart J. 1995;130:195–203.
36. Ohtani T, Ueda Y, Mizote I, et al. Number of yellow plaques detected in a coronary artery is associated with future risk of acute coronary syndrome: detection of vulnerable patients by angioscopy. J Am Coll Cardiol. 2006;247:2194–200.
37. Ishibashi F, Mizuno K, Kawamura A, et al. High yellow color intensity by angioscopy with quantitative colorimetry to identify high-risk features in culprit lesions of patients with acute coronary syndromes. Am J Cardiol. 2007;100:1207–11.
38. Kubo T, Imanishi T, Takarada S, et al. Assessment of culprit lesion morphology in acute myocardial infarction: ability of optical coherence tomography compared with intravascular ultrasound and coronary angioscopy. J Am Coll Cardiol. 2007;50:933–9.
39. Brown MS, Goldstein JL. Atherosclerosis. Scavenging for receptors. Nature. 1990;343:508–9.
40. Shah PK, Falk E, Badimon JJ, et al. human monocyte-derived macrophages induce collagen breakdown in fibrous caps of atherosclerotic plaques. Potential role of matrix-degrading metalloproteinases and implications for plaque rupture. Circulation. 1995;15:1565–9.
41. Bocan TM. Pleiotropic effects of HMG-CoA reductase inhibitors. Curr Opin Investig Drugs. 2002;3:1312–17.
42. No authors listed. Randomised trial of cholesterol lowering in 4444 patients with coronary heart disease: the Scandinavian Simvastatin Survival Study (4S). Lancet. 1994;344:1383–89.
43. No authors listed. Prevention of cardiovascular events and death with pravastatin in patients with coronary heart disease and broad range of initial cholesterol levels. The Long-Term Intervention with Pravastatin in Ischaemic Disease (LIPID) Study Group. N Engl J Med. 1998;339:1349–57.
44. No authors listed. Effect of simvastatin on coronary atheroma: the Multicenter Anti-Atheroma Study (MAAS). Lancet. 1994;344:633–8.
45. Asakura M, Ueda Y, Yamaguchi O, et al. Extensive development of vulnerable plaques as a pan-coronary process in patients with myocardial infarction: an angioscopic study. J Am Coll Cardiol. 2001;37:1284–8.
46. Takano M, Inami S, Ishibashi F, et al. Angioscopic follow-up study of non-culprit ruptured plaques. J Am Coll Cardiol. 2005;45:652–8.
47. Hirayama A, Saito S, Ueda Y, et al. Qualitative and quantitative changes in coronary plaque associated with atorvastatin therapy. Circ J. 2009;73:718–25.
48. Kodama K, Komatsu S, Ueda Y, et al. Stabilization and regression of coronary plaques treated with pitavastatin proven by angioscopy and intravascular ultrasound-the TOGETHAR trial. Circ J. 2010;74:1922–8.
49. Osawa H, Uchida Y, Fujimori Y, et al. Angioscopic evaluation of stabilizing effects of an antilipidemic agent, bezafibrate, on coronary artery plaques in patients with coronary artery disease: a multicenter prospective study. Jpn Heart J. 2002;43:319–31.
50. Crisby M, Nordin-Fredriksson G, Shah PK, et al. Pravastatin treatment increases collagen content and decreases lipid content, inflammation, metalloproteinases activity and cell death in human carotid plaques: implications for plaque stabilization. Circulation. 2001;103:926–33.
51. Takarada S, Imanishi T, Kubo T, et al. Effect of statin therapy on coronary fibrous-cap thickness in patients with acute coronary syndrome: assessment by optical coherence tomography study. Atherosclerosis. 2009;202:491–7.
52. Schartl M, Bocksch W, Koschyk DH, et al. Use of intravascular ultrasound to compare effects of different strategies of lipid-lowering therapy on plaque volume and composition in patients with coronary artery disease. Circulation. 2001;104:387–92.

53. Okazaki S, Yokoyama T, Miyauchi K, et al. Early statin treatment in patients with acute coronary syndrome: demonstration of the beneficial effect on atherosclerotic lesions by serial volumetric intravascular ultrasound analysis during half a year after coronary event: the ESTABLISH study. Circulation. 2004;110:1061–8.
54. Nissen SE, Nicholls SJ, Sipahi I, et al. Effect of very high-intensity statin therapy on regression of coronary atherosclerosis: the ASTEROID trial. JAMA. 2006;295:1556–65.
55. Schoenhagen P, Tuzcu EM, Apperson-Hansen C, et al. Determinants of arterial wall remodeling during lipid-lowering therapy: serial intravascular ultrasound observations from the Reversal of Atherosclerosis with Aggressive Lipid Lowering Therapy (REVERSAL) trial. Circulation. 2006;113:2826–34.
56. Kawasaki M, Sano K, Okubo M, et al. Volumetric quantitative analysis of tissue characteristics of coronary plaques after statin therapy using three-dimensional integrated backscatter intravascular ultrasound. J Am Coll Cardiol. 2005;45:1946–53.
57. Hong MK, Park DW, Lee CW, et al. Effects of statin treatments on coronary plaques assessed by volumetric virtual histology intravascular ultrasound analysis. JACC Cardiovasc Interv. 2009;2:679–88.
58. Kini AS, Baber U, Kovacic JC, et al. Changes in plaque lipid content after short-term intensive versus standard statin therapy: the YELLOW trial (reduction in yellow plaque by aggressive lipid-lowering therapy). J Am Coll Cardiol. 2013;62:21–9.
59. Nissen SE, Tuzcu EM, Libby P, et al. Effect of antihypertensive agents on cardiovascular events in patients with coronary disease and normal blood pressure: the CAMELOT study: a randomized controlled trial. JAMA. 2004;292:2217–25.
60. Nissen SE, Nicholls SJ, Wolski K, et al. Comparison of pioglitazone vs glimepiride on progression of coronary atherosclerosis in patients with type 2 diabetes: the PERISCOPE randomized controlled trial. JAMA. 2008;299:1561–73.
61. Yokoyama S, Takano M, Yamamoto M, et al. Extended follow-up by serial angioscopic observation for bare-metal stents in native coronary arteries: from healing response to atherosclerotic transformation of neointima. Circ Cardiovasc Interv. 2009;2:205–12.
62. Takano M, Yamamoto M, Inami S, et al. Appearance of lipid-laden intima and neovascularization after implantation of bare-metal stents: extended late-phase observation by intracoronary optical coherence tomography. J Am Coll Cardiol. 2009;55:26–32.
63. Higo T, Ueda Y, Oyabu J, et al. Atherosclerotic and thrombogenic neointima formed over sirolimus-eluting stent: an angioscopic study. JACC Cardiovasc Imaging. 2009;2:616–24.
64. Nakazawa G, Otsuka F, Nakano M, et al. The pathology of neoatherosclerosis in human coronary implants bare-metal and drug eluting stents. J Am Coll Cardiol. 2011;57:1314–22.
65. Takano M, Yamamoto M, Mizuno K. Two cases of coronary stent thrombosis very late after bare-metal stenting. JACC Cardiovasc Interv. 2009;2:1286–7.

Index

© Springer Japan 2015
K. Mizuno, M. Takano (eds.), *Coronary Angioscopy*,
DOI 10.1007/978-4-431-55546-9